Diagnostic Radiography

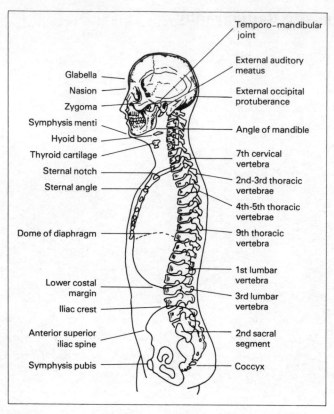

Glabella

Nasion

Zygoma

Symphysis menti

Hyoid bone

Thyroid cartilage

Sternal notch

Sternal angle

Dome of diaphragm

Lower costal margin

Iliac crest

Anterior superior iliac spine

Symphysis pubis

Temporo-mandibular joint

External auditory meatus

External occipital protuberance

Angle of mandible

7th cervical vertebra

2nd-3rd thoracic vertebrae

4th-5th thoracic vertebrae

9th thoracic vertebra

1st lumbar vertebra

3rd lumbar vertebra

2nd sacral segment

Coccyx

Some anatomical features used as radiographic centering points

Diagnostic Radiography

A CONCISE PRACTICAL MANUAL

Glenda J. Bryan
D.C.R., S.R.R.
Superintendent Radiographer
Bristol Royal Hospitals

FOREWORD BY

J. H. Middlemiss
C.M.G., M.D., F.R.C.P., F.R.C.S., F.R.C.R.
Professor of Radiology
University of Bristol

THIRD EDITION

CHURCHILL LIVINGSTONE
EDINBURGH LONDON AND NEW YORK 1979

CHURCHILL LIVINGSTONE
Medical Division of Longman Group Limited

Distributed in the United States of America by
Longman Inc., 19 West 44th Street, New York,
N.Y. 10036, and by associated companies, branches
and representatives throughout the world.

First Edition 1970
Second Edition 1974
  Reprinted 1976
Third Edition 1979

ISBN 0 443 01923 1

British Library Cataloguing in Publication Data
Bryan, Glenda June
   Diagnostic radiography.—3rd ed
   1. Diagnosis, Radioscopic
   I. Title
   616.07'57   RC78   78–40847

Printed in Great Britain by
Butler & Tanner Ltd, Frome and London

Foreword

Miss Glenda Bryan is an experienced Superintendent Radiographer on the staff of the University of Bristol Teaching Hospital which has traditional links with many overseas countries, and during the absence of the proposed Jamaican Principal Teacher she was seconded to the School of Radiography in Jamaica, which has been associated with Bristol for some years and which trains students for the English qualification, the M.S.R. [now D.C.R.].

She had been intimately concerned for several years with the daily supervision of the practical work of students but when she became responsible for classroom teaching and the organisation of students' curricula, she found a real gap in the available textbooks. There is available a superb, monumental and heavy reference book on radiography. There are books on physics and equipment and on radiographic anatomy and darkroom procedures. But there was no satisfactory handbook of moderate cost to which the ordinary student could refer in everyday work and which would provide information on the routine activities which the radiographer has to undertake. And so, in Jamaica, she had to prepare her own notes and lecture material.

On returning to Bristol she developed and systematised the notes which she had prepared and used to considerable effect. The process of elaborating her original notes has gone on now for nearly two years in the department in Bristol with frequent and lengthy discussions among the staff, radiographers and radiologists alike, with trials and practical experiments, with drafts and redrafts of sections and chapters.

What has emerged will, I hope and believe, fulfil a need in practical everyday radiography—a handbook, of modest cost and reasonable size, written by a practising radiographer, providing technical details and practical advice on routine procedures. There is a wealth of experience and commonsense in this book. I commend it to all practising radiographers, junior and senior, and to all student radiographers in the United Kingdom and overseas. The illustrations, both radiographs and line-drawings, have been carefully selected to demonstrate, without being too elaborate, those points of greatest importance in the busy life of a general department. Many specialised departments will have more sophisticated and detailed procedures in certain fields. In this book, however, there is presented a standard practice and a simple approach to most fields of work which, if followed, will provide most departments, most radiologists and most clinicians with the diagnostic criteria required in dealing with the problems that present on most days in every department.

Bristol, 1970   J. H. Middlemiss

Preface to the Third Edition

Since the publication of the second edition, new techniques have been evolved and new equipment has been introduced. In this edition, as in the previous one, the aim has been to deal with these without losing sight of the original concept of the book as a concise practical manual. The descriptions of simple methods and apparatus have of course been retained, as in many departments the latest equipment and instruments are not available.

The text throughout has again been extensively revised and brought up to date and many recent publications will be found in the list of references. Several additional plates and figures have been included but these have had to be restricted in number so as to keep the book within the limits of its self-imposed objective.

In Part I, the chapter on patient care now includes separate sections on infants and children and on elderly patients. Radio-isotope scanning and ultrasonic scanning are becoming increasingly the responsibility of departments of radiodiagnosis and the chapters on these topics have been slightly expanded. At the date of the second edition, C.T. scanning (computerised transverse axial tomography) was in its early days and its use was confined to the examination of the head. Since then rapid progress has been made—now all parts of the body can be examined by this technique, so the short section in the second edition has been replaced by a separate chapter, though this important new technique is rapidly attracting a vast specialised literature of its own.

In Part II, the chapter on the vertebral column now includes a larger section on the cervico-thoracic vertebrae. The section on teeth has also been expanded.

In Part III, the chapter on the gastro-intestinal tract describes the newer methods of investigation but as some of these may not be current practice in some departments, descriptions of the conventional techniques also have been retained. The chapter on arthrography has been rewritten and many other chapters have additional sections, including one on coronary arteriography.

Several improvements in this new edition arise from comments made by colleagues and others who have been kind enough to communicate with me, and from the constructive suggestions contained in the reviews of the second edition, all of which have been given very careful consideration. No change has been made, however, in the methods of centering described. Where appropriate, an anatomical centering point is given in accordance with conventional teaching, but there are many other cases where in practice it is more satisfactory first to place the cassette carefully in relation to certain easily palpable anatomical structures and then to centre the beam to the cassette. Experience shows that in such cases this is not only easier but often a more reliable method of ensuring that the required area is correctly sited on the radiograph.

Those to whom I gratefully acknowledge my ever-increasing debt of gratitude for their help, criticism and encouragement, for this edition and for the previous ones, include Dr H. Baddeley, Dr R. J. Burwood, Mr M. W. Cooksey, Dr E. R. Davies, Dr Z. Davies, Dr M. J. Gibson, Mr D. Gifford, Dr I. R. S. Gordon, Dr M. Griffiths, Dr. M. Halliwell, Mr W. Harrison, Professor J. H. Middlemiss, Dr R. A. Mountford, Dr D. J. Nolan, Dr T. J. T. Privett, Dr F. G. M. Ross, Dr J. Roylance, Dr A. Sargood, Dr J. L. G. Thompson, and Dr I. Watt (all of the United Bristol Hospitals), Dr B. B. Beeson, Dr W. M. Park, Dr B. H. Phillips, Dr J. F. Ryan and many others too numerous to mention individually.

My sincere thanks are due also to Mr E. J. Turnbull for drawing the figures; Mr S. E. Cook, Mr J. Hancock and Miss D. M. Ovendon for making the prints from which the plants were produced; the Department of Anaesthetics, United Bristol Hospitals, for permission to use Fig. 34; the Department of Radiology, University Hospital of the West Indies, for permission to use Plate XLVII; the Department of Radiology, Royal Prince Alfred Hospital, Camperdown, New South Wales, for permission to use Plate L; the Department of Radiology, Robert Jones and Agnes Hunt Orthopaedic Hospital, Oswestry, for permission to use Plates LII and LIV; the Department of Radiology, Radcliffe Infirmary, Oxford, for permission to use Plates XXXII, XXXIII and XXXIV and to the Department of Clinical Research, Royal United Hospital, Bath, for permission to use Plate XI.

I am also extremely grateful to Mr Martin Davies for his constant encouragement and for his help in drafting the manuscript, to Miss Carol Phillips for typing it and to the Publishers for their friendly advice and co-operation in the production of this book.

Bristol, 1979   G. J. B.

Preface to the First Edition

The purpose of this brief synopsis of diagnostic radiography is to provide a practical guide for the day-to-day work in an X-ray department (both plain film radiography and radiological procedures) and to instruct the student in practical as well as theoretical radiography. More detailed treatment of many aspects of the subject will be found in specialised works for which this book does not pretend to be a substitute.

Part I discusses general principles, applicable to many fields of radiography, and a brief mention of the diagnostic use of radioisotopes and ultrasound has been included in this section as these are becoming the responsibility of some diagnostic departments. Part II describes a basic technique for the radiographic examination of each region of the body, though in many cases alternatives are possible and may be employed in some hospitals. Part III deals with radiological procedures. For each of these there are wide possible variations in detail and the method employed will depend on the requirements of the radiologist. One standard method has been described in each case.

For reasons of size and cost, the illustrations have been deliberately restricted in number and basic views taken routinely in most departments have not been illustrated. A consistent order and method of description has been used throughout each section for easy reference and also to encourage the logical approach needed for answering questions on radiographic technique.

Bristol, 1970   G. J. B.

Contents

Part II: Regional Radiography

Part III: Radiological Procedures

Part I

GENERAL RADIOGRAPHY

1

Patient care

The radiographer should make every effort to obtain the willing co-operation of the patient because without this it will seldom be possible to obtain maximum information from a radiographic examination.

By a calm and friendly manner and tone of voice the radiographer can often do a great deal to give the patient confidence that he is in efficient and sympathetic hands and that his examination is both necessary and being performed in a department where his well-being is of real concern and interest to the staff, but a loud, 'hearty' or over-familiar approach must always be avoided.

Patients arriving in an X-ray department are often worried or apprehensive and this may make it difficult for them to understand instructions or may produce an apparently aggressive attitude. In such cases, the radiographer must be especially understanding and tolerant.

At any examination in which the radiologist participates, for example venepuncture, it is often helpful for the radiographer to introduce the patient and the radiologist to one another by name. This will reassure the patient that he is regarded as an individual and not just 'the next case', and that there is no mistake as to his identity or as to the procedure that is being carried out.

Identity. Before any examination is performed, the identity of the patient must be checked by the radiographer (even though in certain cases the radiologist will also do this) as experience shows that occasionally a patient will answer to a name not his own. This is always important but is especially so when specialised radiological procedures are being performed, particularly those involving contrast media.

Waiting. Nearly every patient who attends an X-ray department has to spend some time waiting, if not for the actual radiography then for checking or reporting on the films. An efficient appointments system is essential for keeping the waiting time to a minimum. Waiting is made less tedious if the patient has something to do, so a supply of recent magazines and newspapers, suitable for different tastes and age groups, should be available. Pictures (which are sometimes available on loan from art galleries), a small aquarium, simple toys and so on, all help to lessen boredom whilst waiting. When an appointment is made for an examination that is bound to take a long time, the patient can also be invited to bring something to help pass the time, for example a book or knitting. Patients should always be told in advance the approximate length of time that the examination will take and it is better to over-estimate than under-estimate this.

Flower arrangements in waiting rooms or corridors can have a favourable effect on the patient's peace of mind and contribute to the aesthetic attraction of the department. Such arrangements need not always be of fresh flowers, which are expensive to buy and time-consuming to arrange. An arrangement of dried flowers, leaves and grasses can be very attractive and will often need no further attention for months.

Whenever possible, separate waiting areas should be available for different types of patients, e.g. for the seriously ill or accident cases, for patients who have already undressed and those waiting to do so, for children and for patients waiting for further films. Obviously, the layout of the department determines whether these requirements can be met and in an old department compromises often have to be made. However, a patient should not have to wait for a long time in a small, relatively airless, changing cubicle. Lavatories must be available near the waiting room and their location indicated by clearly visible notices.

Undressing. A clean gown must be provided for each patient and a dressing gown also is required if the cubicle does not lead directly into the X-ray room. Instructions about personal matters, such as which clothes to remove, should be given as privately as possible. It is often helpful to have printed instructions displayed in the cubicle regarding undressing, what to put on and whether to proceed to another waiting room or wait until called. Often patients do not hear or fully understand instructions given too rapidly or too quietly. Some method of safe-keeping for money or valuables must be provided.

Privacy. Radiographic examinations should be carried out in as much privacy as possible. The door of the X-ray room should be closed and only the necessary persons should be present in the room. This is of particular importance in examinations such as hystero-salpingography and micturating cystography, where the patient is required to relax but may find it very difficult to do so without sufficient privacy. The patient should be covered with a light-weight blanket or sheet whenever possible.

Comfort. If practicable, a foam mattress, encased in a polythene cover, should be placed on the X-ray table for the patient to lie on, particularly for any examination where the patient must remain in the same position for a long time. Moving the patient across the table during positioning is facilitated if the mattress (with its polythene cover) is encased in a cotton covering. Sufficient pillows, foam pads and sandbags should be used to make the patient comfortable. A patient who is uncomfortable, or who feels insecure, is likely to move during the exposure.

A sturdy platform, or preferably a small set of steps, must be available so that the patient can climb easily on to the X-ray table. During fluoroscopic examinations, when the patient must be moved from the horizontal to the vertical position, hand-grips and a firm foot-rest must be provided.

A patient must *never* be allowed to descend from a table without someone being at hand to steady him. A nervous patient may try to do so too quickly and fall over. The radiographer should not tell a patient that the examination is finished and that he can get down from the X-ray table unless the radiographer is near enough to assist. A patient with a condition such as Menière's disease or postural hypotension may need a few moments sitting up on the table before getting off. The radiographer must see that the X-ray tube is out of the way so that there is no risk of the patient's striking his head against it when sitting up or getting off the table.

A wheel-chair must always be steadied when a patient is getting into or out of it, and the brake should be on. If there is no brake, the radiographer should put his or her foot behind the wheel to act as a chock. Some modern wheel-chairs are so designed as not to tip up even if someone stands on the step, but others will tip if the patient just puts one foot on the step.

Hygiene. The X-ray room should be tidied immediately after use so that it is clean and tidy when the next patient enters it. If it is not possible to have a clean sheet and pillowcase for each patient who is radiographed lying on the X-ray table, then use should be made of tissues, paper towels or, preferably, large sheets of tissue paper placed over the sheet and pillow and changed for each patient.

There should be a vomit bowl in the X-ray room, visible and within easy reach, particularly for accident patients and for some ward patients for whom a change in position may cause vomiting.

Immobilisation. The patient must remain absolutely still in the required position while each exposure is being made. Any movement during the exposure will cause blurring of the film, necessitating a repeat exposure.

For radiographic examination of the skull, head-clamps or head-bands are used to immobilise the patient's head. For radiographic examination of the extremities, foam pads and sandbags should be used for support and immobilisation. The patient must be made as comfortable as possible because if he is in pain or in an uncomfortable position, it is unlikely that he will be able to keep still for long.

Radiography. The radiographer must see that everything, including any special equipment that must be tested before use, is ready before the patient is brought into the X-ray room. Clear instructions regarding position, respiration, etc. must be given to the patient in advance and it is often advisable to have a practice run without radiation to make sure that the patient arrests respiration for the required length of time.

Positioning of the patient should be efficient, speedy and gentle. The palm of the hand and the palmar surface of the fingers (not the tips of the fingers) should be used for positioning and centering. The patient's skin may be tender as a result of radiotherapy or a recent operation.

Explanation. Although it is usually unnecessary (and often contra-indicated) to give the patient a detailed explanation of the examination to be performed, most patients appreciate being given some information, particularly as to how long the examination will take.

If the procedure is going to cause any pain or discomfort, warning should be given to the patient (usually by the radiologist) so that he will not be surprised or alarmed by it and will be able to keep still when required. But if the examination is unlikely to cause pain or other unpleasant effect, the radiographer should never specifically tell the patient this, as occasionally a procedure (e.g. venepuncture) does unexpectedly cause pain or some other unpleasant effect. If this happens after the patient has been reassured to the contrary, his confidence may be destroyed. This is particularly relevant in the case of a child. Furthermore, the mere mention of some specific sensation may make the patient apprehensive when he would not otherwise have thought of it and the slightest sensation will tend to be magnified.

If apparatus that makes considerable noise is about to be used (as, for example, in rapid serial radiography) or if the X-ray tube is going to move during the exposure (as, for example, in tomography) the patient should be warned of this as otherwise he may move because of surprise or alarm when it happens.

The radiographer must never divulge to a patient a diagnosis or the result of a radiographic examination, for example whether a fracture is present or whether a chest radiograph is normal. Such information must be given to the patient *only* by a doctor. However, when avoiding answering a patient's questions, the radiographer must be careful not to alarm him and this can best be done by explaining that it is because of this general and inflexible rule and not because of anything to do with his particular case that his questions cannot be answered by the radiographer.

A patient must never be allowed to learn his diagnosis or prognosis by reading his notes or case records and therefore must never be given these to hold. Unless the details on the request form are absolutely innocuous, he must never be allowed to read it. For these reasons, notes and case records should always be placed out of the patient's view and the request form should be placed face downwards so that it cannot be read by him.

Consent forms. These are usually signed by adult patients at the commencement of their treatment but many radiological examinations also require the patient's specific consent. For patients under 16 years of age, the consent must be obtained from the parent or guardian. Although it is not part of the radiographer's duties to obtain a valid consent form, he or she should check that one is included with the patient's notes before contrast studies are performed.

After-care of the patient. After-care of the patient for specific radiological procedures is dealt with in Part III. However, care of the patient following plain film radiography must not be overlooked. Patients must be fit to leave the department before they do so and particular care must be taken of diabetic patients to ensure they are not kept waiting long when their meal or insulin is due.

Emergencies. It is important for the radiographer to know how to deal with emergencies that occur from time to time in an X-ray department. When they do occur, it is usually following the injection of contrast medium and therefore the subject is dealt with in Part III (p. 208) to which reference should be made.

The whole subject of patient care is a very large one and is more fully treated in specialised works (e.g. Chesney and Chesney, 1973).

INFANTS AND CHILDREN

Paediatric radiography presents particular problems and is best carried out by staff trained and interested in dealing with infants and children, preferably in a specially designed and equipped department, though every department, especially Accident and Emergency departments, will sometimes have to radiograph infants and children. Even in a busy general department, extra time taken in attempting to gain a child's confidence is well spent. It is also necessary to obtain the co-operation and assistance of the parent, if present, as he or she is often required to hold the child during the examination.

Details about specific difficulties, or special views for children, are given in the appropriate sections throughout the book, usually under 'Modifications', 'Special Circumstances' or 'Supplementary Views'. Further information can be found in specialised books on the subject, e.g. *A Handbook of Paediatric Radiography* by Gyll (1977) and *Diagnostic Radiology in Paediatrics* by Gordon and Ross (1977).

Equipment. High powered equipment should be used for both departmental and mobile examinations. Very fast screens, permitting short exposure times, should be used to avoid unsharpness due to movement or respiratory blur. Specially designed tables, incorporating cradles or trays in which a child can be positioned and immobilised, are available but usually only in specialised paediatric departments.

Even if a room is not specially designed for paediatric radiography, any general room in which it is carried out must have the necessary equipment of the basic kind, e.g. wide compression bands, foam pads and sandbags (some disguised as toy animals), toys (one with a loud squeak to attract a child's attention at a crucial moment), 'Velcro' fastened straps and radiolucent tape.

Waiting. If a child has to be kept waiting before being radiographed, it should be for the shortest possible time. A distressed or unco-operative child is a cause of worry to other patients who are waiting and it is often best to treat a sick or injured child as an urgent case to be dealt with quickly, even if out of turn. Even in a general waiting room it is usually possible to have one corner devoted to children if their examination occurs frequently as in Accident and Emergency departments. It should look friendly and interesting, with some appropriate pictures at a suitable height, toys, perhaps an aquarium and one or two small chairs that children can sit in comfortably.

Undressing. A child should not be undressed unnecessarily, as this produces a feeling of insecurity in many children. If it is necessary for him to be undressed, it should be done by the parent in the X-ray room after the child has become acquainted with the room and the 'camera'. If he objects to taking his clothes off, and is likely to prove unco-operative as a result, it is better to leave them on and move any metal hooks, zip-fasteners, etc. out of the way for each radiograph. A few obvious artefacts on the radiograph of a co-operative child are preferable to blurred or rotated radiographs of an unco-operative child who undressed unwillingly.

Explanation. An explanation must be given to a child, in words that he can understand, as to what is going to happen and what is wanted of him. It is important that a child is told the truth but not necessarily the whole truth. In particular he should not be told that something will not hurt, if it *is* going to, however slightly, e.g. venepuncture. Otherwise he will be very unwilling to allow anything similar to happen again.

Radiation protection. The X-ray beam must be collimated so that only the area being examined is irradiated, e.g. a chest radiograph of a baby must not include half the abdomen as well. The beam must be collimated so that the hands of the person holding the child do not appear on the radiograph. There must be enough lead coats, gloves and protective screens for persons holding a child for radiographic examination to be adequately protected. The radiographer must ask the mother or nurse who is with the child if she is pregnant. If so, someone else (but not a radiographer) must hold the child. The same person must not assist too often. A notice should be displayed in the waiting room to the effect that if a woman accompanying a child for X-ray is pregnant she must tell the radiographer before the child is X-rayed. As such a notice fails if there are language or literacy problems the radiographer should always ask.

A helper may find that wearing lead rubber gloves makes it difficult to hold a child in the required position. Instead, it is often easier, once the helper is holding the child correctly, for the radiographer to place pieces of lead rubber over the helper's hands.

Gonad protection should be used whenever possible. In radiography of the hip joints, protection of any sort is difficult to maintain in position even with radiolucent tape. It is therefore not advised for an initial examination because repeat films will be necessary if essential detail is obscured as a result of the protection device having moved.

Radiography. Two radiographers working together as a team can set up a routine which greatly reduces the time for the examination and which, if the child is unco-operative, results in a less exhausting experience for everyone. One radiographer positions the child and shows the parent or nurse how to hold him and the other radiographer changes the cassettes, sets the exposure factors and makes the exposure. The easiest, or least uncomfortable, view or position should be done first, e.g. a lateral view of the elbow before attempting an antero-posterior view. If the first 'picture' is easy for the child and he is praised and encouraged, subsequent examination is more likely to succeed.

Exposure factors should be correct first time. If the exposure is not perfect but the child was still and in the required position, it is advisable to seek the advice of the radiologist who will report on the radiographs, as it may be possible for a diagnosis to be made on a less than perfect radiograph and so avoid extra radiation to the child. Exposure charts for all parts of the body and for all ages and physique types of infants and children should be by the control table. It is essential to take into consideration physique as well as age because a stocky 9 or 10 year old child may need as much exposure for a radiograph of the chest or abdomen as would a slim adult. A thick-set 2 or 3 year old child needs as much exposure for a chest radiograph as does an average 7 or 8 year old. Exposures should be set, or provisionally decided on, before the child is brought into the X-ray room so that there is no delay once the child is positioned.

The X-ray tube should be centred and the beam collimated to the cassette before the child is positioned. It is very important that the tube height for over-couch views is fixed *before* the child is positioned and it must never be lowered over him. The fright caused by lowering the tube may result in further radiography being very difficult and the child may remember this fear if he needs to be radiographed again.

Co-operation. Usually children of school age will co-operate if they are told and shown what is going to happen and if, for example, they are allowed to place their injured limb into position themselves. The exceptions to these co-operative schoolchildren are the mentally handicapped or those who are too frightened to co-operate. Tiny babies can usually be held successfully, though they are quite surprisingly strong. The difficult children to radiograph are those aged between 9 months and about 5 years, when they may be too young to understand but rather strong to be held against their will. If it becomes obvious that despite encouraging yet firm persuasion the child is not going to co-operate, he must be held firmly by the parent or nurse and the examination carried out as quickly as possible.

Whatever method of immobilisation is chosen it must be effective and gentle and the child must not be frightened by it. He should be chatted to the whole time to encourage him. For radiography of the skull, one of the best methods of immobilising a struggling child is to wrap ('swaddle') him firmly but gently in a small blanket and put a wide compression band over the abdomen and knees. His head is then held between foam pads by the parent or nurse. A wide compression band (without the swaddling) over the abdomen and knees can be used when views of the chest are being taken, or over the knees and legs for views of the abdomen, in each case the child's hands being held over his head by the helper. Radiography of the hands and feet can be difficult because it is almost impossible to persuade a tiny child not to curl his fingers or toes. Radiolucent adhesive tape, applied at the last moment, will keep them still during a short exposure.

The age at which a child can co-operate in holding his breath varies but if a very short exposure time is used the child's breathing should be observed and the exposure made at the correct moment.

A gentle but firm voice helps to give confidence to a frightened child but it may be impossible to communicate if he is making too much noise to hear. The radiographer must always try to keep the situation under his or her control because a child can sense stress and lack of confidence and will take advantage of it. The radiographer must never shout at a screaming child as this will only make a difficult situation worse.

Tiny babies are usually easiest to radiograph immediately after a feed, when they may sleep through it all. Arrangements should be made with the ward, or the mother, so that feed and examination can be synchronised.

Sedation. If all efforts to achieve the required radiographs fail it may be necessary for the child to be sedated. This will be decided by the radiologist or clinician. Facilities must be available for the sedation to be given, for the child to remain quietly while it takes effect and for him to remain afterwards while it wears off. This is both time- and space-consuming and is therefore carried out only when unavoidable. The sedation must be given at a time appropriate for the examination and must last long enough for it to be completed.

For examinations where a child has to remain still in the same position for a long time, sedation is usually necessary and children under 12 usually receive a general anaesthetic for the more complicated or unpleasant examinations involving injections of contrast media.

Multiple injuries. A child with multiple injuries must be either radiographed on the casualty stretcher or, if he can be moved, lifted on a canvas. Although it is easy to lift a child, he should be moved as little as possible and lateral views should be taken using a horizontal beam.

Non-accidental injury in the young ('Battered baby'). When this condition is suspected, the following views are taken:

  (i) Antero-posterior view of the pelvis
 (ii) Antero-posterior view of the thorax
(iii) Antero-posterior views of all long bones
(iv) Lateral view of the skull

Extra views are taken of any areas showing bruising, or as required by the radiologist or clinician. Sometimes the radiographer may need to exercise considerable tact if a parent objects to such extra views being taken.

ELDERLY PATIENTS

Patients aged from about 60 years who are acutely or chronically ill are usually termed geriatric patients. Such patients are not necessarily senile or irremediably chronically ill, but they often present problems not usually associated with younger patients.

Many general X-ray departments are becoming increasingly involved in the radiography of geriatric patients and the main essentials are (a) allowing sufficient time and (b) versatility of radiographic technique. Most such patients try very hard to co-operate but usually they cannot be hurried and often need a lot of assistance.

When the patient attends for radiographic examination, there is some conflict of interest between completing the examination as quickly as possible and allowing the patient to do as much as he can for himself. It is important in geriatric medicine that the patient retains maximum independence for as long as possible but if he is acutely ill he obviously requires much help and support.

It must never be assumed that because a patient is elderly he is also deaf and probably senile as well. Unfortunately this assumption is often encountered in hospitals and is much resented by the patients. The patient should be treated with respect and not with over-familiarity. A radiographer from the start of training should make an effort to remember the name of the patient with whom he or she is dealing and *use* it.

Some conditions make any sort of movement painful, and considerable gentleness is needed. Frail old people have very delicate skins and care must be taken not to hurt them. The possibility that he or she may have pressure sores must be remembered when lifting a bedridden patient.

The timing and method of examination and the views needed will vary with the clinical requirements and with the staff, equipment and space available in each department.

Appointments. It is often preferable to make appointments for the late morning or mid-afternoon to avoid the patient's having to rush to get ready in the morning and to avoid crowded public transport, if used. It is also desirable to avoid times when the department is particularly busy. However, if hospital transport is needed, the appointment will probably have to be made to coincide with existing transport arrangements and routes. Sometimes patients are admitted to hospital for the night preceding some radiological procedures to ensure that preparation (such as taking drugs, or abstaining from food and/or drink) is carried out. Appointments and preparation instructions must *always* be written and not just given verbally and it must be certain that they have been understood.

Undressing. Sufficient time must be allowed for the patient to undress and careful instructions must be given as to exactly what is required. The patient should not be told to take off all his clothes and put on the hospital gown if it is not really necessary for all clothes to be removed. It is often sufficient to remove some garments only, or the patient may have come prepared for the examination and be wearing underclothes perfectly suitable for radiography so that only the outer garments need to be removed or raised. Unnecessary undressing should be avoided as it is time-consuming and is tiring for the patient. If a gown is needed, it may be better to provide one that opens down the back as it is easier to put on than one that needs to go over the head. A dressing gown should be provided or the patient should wear his coat. He must not be allowed to get cold while waiting, wearing just a thin gown. He should not be left to wait in a relatively airless cubicle.

Privacy. Elderly patients appreciate (and should be given) privacy and modest treatment. The door to the X-ray room must be kept closed during the examination and the patient covered with a sheet or light-weight blanket. When a lateral view of the neck of the femur is being taken, the pelvis should be covered with a dressing-towel or large piece of tissue paper and not left exposed. A patient on a trolley should be covered before returning to the waiting area.

Explanation and instructions. The patient should always be told what is going to happen and what he is expected to do, so that he can co-operate as much as possible. The radiographer will then know how much or how little he can do for himself. The patient is usually apprehensive and although detailed explanation is not always advisable (p. 6) he usually appreciates being told what is involved. Instruction regarding breathing or swallowing should be given clearly and rehearsed to ensure that the patient does hold his breath or swallow when required to do so.

The radiographer should find out as early as possible whether the patient is deaf and, if so, instructions must be given clearly enough to be heard and understood. If the patient is very deaf it may be necessary for him to lip-read or for hand signs or written instructions (e.g. a card with large print) to be given. The radiographer must find out how to communicate with the very deaf patient sympathetically and without making him feel inadequate. It is often unnecessary to ask a patient to hold his breath for chest or abdominal radiography if a very short exposure time is used and his breathing rhythm is observed. Patients who have impairment of vision as well as of hearing need particular care and sympathy, especially when these conditions are in addition to their main presenting illness.

When calling a patient who is sitting in the waiting room, it must be remembered that he may need help in getting up from the chair and support when walking. A radiographer should not call a patient's name and expect him to rise and follow. He must be allowed time to walk without being hurried. In a busy department, it is very easy to become intolerant with patients who need a lot of time to move, to get undressed or to carry out instructions, but the radiographer must allow the time. In some departments that deal frequently with geriatric patients there are helpers or auxiliaries who are able and experienced in helping patients to get undressed or to move from place to place.

Problems associated with geriatric patients. These include:

1. Co-ordination problems, particularly after a cerebro-vascular accident ('stroke'), making movement and co-operation difficult.
2. Chronic cardio-vascular disease, causing dyspnoea and circulatory problems, making movement and effort difficult.
3. Chronic bronchitis or emphysema, causing dyspnoea and difficulty in holding breath.
4. Impaired hearing and/or vision, making understanding and co-operation difficult.

5. Early dementia, causing difficulty in remembering or carrying out instructions.
6. Arthritis, making movement difficult or painful.
7. Postural hypotension, or Menière's disease, causing difficulty in balance.
8. Obesity, making movement difficult and causing radiographic problems.
9. Involuntary movement, e.g. in Parkinson's disease.
10. Incontinence, e.g. in carcinoma of the bladder or colon, or from senility.
11. General frailness, caused by osteoporosis, metastases, post-operative conditions, emaciation in the elderly, etc.

Radiographic considerations. Radiographic technique should be modified so that maximum information is obtained with minimum disturbance, movement or discomfort to the patient.

1. A floating-top table allows a number of views to be taken without moving the patient.

2. The X-ray tube must be capable of being lowered sufficiently for lateral views of the knees, ankles or feet to be taken with a horizontal beam and with the patient sitting in a wheel-chair or lying on any type of stretcher or trolley.

3. Antero-posterior views of the knees, legs and ankles can be taken with the patient sitting in a wheel-chair and with the limb supported on a foot-rest. There is no need for a patient to climb on to an X-ray table for these views.

4. Views of the feet should be taken with the patient sitting in a chair and with the film placed on the floor.

5. If a patient cannot stand easily for views of the chest, he should remain in the wheel-chair and antero-posterior and lateral views can be taken with him sitting comfortably. Such views will be straight and without respiratory or movement blur. They should be clearly marked so that the radiologist knows an antero-posterior view has been taken.

6. Wheel-chairs should have removable arms so that lateral views of the chest or thoracic spine can be taken with the patient sitting in the wheel-chair.

7. A small set of steps with a hand-rail is useful when a patient has to get up on to the X-ray table.

8. A canvas and lifting poles should be used to lift a patient from a bed or trolley on to the X-ray table.

9. Plenty of pillows, foam pads and sandbags should be ready to hand, for support and immobilisation.

10. Very fast screens which allow short exposure times help to minimise unsharpness due to movement or respiratory blur. Very fast screens also allow more frequent use of the fine focus for optimum bone detail.

11. If grid cassettes are used, they can be placed to suit the patient's position rather than positioning the patient to the X-ray table or vertical Bucky.

12. Previous radiographs should always be studied before the patient is radiographed to see if conditions such as pneumonic consolidation, osteoporosis, or Paget's disease are present as these will influence the selection of exposure factors.

13. If several views are required, a plan of work should be thought out in advance to avoid delay or needless movement of the patient. Such a plan is described for skeletal survey (pp. 199 and 200).

Kindly reassurance helps allay fears of a strange environment and frightening equipment which those who work in the department take for granted. A friendly, sympathetic smile and gentle manner will make the examination less of an ordeal for the patient. A relative waiting with the patient (particularly a husband or wife who is also elderly and who may be very distressed) must also be treated with kindness and consideration and their offers of help received courteously and, if not acceptable, declined tactfully.

2

Radiation protection

The ionising radiation used in diagnostic radiography is potentially harmful but if proper protective measures are taken the risk is small compared with the benefit to the patient. It is essential to ensure that the radiation dose received by the patient is the minimum required to provide the necessary diagnostic information, but at the same time this consideration must never be allowed to make an examination inconclusive through being incomplete.

All radiation which is outside the area of diagnostic interest or which is absorbed in the superficial layers of the patient, contributes nothing to diagnostic detail and involves unnecessary irradiation. The amount of scattered radiation depends both on the dose and on the area irradiated and so the reduction of unnecessary dose to the patient also results in reduction of the dose received by the staff (Adrian Report, 1960).

The radiographer must always aim to produce a perfect result at the first attempt as the greatest source of unnecessary irradiation of a patient is the repeat film. Even low doses are of great statistical importance because of the large number of patients who receive them and the fact that the exact relationship between dose and effect at low doses has not yet been established. It is not possible to rely upon the existence of a threshold level of dose, below which no genetic effects occur.

There are three main reasons for continued efforts to minimise the radiation dose received by both patient and staff.

1. To reduce the gonad dose to the general population. In examinations carried out on a large percentage of the population annually, such as routine chest examinations, mammography and dental examinations, the gonad dose per film is small but, because of the extremely large numbers of such examinations, the doses received are of statistical importance owing to the possibility, however remote, of gene mutations. This is called the 'genetic effect', i.e. it is observed only in the descendants of those irradiated.

2. To protect from damage tissues that are particularly susceptible to irradiation. These include the gonads, the eyes and tissues containing a large number of cells undergoing division, such as the bone marrow and foetus. Effects observable in the individual irradiated are called 'somatic effects'.

3. To ensure that the radiation dose received by staff working in X-ray departments is kept at a level at which it is of negligible significance. With modern standards of X-ray protection in the tube housings, etc., and with modern protective devices such as light beam diaphragms, lead aprons and protective screens, this is quite possible without restrictions being applied to the number and type of investigations carried out. This leaves a safety margin so that in the event of an accidental exposure (even if this results in a significant dose) the maximum permissible doses for a calendar quarter, or for a year, may not in fact be exceeded.

It has been considered for some years that there is no tolerance level of radiation dose. The concept of tolerance has been replaced by that of Maximum Permissible Doses for various parts of the body, which are continually reviewed as greater knowledge of the effects of radiation is obtained. Better equipment and techniques have made it possible to keep pace with the higher standards required.

General measures for radiological protection are laid down in the 'Code of Practice for the Protection of Persons against Ionising Radiations arising from Medical and Dental Use', a copy of which should be available in every X-ray department. Every member of the staff to whom this Code applies is required to read the sections which affect his or her work and well-being and also the local rules drawn up by the Radiological Safety Committee for the particular department and must sign a statement that he or she is aware of, and understands, the responsibilities laid down in the Code and the local rules.

The relevant provisions of the Code of Practice must always be implemented. For example, all departments must have a safety officer, X-ray sets must be checked for any radiation leakage, the appropriate filters must always be used and radiation monitoring films, thermo-luminescent dosimeters or personal ionisation chambers must be worn by all members of the staff who are 'designated persons'. But staff should not be designated unnecessarily.

The staff of an X-ray department should always be aware that the dose they themselves receive is affected by the way in which they carry out their work, and the following points must always be remembered:

1. Never stand in the direct beam.
2. Collimate the beam accurately, to reduce the area irradiated.
3. Never support or hold patients during radiography.
4. Always stand behind the lead protective screen round the control console or leave the room while the exposure is being made. If this is not possible, a lead apron must be worn.
5. Protective coats, aprons, gloves and gonad shields should be checked for cracks—visually at frequent intervals and radiographically at least annually. Coats and aprons should be hung on hangers or on a rail and never folded.

Examinations entailing the risk of a high gonad dose (e.g. examinations of the pelvis, lumbar spine and hip joints) must be carried out with zealous attention to protection against irradiation.

For male patients, gonad protection must be used whenever possible.

For female patients of child-bearing capacity, the 10-day rule should be observed, i.e. radiographic examination of areas between the diaphragm and the knees should be carried out, if possible, within 10 days after the first day of the menstrual period so as to reduce the likelihood of irradiating an early stage of pregnancy. It is the duty of the referring clinician to enter the date of the last menstrual period on the request form and state if, on grounds of clinical urgency, the 10-day rule should *not* be observed (Code of Practice, 1972; Royal College of Radiologists Recommendations, 1975).

For female patients undergoing pelvic or gastro-intestinal examinations, it is not possible to use any form of gonad protection and great care must be taken to restrict irradiation as much as possible and to avoid the need for repeat films. The possibility should be considered of taking postero-anterior views, rather than antero-posterior views for the sacrum, sacro-iliac joints, etc., particularly if frequent follow-up examination is likely.

During excretion urography, female patients should be protected with a lead shield across the pelvis when the kidney area is being examined. Such a protective shield is often incorporated in the compression device.

Infants and children present special problems which are mentioned in the previous chapter (p. 9).

The highest gonad doses to men are received in the examination of the hip and upper femur (1,200 mrad) while the highest gonad doses to women are received in cystography (1,500 mrad) (I.C.R.P.,

1970). The highest skin doses are received in an examination such as a lateral view of the lumbar spine in an obese patient.

It is not within the scope of this book to discuss in detail all methods of reducing radiation dose to patient and staff but the points to which particular attention must be paid may be summarised as follows:

IN RADIOGRAPHY

1. Correct positioning, kilovoltage, exposure and film-screen combination must be used so as to prevent the necessity for repeat films. The part under examination should be immobilised. When radiographing very large patients, consideration should be given to increasing the focus-film distance, to reduce the incident skin dose. Attention must be paid to efficient dark-room technique to avoid the possibility of films being double-exposed or their being spoilt through faulty handling. Careful monitoring of processing solutions, fresh chemicals and appropriate replenishment must be carried out to maintain constant exposures.

2. The primary beam must be accurately limited with cones, apertures or, preferably, light beam diaphragms, so that only the exact area to be investigated is irradiated. The beam must never extend beyond this area or beyond the cassette.

3. Light beam diaphragms must be checked as soon as possible after they are installed, and after any servicing procedures, to ensure that the area covered by the X-ray beam is identical to that covered by the light beam.

4. Gonad dose should be controlled by placing lead rubber over the gonads whenever possible and by ensuring that the gonads are never irradiated unnecessarily. The primary beam must be directed away from the gonads whenever possible, e.g. in radiography of the extremities.

5. The fastest film/screen combination consistent with satisfactory diagnostic quality should be used. Rare earth screens or very fast tungstate screens should be used whenever possible for examinations entailing a high dose to the gonads or eyes or where there is probability of movement blur.

6. When the thicker parts of the body are being radiographed, the skin dose can be reduced by using high kilovoltage technique. It is also of advantage for infants or unco-operative adults because the high output and correspondingly short exposure times possible help to prevent movement blur.

7. Notices should be displayed in waiting rooms and changing

cubicles instructing patients to inform the radiographer *before* they are radiographed, if they are, or think they may be, pregnant.

8. Radiography of a pregnant patient should never be undertaken unless it is absolutely essential, and when it is carried out care must be taken to avoid, whenever possible, irradiation of the foetus. Mass miniature radiography should be avoided, because of the higher doses involved.

9. When tomography is being carried out, consideration should be given to the use of multi-section cassettes.

10. Lead eye shields should be used during tomography (particularly hypocycloidal tomography) of the petrous bones.

11. Short distance techniques must be avoided because of the high skin doses involved.

12. The appropriate grid should be used, as too high a grid ratio may lead to an increase in the dose received by the patient. Consideration should be given to the use of the air gap technique (p. 27), instead of a grid for examinations such as orbital phlebography and cerebral angiography.

13. Under the Health and Safety at Work etc. Act 1974 patients who are not themselves being examined or treated by radiation are regarded as members of the public. Thus, when a mobile unit is used in a ward, measures must be taken to ensure that no-one is irradiated other than the patient being examined. Mobile lead screens should be used to protect patients in adjacent beds, visitors and staff.

14. Patients undergoing treatment with radium or caesium insertions should not be taken into a waiting room or lift, or other areas where there are other patients, hospital staff or visitors.

15. If the services of a department of medical physics are available, X-ray tubes should be checked (for output, quality, timer accuracy and effective kilovoltage) on installation and thereafter annually or more often if required. Also, image intensification systems should be checked for output on installation and thereafter at frequent intervals.

IN FLUOROSCOPY

1. Because of the high doses involved (particularly to the patient's bone marrow and to the staff carrying out the procedure) fluoroscopy should never be undertaken if the same information can be obtained radiographically.

2. Image intensification should be used whenever available. Sophisticated techniques such as cardiac catheterisation should never be carried out without an intensifier, as the doses otherwise received by the staff and patient are too high.

3. When image intensification is not available, adequate dark adaptation is essential. Increased screening factors must not be used to compensate for inadequate dark adaptation. Sudden lights should be avoided during screening sessions.

4. Any X-ray tube used for fluoroscopic examinations must be under the control of a spring-biassed switch, so that release of the switch automatically terminates the exposure. A timing device with a maximum setting of ten minutes is also required by the Code of Practice.

5. A lead apron not less than 45×45 cm (18 in $\times$ 18 in) and with a lead equivalent of at least 0·5 mm, should be attached to the bottom of the screen and, if possible, additional protection should be fitted to the side of the couch.

6. In training establishments it is important to emphasise the significance of the area of the beam as a factor in determining the integral dose, particularly to the bone marrow. The Code of Practice recommends that an instrument should be available for measuring the surface integral of exposure (i.e. the product, in Rcm^2, of the exposure and the area).

SEALED RADIOACTIVE SOURCES

In departments where radiography of patients undergoing treatment with sealed radioactive sources is carried out routinely, special attention should be paid in the local rules to the procedure for such patients.

The examination should be carried out speedily. Everything needed for the examination should be ready in advance. Nursing staff and porters should be instructed where to stand when they are with such patients in the recovery room and when taking them to the X-ray department and back to the ward. Nurses should be aware of the inverse square law, i.e. the increasing safety of distance.

RADIONUCLIDES

In general, there are few hazards associated with the handling of diagnostic quantities of radioactive materials but special attention should be paid to the dispensing procedures and to the disposal of radioactive waste. The latter must conform with the terms of any authorisation granted to the hospital by the relevant authorities. All procedures concerning the handling of radioactive materials should be listed in the local rules with particular attention to any special hazard.

3

Exposures

Introduction. When a radiographic exposure is made, X-rays of a selected quality and quantity, determined by the kilovoltage (kV) and milliampere-seconds (mA.s) are emitted from the tube from a source of finite area. They diverge uniformly, so that the area covered is directly proportional to the square of the distance travelled. The beam is attenuated by the inherent filtration of the tube and any added filter, and it is collimated by a diaphragm or cone.

The X-ray beam passes through the patient and is differentially attenuated by the various structures present. This attenuation depends on the atomic weight of the constituent material and upon the kilovoltage employed. Secondary radiation resulting from photo-electric absorption and scattering arises in the patient during the course of attenuation of the primary beam and is emitted in all directions. Thus variations of intensity are produced across the plane of the emergent beam. This may then be passed through a grid which absorbs predominantly the secondary radiation and the image is recorded when the final beam passes through a film or film-screen combination. The film is then processed.

Over a wide range, the response of the film to radiation is a function of the logarithm of exposure. Thus, equal increments in density are produced by successive doubling of the exposure.

The diagnostic value of the film depends on adequate definition and contrast of the image. The aim of the technique employed is to produce a sharp image with the densities spread evenly along the straight line part of the characteristic curve of the film, at the same time keeping to the minimum the radiation dose to the patient. Maximum sharpness is obtained when geometric blur, movement blur and photographic blur are all minimal. Any increase in the level of one of these types of blur above that of the other two will produce an almost equal decrease in sharpness, whereas reduction in the level of one below that of the other two will have no appreciable effect. It is therefore important to keep all uniformly low.

All these effects must be taken into consideration when selecting a suitable radiographic exposure. Although they are all interrelated, they are perhaps best considered individually.

Kilovoltage. Because of the complex and variable nature of the waveform of the voltage applied to the tube, it is customary to state the peak value of the potential applied, rather than attempting to define any effective value. The peak value is referred to as the kVp or, more usually, just as the kV.

An increase in kilovoltage has four effects:

1. Increase in the energy of the beam, so that greater film blackening is achieved. In the 50 to 80 kV range, an increase of 10 kV approximately doubles the exposure. At higher kV, similar increases have less effect and an increase of 15 kV is required to double the exposure.

2. Reduction of subject contrast, mainly because attenuation of the beam in dense structures such as bone is reduced and (to a lesser degree) attenuation in less dense structures such as fat is increased. Thus at higher kV levels the image contrast is less and a wider range of densities can be visualised on one exposure. The exposure factors are less critical because the densities do not occupy the whole of the straight line part of the characteristic curve.

3. Reduction of the skin and integral dose to the patient for any given degree of film blackening. But the gonad dose may be increased because of increase in secondary radiation.

4. Increase in secondary radiation. A high ratio grid is therefore needed to keep to a minimum the scattered radiation reaching the film.

The optimum kilovoltage is that which enables detail of all the structures of interest to be clearly shown.

Milliampere-seconds (mA.s). The total quantity of electrical energy passed through the tube is determined by the product of the tube current, usually measured in milliamperes, and the duration of the exposure. The radiation emitted is a function of the electrical energy incident at the target.

A satisfactory radiograph is obtained when the milliampere-seconds factor, for the kilovoltage employed, is sufficient to produce a density of 1·6 to 2·2 at the darkest point on the film. Normally the highest current available is used, so that the exposure time is as short as possible, thus avoiding movement blur. Only in special circumstances, including auto-tomography, is a long exposure time deliberately selected.

Filtration. All diagnostic tubes have an inherent filtration to which must be added a further filter of aluminium to give total filtration of 2 mm Al for voltages between 70 and 100 kV, and 2·5 mm Al for voltages over 100 kV (Code of Practice, 1972). This filtration selectively removes the softer radiation of the beam and therefore reduces the skin dose to the patient without greatly affecting film density.

When very low kilovoltage is required (as in mammography) additional filtration is a disadvantage. When very high kilovoltage is required, added filtration is an advantage.

Field size. Reducing the field size decreases the amount of scattered radiation. This decrease improves the contrast in the radiograph and reduces the integral dose to the patient but the exposure must be increased to produce an image of similar overall density. It is always important to use the minimum acceptable field size.

Distance. Increasing the focus-film distance has four effects:

1. Reduction of geometric blur, by reducing the effect of the finite focal spot size. This is of particular importance when the object of interest cannot be placed next to the film, as for example in a lateral view of the cervical spine.
2. Reduction in magnification, when the object cannot be placed next to the film. This is of particular importance in chest radiography.
3. Increase in the required exposure, which must be proportional to the square of the distance.
4. Reduction of the skin dose to the patient, by increasing the distance between the tube and the patient.

In practice, a standard optimum distance, often 90 cm (36 in) or 100 cm (40 in), is used for each radiographic examination. Other distances (120 cm, 150 cm or 180 cm) are employed in certain examinations, for example radiography of the chest and lateral views of the cervical spine.

Focal spot size. A small (0·3 mm^2) focal spot causes little geometric blur but the loading on the tube is such that usually only 25 mA is permissible and thus a 0·3 mm^2 focal spot is impracticable for most radiography. A 0·6 mm^2 focal spot is a useful compromise and usually allows at least 50 mA to be used. Often 1,000 mA can be used with a 2 mm^2 focal spot.

In general, the smallest focal spot should be used, taking into consideration tube loading and the possibility of movement blur.

Films and screens. The film-screen combination selected will be a compromise between the need for (*a*) optimum recording of detail and contrast (*b*) low radiation dose and (*c*) minimum photographic and movement blur. Non-screen film provides maximum detail, particularly in radiography of the extremities. High definition screens have a very small grain size and give admirable detail but require a longer exposure time, thus making movement blur more likely. Recently, some calcium tungstate screens have been introduced that are twice as fast as conventional 'fast tungstate' screens but with no significant increase in grain size. Rare earth screens (whose phosphors are terbium activated gadolinium or lanthanum oxysulphide) are several times more efficient at converting X-ray quanta into light than are conventional calcium tungstate screens.

The use of very fast screens (so-called 'new generation' screens) allows either:

(i) reduction of exposure time (to prevent unsharpness due to movement), or

(ii) reduction of kilovoltage (to improve contrast), or

(iii) reduction of milliamperage (to allow use of lower powered equipment and extend equipment life), or

(iv) use of the fine focus (to improve definition and for macroradiography).

Grids. The secondary radiation reaching the film can be as much as eight times greater than the amount of radiation due to the primary beam. This results in decreased contrast and loss of diagnostic detail. The amount of secondary radiation reaching the film can be reduced by the use of a grid, which consists of alternate strips of radiolucent and radiopaque material so arranged that they lie along the direction of the primary beam so that photons travelling in other directions are greatly reduced in intensity.

Grids can be either stationary or moving. Fine-line stationary grids are invaluable in accident radiography and many other examinations. They are conveniently used in the form of a grid-cassette. Moving grids are incorporated into Bucky trays and may be either oscillating or reciprocating in movement, or may have a single-stroke mechanism which needs to be set manually before use.

The use of a grid is essential for thicker parts of the body and for high kV radiography. However, it removes not only most of the secondary but also some of the primary radiation from the beam emerging from the patient and therefore inevitably leads to a reduction in the exposure reaching the film for a given value of kVp and mA.s.

To produce a radiograph of the required density, the missing exposure must therefore be restored. The consequent increase in dose to the patient can be minimised by increasing the kV (which will result in a slight decrease in contrast) rather than increasing the mA.s, which would result in a greater increase in dose to the patient.

Air gap technique. Instead of a grid, the air gap technique can be used for many examinations. The patient is positioned a little distance, usually about 15 cm, away from the cassette and the resulting air gap avoids the necessity for using a grid because the oblique scattered radiation fails to reach the film. Unless magnification is required, as in macroradiography, the focus-film distance is increased to compensate for the increased object-film distance. The exposure must be increased in proportion to the change in FFD (the inverse square law) but it will still be significantly less than that required when a grid is used.

Subject. The exposure factors chosen for a particular examination depend on the region of the body being examined, the structures to be demonstrated and the physique of the patient. When a contrast medium is used, the kilovoltage required depends on the intrinsic density of the contrast medium. Thus, in excretion choledochography the low density of the contrast medium demands low kilovoltage, while examinations with barium (which has a high intrinsic density) permit a high kilovoltage to be used. When contrast medium is not being employed there is usually considered to be an optimum range of kilovoltage for all parts of the body.

Exposure times are determined most efficiently by the use of a photo-timer. This measures the radiation emerging from a preselected area in the field and terminates the exposure when a predetermined level has been reached. When a photo-timer is not available, the exposure factors are selected after a general assessment of the patient, the clinical problem and the investigation required. It is helpful to have charts of satisfactory exposures at the control panel of each machine, so that a constant technique can be maintained. The chart should have exposure factors for average and large patients, for children and infants. When assessing a large patient, it is important to take his build into consideration as an obese patient requires less increase in exposure than a muscular patient of the same general size. These charts must be compiled on the basis of experience with each individual machine.

Refinements of non-automatic exposure selection which make for standardisation of technique are based on the weight of the patient and the thickness of the site under examination (Dawson *et al.*, 1966), or the Unit-step technique (Schwarz, 1961). The weight/thickness method is usually in the form of a table of kV per weight and thickness of patient for a constant mA.s and fixed focus-film distance. The Unit-step technique allows either the kV or mA.s to be changed. The part being examined is measured by calipers graduated in specially determined units. Unit numbers are assigned to the kV and mA.s (or separate mA and time) controls. A whole number is used for each doubling of radiographic effect. The controls are correctly set when the sum of the control numbers equals the caliper measurement.

Each of these methods requires considerable preliminary experiment but once the charts, or the calipers and marking of the controls, are established these methods each give very reliable results.

Variation from standard exposure. Variation from any of these three methods of determining the exposure factors must be made in certain circumstances. For example, if a limb is encased in plaster of Paris the exposure required is twice (for wet plaster, three times) the normal exposure. This usually necessitates a change from non-screen to screen film in order to reduce exposure time and the radiation dose. The use of a 6:1 grid requires four times the exposure needed without a grid, and a high-ratio grid requires correspondingly more.

Occasionally the optimum exposure factors may have to be sacrificed to other considerations, including the reduction of radiation dose and the prevention of movement blur in patients who cannot keep still.

Differing opinions are held as to whether it is better to vary the exposure factors when certain pathological conditions are present or to use a standard exposure so that the pathology is more obvious. For example, if a patient suffering from osteoporosis (decreased bone density) is radiographed with reduced kilovoltage, the final radiograph may approximate to normal, whereas if standard technique is employed, the film will appear greatly over-exposed and the condition will be made more obvious. On the other hand, with a patient suffering from osteopetrosis (increased bone density) if increased kilovoltage is used to show bone detail more clearly, the severity of the condition may be less obvious on the resulting radiograph. Whether or not the standard exposure factors are to be varied in such cases will be decided by the radiologist.

Processing. Each film has a correct processing technique and this information is available from the manufacturers. Ideally, automatic processing should be used but when hand processing is used a standard procedure must be employed. If the processing is varied to compensate for incorrect exposures, the final quality of the film is inevitably impaired and the accurate assessment of subsequent exposure factors becomes more difficult.

When an automatic processor is used, the replenishment rates and temperature must be carefully monitored. The machine must be kept scrupulously clean to avoid contamination and to prevent scratches and roller marks on the radiographs.

Conclusion. Not only is the selection of exposure factors governed by many conflicting considerations, making compromise necessary, but the choice of exposure factors is made more difficult by the fact that no two X-ray machines produce the same quantity of radiation with the same control setting, though each individual set is consistent in its own output. Furthermore, there is a wide range of preference among radiologists regarding the quality of the desired image.

It is therefore impossible to determine accurate exposure factors without taking into account all the considerations mentioned earlier and for this reason no lists of general exposure factors are given in this book. When a particular exposure technique is recommended, indication of this is given in the text.

4

High kilovoltage technique

Contrast in a radiograph is the difference in density between adjacent or superimposed shadows and this is produced by the difference in attenuation of X-rays by different tissues. The absorption of X-rays in different kinds of tissue varies with increase in kilovoltage, increasing slightly in soft tissues and decreasing sharply in bone. The difference in density between soft tissues and bone is therefore much less at 120 kV than it is at 60 kV.

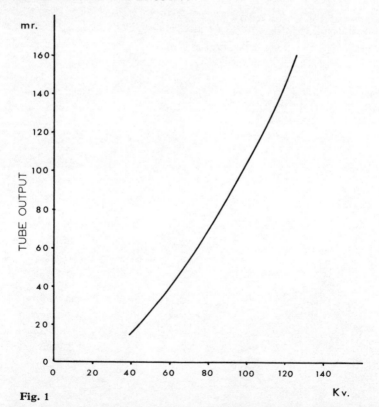

Fig. 1

In radiography, the main advantage of this phenomenon is that the use of high kilovoltage will increase the range of tissue densities that can be shown on a single radiograph.

The output of the X-ray tube is considerably increased at high kilovoltage (Fig. 1). The fluorescent yield from intensifying screens also increases rapidly with increase in kilovoltage, thus allowing the exposure factors to be considerably decreased. But, as the relative effect of scattered radiation greatly increases with higher kilovoltage, an effective grid (i.e. higher grid ratio) is required. Alternatively, the air gap technique (p. 27) can be used. The area irradiated should be reduced to the minimum by accurate collimation.

Advantages

1. A wide range of tissue density can be visualised on one film.
2. Reduction in milliampere-seconds (mA.s) allows a shorter time factor to be used, thus reducing the possibility of movement blur.
3. The heating of the X-ray tube is reduced. This is especially useful in rapid serial radiography.
4. There is greater exposure latitude.
5. The use of lower mA.s allows more frequent use of fine focus.
6. The radiation dose to the patient is reduced.

Disadvantages

1. Special equipment is needed.
2. Scattered radiation is increased and therefore a high-ratio grid is required. Lead backing to the cassette is also required.
3. There is loss of detail, and poor contrast, in soft tissue structures, e.g. the gall-bladder.
4. The gonad dose in chest radiography is higher.
5. There is risk of over-penetration, e.g. in small peripheral vessels.
6. Bone detail in skeletal work is poorly rendered.
7. Poor contrast is obtained in tomography.

Uses

1. In obstetric radiography, because of the reduction in dose to the mother and foetus.
2. In hystero-salpingography, because of the reduction in gonad dose.

3. In barium examinations and rapid serial examinations, because of the shorter exposure times possible, with less heating of the tube.
4. In lateral views of the lumbo-sacral spine, because of the greater range of densities that can be shown.

High energy technique

In the range of energies used in 'conventional' radiography, contrast is produced entirely from differing degrees of attenuation of the primary beam due to the photo-electric effect. This depends on the third power of the atomic number of the various elements present in the absorbing material, e.g. calcium in bone. At high energies, contrast is due entirely to the Compton effect which is independent of atomic number but proportional to density. This leads to the possibility of obtaining radiographs of diagnostic value with high energy radiation, e.g. radiographs of lungs and air-filled spaces, using cobalt[60] gamma radiation.

Some high energy equipment, e.g. a betatron, incorporates a diagnostic tube which gives an X-ray beam whose axis is parallel with that of the treatment beam and which may be used to obtain radiographs of the field treated, *in situ*, under geometrically similar conditions.

5

Soft tissue radiography

The individual tissues, such as muscle and fat making up soft tissue, have a low intrinsic density and there is very little difference in density (i.e. contrast) between adjacent structures. When radiographing soft tissues, a technique must be used that makes maximum use of this small degree of contrast.

When the apparatus is available, xeroradiography (p. 77) is the technique of choice, but when this is not possible, the usual conventional radiographic method is to use the lowest kilovoltage that will penetrate the part adequately. The kilovoltage chosen is 15 to 20 less than that required for bone detail of the same part. In some examinations, the most important of which is mammography, the kilovoltage required may be as low as 25. Modification of existing apparatus is therefore necessary. Specialised equipment for mammography, capable of giving very low kilovoltage combined with a high milliamperage and incorporating a photo-timer, has been developed. The rating charts of conventional, but modified, apparatus must be consulted to avoid overheating the tube by giving repeated exposures at low kilovoltage and high milliamperage.

When low kilovoltage technique is being used, materials that are radiolucent at higher kilovoltage values may be visible and may result in misinterpretation. For this reason, the part being examined should not be covered with a gown or other clothing, skin folds must be avoided by careful positioning and the presence of warts, moles, cysts or other skin lesions should be noted for the radiologist's information. Immobilisation and comfortable positioning are essential because the exposure may be of several seconds, especially if a fine focus is used.

Non-screen film will give optimum detail of soft tissue structures but may be impractical for thicker parts of the body, owing to the long exposure time that would be required. Industrial non-screen film gives even greater detail but is several times slower than medical non-screen film. A non-screen film placed on top of a cassette provides useful information regarding the soft tissues of the skull and face, particularly in the lateral view. This technique can also be of value in the case of patients with Paget's disease where, to obtain adequate penetration of dense bone, the soft tissues are greatly over-exposed. For investigation of soft tissue masses on the skull or limbs, the part if positioned so that the lesion is in profile.

Radiation protection

The use of low kilovoltage technique greatly increases the radiation dose to the patient, so zealous attention *must* be paid to protection of the gonads.

Uses

1. For mammography
2. To demonstrate:
   (a) Low-density foreign bodies
   (b) The larynx and soft tissue structures of the neck in a lateral view (Fig. 30, p. 176 and Plate XXII)
   (c) Cysticercosis (parasitic calcification)
   (d) Calcification in tendons and arteries
   (e) Soft tissue ulceration
   (f) Subcutaneous fat in nutrition surveys
   (g) Soft tissue signs following dislocation or subluxation of the acromio-clavicular joint (Weston, 1972)
   (h) Subdeltoid fat layer changes in peritendinitis or bursitis of the shoulder (Deichgraber and Olsson, 1975).

Multiple radiography

Principles. In multiple radiography, two or more radiographs are produced by a single exposure, the radiographs being either of different radiographic densities or replicas of each other. The procedure depends on the use of a series of intensifying screens, graded in speed so as to give a certain density on each film, either 'wide range' or duplication, the range of the former usually covering the difference between density for bone and that for soft tissues.

In general radiography, two or sometimes three pairs of screens are used which are graded in speed to achieve the required results. If radiographs of different densities are required, the screens are reversed in order, so that the fastest screens are nearest to the tube to give a radiograph with good bone detail, and the slowest screens are placed behind, to give a radiograph with soft tissue density. If duplicate radiographs are required, the sensitivity of the screens is increased progressively backwards, i.e. away from the tube, to compensate for the filtration afforded by the film, or films, in front.

The main advantages of this technique are that films of excellent definition throughout a large range of densities can be obtained on one exposure and that duplicate radiographs for teaching or research purposes are easily obtained (when more sophisticated methods of copying are not available) without additional radiation dose to the patient.

Uses. The uses of multiple radiography include:

1. Demonstration of the trachea, both suprasternally and retrosternally, in a lateral view of the thoracic inlet.
2. Investigation of placental site.
3. Demonstration of the thoraco-lumbar region, in a lateral view, where the difference in density above and below the diaphragm makes difficult the choice of exposure factors.
4. Any examination where both bone and soft tissue detail is required.
5. Duplication of radiographs.
6. Multi-section tomography (see under Tomography, p. 51).

Stereography

Stereography is the technique by which a three-dimensional image is produced by two radiographs. To achieve this third dimension in a two-dimensional plane, a pair of radiographs is taken, the X-ray tube being moved a certain distance between the exposures.

The total tube shift used is usually 6 cm, which is the normal inter-pupillary distance. The patient and cassette tray remain in exactly the same positions and only the tube is moved. Theoretically, the optimum focus-film distance used is ten times the total tube shift but in practice this is too short and in many cases would give an excessively high skin dose to the patient. However, it is important that the film be viewed from the same distance as the focus-film distance.

Usually the direction of the tube shift is at right angles to the long axis of the part under examination, e.g. a transverse shift is used for the spine and a longitudinal shift for the ribs.

Stereoscopic views in two planes are taken when accurate measurements are required, e.g. of the position of a radium implant. In these cases a cassette tunnel is used so that the two sets of radiographs may be taken with no movement of the patient. Shift markers are placed on the cassettes to indicate the direction of the tube shift. Exact measurements are obtained by the use of the mathematical formula of similar triangles.

Marking of radiographs. Stereoradiographs should be carefully marked to indicate (*a*) the anatomical left or right and (*b*) the direction of the tube shift. The markers should also show whether the radiographs are antero-posterior or postero-anterior views.

Viewing. Stereoscopic radiographs are viewed using stereo-binoculars or a stereoscope. In each method the radiograph taken with the left shift is viewed by the left eye and that taken with the right shift by the right eye. If it is not certain which radiograph is which, they should be superimposed on a viewing screen with their tube aspect away from the observer. The radiograph showing an image to the left of the other is the one that has been taken with the left tube shift and must be viewed with the left eye. The one showing an image to the right of the other is the one taken with the right tube shift and must be viewed with the right eye.

If a stereoscope or stereoscopic binoculars are not available, stereoradiographs can be examined by direct viewing. In this case, as there is no mirror system involved, the radiographs are placed side by side on a viewing screen with their tube aspect towards the observer. The right shift radiograph is placed to the observer's left and is viewed with the right eye, and the left shift radiograph is placed to the observer's right and viewed with the left eye.

Uses. Although stereography obviously doubles the radiation to the patient, the third dimension it affords may give added information in certain cases of doubtful diagnosis. Its most frequent use is probably for the sacro-iliac joints, particularly when overshadowed by bowel contents. It is also of use in certain views of the skull and can be used for direct measurement in any part of the body.

The technique of stereography may be included in some special procedures, such as angiography. Two X-ray tubes are mounted so that rapid exposures, alternating from one tube to the other, produce stereo pairs without moving the tubes.

8

Macroradiography

Macroradiography is the production of an enlarged image by X-ray magnification. The divergence of the beam from a small source is used to magnify the image geometrically.

Requirements. Successful macroradiography is governed by two conflicting requirements:

1. A fine focus tube is essential to reduce geometric blur. A focus of $0.1 \, mm^2$ or less is ideal, but in practice a $0.3 \, mm^2$ or $0.6 \, mm^2$ focus can produce perfectly acceptable macroradiographs.

2. A short exposure time is needed to avoid movement blur but, as the fine focus is being used, the tube rating will allow a maximum of only about 20–50 mA, unless a high speed tube is available.

Photographic blur, caused by the grain size of the film and intensifying screens, if used, is of little importance in macroradiography as only the image detail, and not the grain size, is magnified and resolution is increased (Hungerford, 1975).

Principles. The degree of magnification obtained by macroradiography depends on the ratio of the focus-film distance to the focus-object distance. Thus:

$$\text{magnification} = \frac{\text{size of image}}{\text{size of object}} = \frac{\text{focus-film distance}}{\text{focus-object distance}}$$

If the object is mid-way between the tube focus and the film, the size of the image is twice that of the object. In practice, magnification factors of $\times 1\frac{1}{2}$ or $\times 2$ are most commonly used. Geometric blur usually becomes unacceptable at values higher than $\times 2$ unless a microfocal tube is used.

Equipment. Although specialised equipment is available, successful macroradiographs can be produced using a variety of equipment:

1. A radiolucent table-top, such as the sliding top employed in angiocardiography, can be used. The patient is positioned on the table-top and the film is placed on the floor under the table. The

position for the centre of the film, to coincide with the central ray, is marked on the floor, immediately below the centre of the table.

2. The film may be placed on the table, with the part to be examined on a radiolucent box or platform placed on the table at the required height.

3. When a skull unit is used, the Bucky tray and mirror device are removed and the film is placed on the curved cross-arms of the tube, directly under the centre of the table. The object-film distance is usually such that the magnification is less than × 2.

4. An under-couch tube and serial film-holder may be used.

Technique. Depending on the apparatus used, the part to be examined is placed on a radiolucent surface and the film placed at a pre-determined distance below it or, if the under-couch tube is used, above it.

Accurate centering and collimation of the beam are essential, as any error will be geometrically magnified. The part under examination should be immobilised, as relatively long exposure times are required for all but the thinnest parts of the body.

The exposures required for macroradiography are determined by the focus-film distance. If fast film or screens are used, the exposure is reduced accordingly.

When rare earth screens are used, the effective 'noise' in the rare earth system is reduced as magnification increases and detail of small structures is much improved (Doi and Imhof, 1977). A single screen/ single emulsion film in a vacuum pack, used with a $0.1 \, mm^2$ focus and × 3 magnification gives fine detail of extremities and long bones (Genant *et al.*, 1977).

A short focus-object distance must not be used to reduce the exposure, because this would increase the radiation skin dose.

The use of a secondary radiation grid is never necessary in macroradiography, because the large air gap between the object and the film ensures that oblique scattered radiation fails to reach the film. Contrast is improved on macroradiographs because of the decrease in scattered radiation.

Radiation dose. In examinations that would otherwise require a secondary radiation grid, the radiation dose to the patient is substantially reduced in macroradiography. This reduction in dose is particularly important and can be as much as 40 per cent (Lloyd and Ardagh, 1972) in examinations where the dose to the eyes can be high, e.g. orbital phlebography, cerebral angiography and dacryocystography.

Uses. The main uses of macroradiography include:

1. Demonstration of skeletal structures, particularly the carpal and tarsal bones, ankles, elbows and distal long bones (Genant *et al.*, 1977).
2. Investigation of the chest, particularly in the diagnosis of pneumoconiosis (McLaughlin, 1965), and in distinguishing fine vascular branches or thickened interlobular septa from miliary or lobular areas of consolidation or collapse (Gordon and Ross, 1977).
3. Sialography.
4. Dacryocystography (Campbell, 1964).
5. Investigation of the temporal bones (Weller, 1964).
6. Lymphography (Isard *et al.*, 1962).
7. Orbital phlebography and cerebral angiography (Lloyd and Ardagh, 1972; Hungerford, 1975).
8. Investigation of small renal vessels during arteriography (Sidaway, 1972).
9. Investigation of neo-natal heart disease (Cremin, 1972).

9

Subtraction

In the subtraction technique, a positive image of one radiograph is superimposed over the negative image of another radiograph taken following injection of contrast medium but otherwise under identical circumstances. All images common to both radiographs are thus eliminated and a separate image of the differences between the two (i.e. the contrast medium) is produced, all other structures having been cancelled out (Plate II).

There should be as little delay as possible between the two exposures, so as to minimise the possibility of change in the position of the patient. The plain film is usually taken first, immediately before the injection of contrast medium, but in some cases it may be taken after the contrast medium has dispersed. In rapid serial radiography, the first film of the series, without contrast medium, is used for the plain film.

Firm immobilisation and marking of centering points help to ensure that the position of the patient is as nearly identical as possible for all the films. When relevant, the phase of respiration or of the cardiac cycle at which the films are taken must also be the same.

There are several methods of producing subtraction films including (a) photographic (b) colour and (c) electronic. Of these, the simplest and most commonly used is the photographic method and this will be described in detail, with brief comments on the two other methods.

PHOTOGRAPHIC SUBTRACTION

Either manual or automatic processing can be used. As many X-ray departments now use automatic processing only, the long-established method of hand-processing industrial film for subtraction has been superseded by automatic processing of film suitable for high temperature rapid processing. This and the automated apparatus that has been introduced for exposing the subtraction films, make the density of the radiographs to be subtracted more critical if optimum results are to be achieved.

The radiographs to be subtracted should have low contrast and a limited density range. The smaller the density differences between the structures to be subtracted, the better is the equalisation of contrast in the final subtraction image (Hardstedt *et al.*, 1976). All parts to be subtracted should be exposed within the straight part of the characteristic curve.

Manual processing

Although a printing frame is usually recommended, no special equipment is essential, other than a sheet of opaque black paper and a sheet of glass. Some authorities (Kimber, 1967) recommend the use of a 25 W pearl bulb in conjunction with a small aperture at a distance of four feet. However, in practice the ceiling light in the dark-room is usually quite satisfactory. A stop-watch is useful to time the exposure accurately. For processing, Kodak DX80 developer is the usual choice.

Plain film. The cassettes, screens and films used for this and for the views taken following the injection of contrast medium must be standardised.

Intermediate positive film ('mask'). A sheet of black paper is placed on the dark-room bench with a commercial fine grain film, e.g. Gevaert N31 or Kodak CF7, on top of the paper. (As commercial film has emulsion on one side only, it must be placed with this side uppermost.) Over this is placed the plain film and finally, above that, a sheet of glass.

If the ceiling light is being used (probably about 100 W at 5 ft) the exposure is made for approximately 10 seconds. The film is then developed for about 40 seconds (in Kodak DX80 developer) with constant agitation. The film is then fixed, washed and dried as quickly as possible.

The contrast should be low. There is a wide latitude for this exposure and a satisfactory combination of exposure and developing times can usually be determined with experience.

Contrast film. From the contrast series, a film is selected which best demonstrates the area of particular interest. Several subtraction films can be produced for different phases when required, the same intermediate positive film being used each time.

Superimposition. When the positive film is dry, it is superimposed over the contrast film which is required to be subtracted. It is easier to superimpose if (a) a bright light is used (b) the viewing box is horizontal and (c) the positive film is smaller than the contrast film. Unnecessary film should therefore be cut off.

The two films are moved relative to each other until a position is reached when the normal bone and soft tissue in each film mutually cancel each other leaving a clear image of the contrast medium. When the subtraction is perfect, the films are taped together. It may happen that the whole image cannot be subtracted, due to slight differences in projection. However, the area of greatest interest can usually be subtracted, sacrificing some of the rest of the film image, e.g. ophthalmic arteries may be satisfactorily subtracted but it may be impossible at the same time to cancel out the teeth on the same film.

Second order subtraction. If perfect subtraction is not obtained, second order subtraction is recommended (Zeides des Plantes, 1970). For this, the intermediate positive film is superimposed on the plain film and a second intermediate positive film is produced. This second intermediate positive is superimposed on the first one and the two films are used as one, perfect, mask.

Final film. Commercial fine grain film (e.g. Gevaert N31 or Kodak CF7) is most frequently used. The exposure is made in a similar way to the intermediate film, and again the dark-room ceiling light can normally be used quite satisfactorily. The film is placed, emulsion side up, on the black paper. The superimposed films are placed above, with the positive film uppermost, and the glass is then placed on top. The exposure is made for about eight seconds and the film is developed for about one and a half minutes, again with constant agitation. The exposure and developing times can be varied to get the best result. Fixing of the commercial film takes about three minutes, and it is then washed and dried.

A variant of this method uses intensifying screens as a light source (Tucker, 1967).

Automatic processing

The procedure is much the same as for manual processing but special film suitable for rapid processing must be used. Kodak RPSU, Dupont and Agfa subtraction film have emulsion on one side only, as for the commercial film used in manual processing. The use of copying film for the final film is sometimes recommended.

A simple technique, similar to that described under manual processing, can be used, but it is more satisfactory, especially if subtraction is performed frequently, to use a more reliable method of timing the exposures. The apparatus usually consists of a light-proof box, fitted with tungsten lamps which are controlled by a timer that can be set to terminate the exposure after the required time. It can be used also for copying radiographs, in which case ultraviolet light is used.

The exact exposure time required for the mask can be calculated from the plain film by using a densitometer or, if this is not available, by radiographing a step-wedge using a series of exposure times and using the resulting step-wedge film strips to match the densities of the radiograph to be used as the mask (Jenkins, 1976).

COLOUR SUBTRACTION

A coloured image gives added depth to a two-dimensional image. One system of colour subtraction works on the principle of prismatic analysis of white light and its converse addition of most of the colour spectrum to give neutral, if not white, tones (Tucker, 1967).

Opposing colours of equal density combine to produce neutral or white light, i.e. yellow, red and orange neutralise blue and green and vice versa. Thus, where there is no opposing colour of equal density, that area is not cancelled out and is visible in colour.

An incandescent source (emitting red and yellow light) is used behind a red filter, and a fluorescent source (emitting blue and green light) is used behind a blue filter. The plain film is placed behind the red filter and the contrast film is placed behind the blue filter. A semi-transparent beam-splitting mirror (usually a two-way mirror, 70 per cent transmission and 30 per cent reflection) is placed at 45° to the two films and the films are viewed at right angles to the mirror. The films are adjusted relatively to each other until there is perfect superimposition of the images. The colour addition of the parts of the films which are identical will produce a neutral colour and the difference between the two films (usually the contrast medium) will stand out clearly in red.

For cerebral angiography, another method of colour subtraction produces final films in colour (Chehata and du Boulay, 1975). The previously described method of producing black and white subtraction films with automatic processing is used. Subtraction films of the arterial, capillary and venous phases are obtained. Colour subtraction films are then obtained using Diazochrome film which is developed in ammonia gas and a coloured transparent dye image results. The arterial phase is usually shown in red, the capillary phase in blue and the venous phase in yellow.

ELECTRONIC SUBTRACTION

Usually two television (vidicon) cameras are used in this method. One camera scans the plain film and gives a positive signal, the other scans the contrast film and gives a negative signal. The signals are mixed and fed to a monitor. A polaroid camera records the subtracted image (Tucker, 1967).

However, because of the difficulty in producing two television cameras that will give perfect superimposition of the radiographs, other methods have been devised. In one of these, a single camera is used which scans the plain film and the video signal is conveyed to a magnetic disc and reversed. The camera scans the contrast film and the signal is mixed with the stored reversed signal. The resulting signal is passed to a television monitor as a subtracted image.

SHIFT SUBTRACTION

In shift subtraction, the difference between the two radiographs is not the presence of contrast medium in one of them but the differing position of the structure or object being examined, e.g. the borders of the heart during different phases of the cardiac cycle in suspected myocardial infarction or a foreign body in the eye when the patient looks in different directions (Zeides des Plantes, 1970; Cowley, 1975) or the larynx in phonation and respiration (Hemmingsson, 1972).

An intermediate positive film is made of one of the radiographs and it is superimposed over the other radiograph. On the resulting final film, one image of the foreign body, or heart border, will be black and the other will be white (i.e. one is a positive and the other a negative image).

USES OF SUBTRACTION

1. Angiography. Although used in angiography generally, it is of greatest importance when small vessels are obscured by dense bone, e.g. in the orbital region, the base of the skull and posterior cranial fossa. It is used in arch aortography and in peripheral arteriography

to demonstrate abnormal vessels and 'tumour blush'. In cerebral angiography, it is of value too in demonstrating early filling of veins, indicating an arterio-venous shunt. In this case the venous phase film is used for the mask and superimposed over the arterial film (Habel, 1970).

2. Any contrast medium examination where the structure of interest is obscured by other structures, e.g. excretion urography in a patient with (*a*) severe kyphoscoliosis, where the kidneys are obscured by the vertebral column or (*b*) large staghorn calculi.

3. Encephalography and gas myelography
4. Sialography
5. Dacryocystography
6. Lymphography
7. Localisation of foreign bodies in the eye

10

Tomography

Conventional radiography produces a two-dimensional image of all the structures between the X-ray tube and the film. This results in the superimposition of the images derived from structures at all levels. Tomography provides a radiographic demonstration of the structures in a pre-selected plane by blurring out the images of structures above and below this plane. This is achieved by arranging that the images of the structures outside the plane of interest are moved across the surface of the film during the exposure and are thus blurred out, whilst the image of each structure within this plane is projected in a constant size and shape on a fixed position on the film. The image of these latter structures therefore remains sharp.

Tomography is always preceded by, and is no substitute for, adequate plain films. Throughout this book, the applications and value of tomography are indicated, both in regional radiography and in radiological procedures, but detailed description of its principles is not within the scope of this book. Reference should be made to the many works which deal fully with the subject (e.g. Clarke, 1964; Meredith and Massey, 1977).

Indications. Tomography is particularly indicated:

1. When overlying structures obscure radiographic detail, e.g. to demonstrate the odontoid peg in a patient with a fixed cervical flexion, or to demonstrate the cervico-thoracic junction if it has not been adequately seen on plain films.

2. To produce positional information where views at right angles cannot be obtained, e.g. in a patient with bilateral hip injuries.

3. To determine accurate measurements both of size and depth, e.g. of the pituitary fossa. In some tomographic apparatus the magnification factor is constant whatever the level of the plane but if this type of apparatus is not available, accurate measurements can still be obtained because the tube/plane and the plane/film distances can be measured directly.

Mechanics. Image blur is achieved by relating the movement of any two of three components (namely the tube, the patient and the film), the third component remaining still. Usually it is the tube and film that are moved and the patient is kept still. In the simplest form of tomography, the tube and film are moved in opposite directions with the same angular velocity. This is known as linear tomography. Sophisticated apparatus is available by means of which more complicated movements can be obtained and the choice now includes the following movements:

1. Linear
2. Circular
3. Elliptical
4. Multi-directional (hypocycloidal)
5. Asymmetrical
6. Transverse axial
7. Rotational

Blur. The most important element in tomography is the dispersal of the unwanted images of the structures outside the plane of sharpness. The more efficiently this is done, the clearer will be the image of the structures within the plane in focus. The dispersal depends upon the distance of the structures from this selected plane and the direction in which these images travel during dispersal. Particularly dense structures will leave blurred but distinct opacities on the film unless the movement is sufficiently complex. Linear objects will be blurred most efficiently when the major component is at right angles to the long axis of the object. Similarly, maximum blur of curved structures will occur when the movement is along a path different from the main arc of the object. In linear tomography, any dense structure that is parallel with the tube movement, however far from the plane in focus, will cause a perceptible linear shadow on the film, producing the well-known 'tomography lines' which detract from the quality of the final tomographic image. The crucial factor is the angular displacement of the tube during the exposure, i.e. the further it travels, the more efficiently will the blur be dispersed.

The tomographic image. In addition to the effective dispersal of the blur, the quality of the tomographic image depends upon the accurate delineation of the various shadows of the structures within the plane in focus in their individual parts of the film during the exposure. The main technical requirements are:

1. Tube-film alignment must remain constant throughout the exposure. In particular, there must be no vibration within the apparatus and no component must stray from the common axis.

2. The selected exposure angle must remain constant, independent of any alteration of the selected plane.

3. The centering of the tube must remain constant throughout the exposure.

4. The film must remain in a constant plane throughout the examination.

5. The patient must remain motionless during the exposure.

The thickness of the selected plane is governed by the total angular displacement of the tube during the exposure. The greater the angle traversed by the tube, the thinner will be the section recorded. The desired thickness will depend on the diagnostic problem presented. Sections about 1 mm thick are invaluable for the demonstration of minute structures such as those in the ear (Plate IA). Thick sections produce excellent demonstration of large subjects with improved contrast but they suffer from poor blurring of neighbouring structures. The technique of thick layer tomography is generally called zonography and is of particular value in the examination of the kidneys (Dombrowski, 1968), the sternum (Korach *et al.*, 1966) and the biliary tract (Sutherland, 1970). Intermediate thicknesses are commonly used, e.g. in the demonstration of intra-thoracic lesions.

The level of the plane demonstrated is determined by the height of the effective fulcrum. The selected plane is parallel with the film which is usually horizontal but it may usefully be inclined to demonstrate oblique structures, e.g. the tracheo-bronchial tree (Mayall, 1965) (Plate IB), the kidneys (Sutherland, 1970) or the sternum (Plate XXVI) more completely. A curved film will record a curved section and this principle is employed in tomography of the mandible, e.g. pan-oral tomography (page 171 and Plate XXI).

Exposure factors. The exposure time is determined by the interval required by the machine for the completion of its movement and this will vary with the differing angles and movements. The tube current (mA) must then be adjusted to give the necessary film blackening during the selected exposure time.

An appreciable loss of contrast over that obtained by conventional radiography is inherent in tomography. The kilovoltage must therefore be kept as low as possible in order to reduce this effect. The optimum film-screen combination must be selected to suit the individual examination. Consideration must be given to the need for low dose, high definition and high contrast. Rare earth screens, or very fast tungstate screens, should be used when thicker parts of the body are being examined or when the gonads or the eyes cannot be protected.

Immobilisation. Tomographic examinations usually take a long time to complete and it is important that the patient does not move during the whole examination and must be made as comfortable as possible to help achieve this. Each exposure is long (up to six seconds for hypocycloidal movement) and absolute immobility is essential during the exposure. When appropriate, head-clamps, compression bands, etc., must all be used to help the patient remain in the required position between exposures. The position used should be easily reproducible. Thus simple antero-posterior and lateral views are most frequently employed.

Small children require heavy sedation or even general anaesthesia to keep them absolutely immobile.

Serial sections must be taken consecutively and not intermittently to make sure that the position of the patient is unchanged. This is particularly important when very thin cuts, at 1 to 2 mm intervals, are being taken.

Cassettes. The cassettes used must be standardised so that the film lies in exactly the same plane for each tomographic cut. Alteration of the level of the film in the cassette will alter the level of the plane in focus. This is of greatest importance when thin cuts at narrow intervals are being taken.

Identification of level. Usually each film is marked with a lead number to indicate the level of the plane in focus as indicated by the fulcrum scale.

Filters. In hilar or whole lung tomography, the use of aluminium wedge filters allows simultaneous demonstration of hilar and lung detail. Two such filters, increasing in thickness from 0 to 1 cm, are fixed on an aluminium plate which slides into channels on the front of the light beam diaphragm. They are angled and spaced so that the area between them covers the hilar region and the wedge filters cover the lung fields. High kilovoltage can be used to advantage (Harris, 1975).

Radiation dose. Tomography is potentially a high dose examination and care must be taken to avoid unnecessary irradiation. Adequate filtration, a well-collimated beam and additional lead protection for the patient's gonads—and for the eyes during petrous tomography—are all essential.

Preliminary films

1. Adequate plain films must first be taken to establish whether the lesion originally seen and for which tomography was requested is still

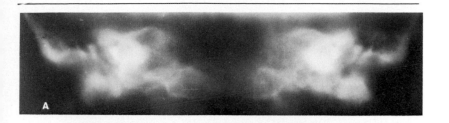

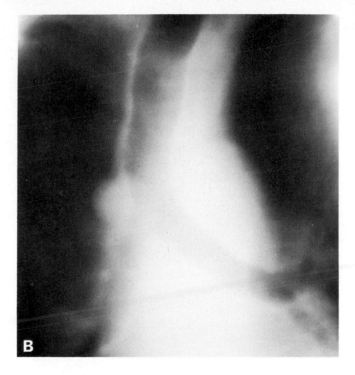

PLATE I. Tomograms. A. Hypocycloidal tomogram of the petrous bones (p. 49 and p. 100). B. Inclined hilar tomogram (p. 49), showing the normal tracheobronchial tree.

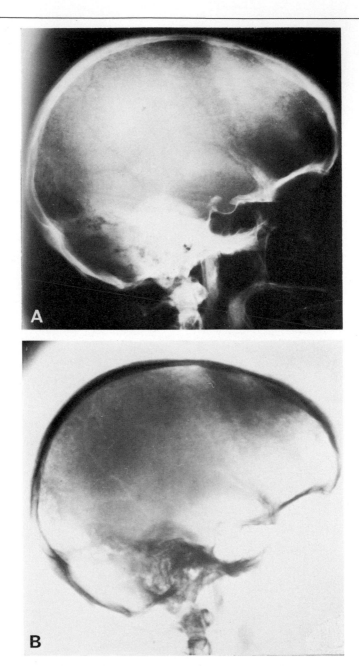

PLATE II. Subtraction series (p. 41). A. Plain film. B. Intermediate positive film.

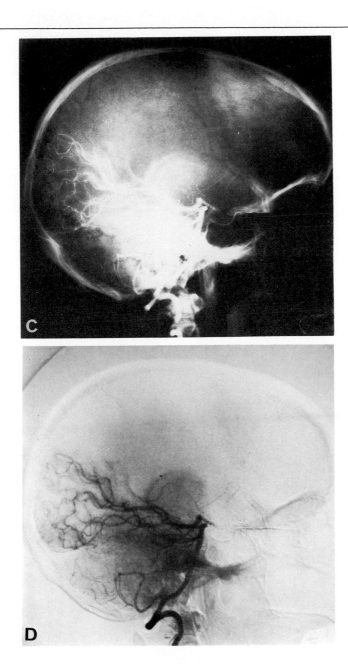

PLATE II. Subtraction series (p. 41). c. Contrast film. d. Final film.

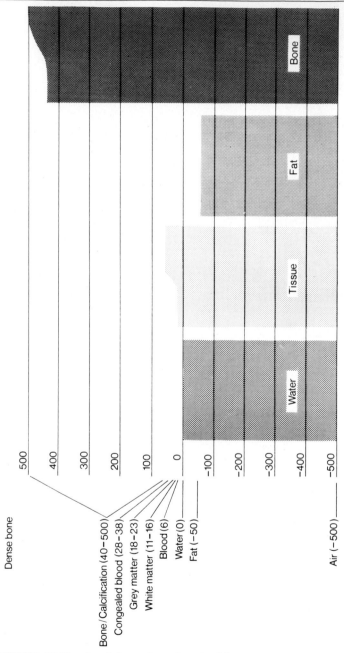

PLATE III. EMI scale of absorption values (p. 54).

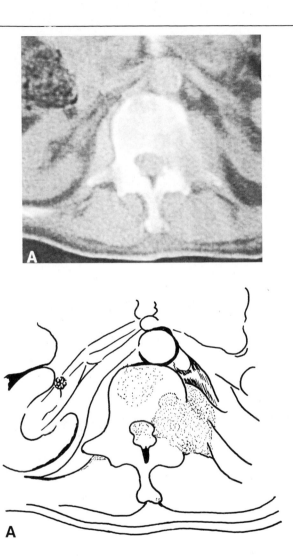

PLATE IV. C.T. scans. A. Magnified view (p. 53), showing metastatic destruction of the pedicle and part of the vertebral body.

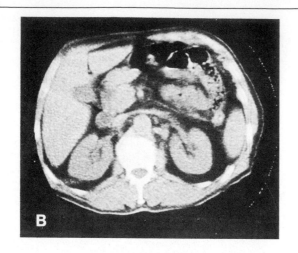

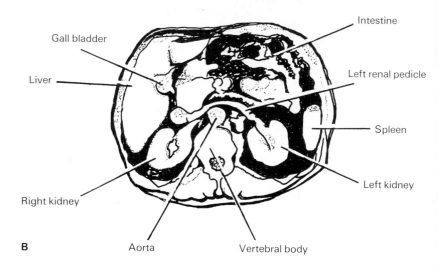

PLATE IV. C.T. scans (contd) B. Abdominal scan (p. 56), taken at C6 level—91 mm below xiphisternum.

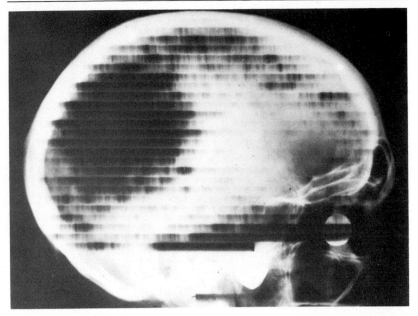

PLATE V. Linear scanner scintigram (p. 66), showing a large area of high uptake in the occipital region due to a glioma.

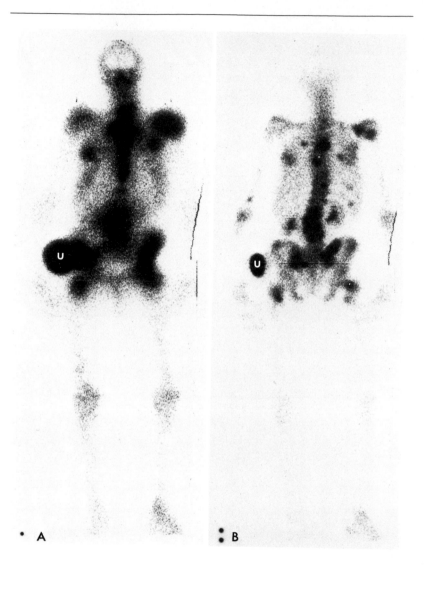

PLATE VI. Skeletal scan (p. 66), using $^{99}Tc^m$ methylene diphosphate. Carcinoma of the prostate with multiple skeletal metastases showing as areas of increased activity. Activity at 'U' is in a urinary drainage bag. A. Anterior scan. B. Posterior scan.

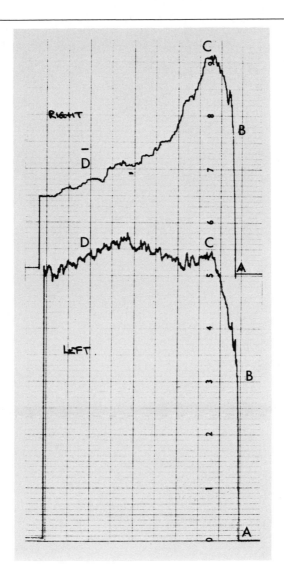

PLATE VII. Renogram curves (p. 68), showing obstructed drainage of the left kidney. Normal right kidney.

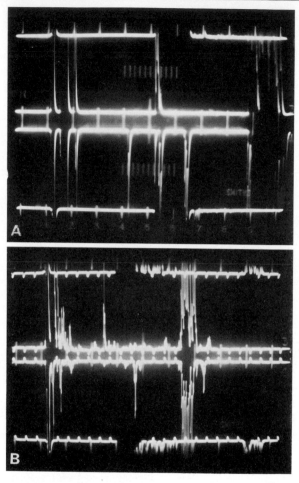

PLATE VIII. Echo-encephalograms (p. 71). A. Normal. B. Showing mid-line shift.

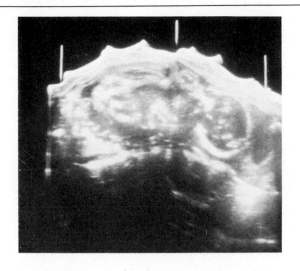

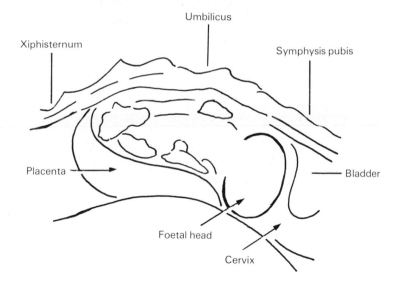

Xiphisternum   Umbilicus   Symphysis pubis

Placenta

Bladder

Foetal head

Cervix

PLATE IX. Ultrasonic scan (p. 72). Longitudinal scan of 30-week pregnancy. Vertex presentation.

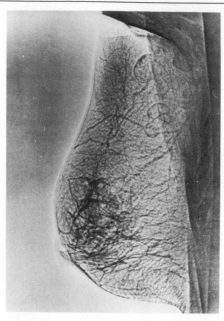

PLATE X. Xeroradiogram (p. 79), showing normal appearances in a breast.

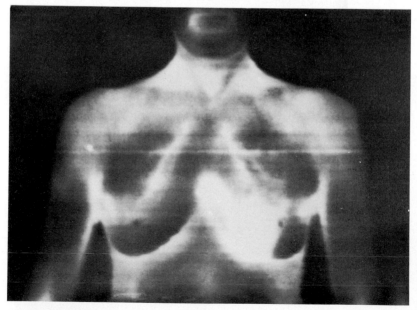

PLATE XI. Thermogram (p. 81), showing carcinoma in the left breast.

present and, if so, to demonstrate its present position preferably in two planes.

2. If a series of tomograms is being taken, a preliminary tomogram, if possible in the centre of the lesion (as determined by the plain films), must be taken to check such things as exposure factors, centering, collimation and size of angle or circle.

Multi-section tomography. This employs a multi-layer cassette which usually contains five pairs of screens, thus allowing five films to be exposed simultaneously. The cassette is in the form of a light-proof box which replaces the conventional Bucky tray. The screens are of differing speeds and are separated by radiolucent spacers of known thickness. The sets of screens are arranged to give uniform density to each of the films. A typical arrangement is that described by Couch and Brodie (1966):

1	High definition High definition	Nearest tube
2	High definition Standard	
3	Standard Standard	
4	Standard Fast tungstate	
5	Fast tungstate Fast tungstate	Furthest from tube

When the patient is positioned for multi-section tomography, the image recorded by the top film in the cassette is usually that of the height set by the fulcrum.

The advantages of using multi-section tomography are (a) the time taken for the examination is reduced (b) the radiation dose to the patient is reduced by approximately a third and (c) all layers are recorded at exactly the same phase of respiration and in exactly the same position. However, many authorities (e.g. du Boulay and Bostick, 1969) consider multi-section tomography an inadequate substitute for single cuts in the investigation of the anatomy of the ear.

A thin layer cassette has been described (Kimber, 1969) for examination of the temporal bone. This retains the advantages of multi-section tomography while the quality of the individual radiographs thus obtained may be as good as that obtained by single cuts. The cassette covers selected sections of cut over a range of 1 cm.

Multi-section tomography using non-screen film is of value in localising foreign bodies in the eye (p. 62).

11

Computed tomography

(COMPUTERISED TRANSVERSE AXIAL TOMOGRAPHY *OR* C.T. SCANNING)

This technique (Hounsfield, 1973) requires highly sophisticated equipment. Originally its use was confined to the investigation of the brain. Equipment for brain scanning is now widely used and has resulted in a considerable increase in very precise diagnostic information and a decrease in more taxing and less tolerable radiological examinations such as encephalography and cerebral angiography.

Improvements in the design and function of the scanners have resulted in the production of even finer detail and also have reduced the scanning time to a level that enables the trunk to be scanned while the breath is held.

The scanner uses sensitive X-ray detectors and a rapid digital computer to evaluate absorption of X-ray photons. Thus very much smaller differences in density can be distinguished than by conventional radiography and the depth of structures beneath the surface of the body can be demonstrated.

Several scanners made by different manufacturers are currently available, each differing slightly from the others. In this chapter, the technique using the EMI 5005 is described.

The scanner consists of (*a*) the scanning unit, comprising the X-ray source, 31 detectors of crystals of sodium iodide (one of which is a reference detector) and photo-multipliers (*b*) the examination couch (which has a microphone-loudspeaker assembly for radiographer-patient communication) (*c*) the control unit, comprising the X-ray console, keyboard and operator's viewing console (*d*) the computer and disc storage unit (*e*) electronics control unit (*f*) line printer (*g*) magnetic tape unit (*h*) diagnostic viewing console and (*i*) independent viewing console.

The patient lies on an adjustable table which extends through the aperture of the scanning gantry and which can be moved so that any part of the patient can be examined. The X-ray source and detectors are mounted in this gantry which traverses and rotates about the patient. A well-collimated fan-shaped beam of X-rays scans the patient in a series of tomographic cuts each 13 mm thick. For each cut, the scanner traverses linearly across the patient and at the end of each traverse it rotates 10° and traverses again. This process of traversing and rotating is performed 18 times in all, i.e. through 180°, and takes 20 seconds to complete. When traversing (i.e. during the exposure) the X-ray source and detectors move in the same direction as each other, instead of in opposite directions as in conventional tomography.

During each traverse, 18,000 readings of the intensity of the emergent X-ray photons are recorded by the 30 detectors. At the end of 18 traverses, approximately 324,000 readings of the coefficients of absorption will have been taken. These readings are automatically fed into the computer while scanning is taking place and a picture is built up in the form of either a 160×160 or 320×320 matrix, an absorption value being given to every point on the matrix. These picture points are known as 'pixels' (picture elements) and each has an area on the 160×160 matrix of 1.5×1.5 mm (for a 24 cm scan field) or 2.5×2.5 mm (for a 40 cm scan field). On the 320×320 matrix, each pixel has an area of 0.75×0.75 mm (for a 24 cm scan field) or 1.25×1.25 mm (for a 40 cm scan field). The absorption coefficient accorded to each pixel is the mean for the 13 mm depth of the section and thus (in the first of the four sets of dimensions just mentioned) it refers to a volume (known as a 'voxel') of $1.5 \times 1.5 \times 13$ mm.

The output of the computer can be obtained (a) as a numerical print-out of the absorption value of each pixel (from +500 to −500 EMI units) or (b) as a grey scale representation on the viewing monitor.

Usually a series of eight scans is taken and these scans can be processed and archived on tape in 5 minutes by two computers, after which they can be viewed on the diagnostic viewing monitor and photographed. Up to eight scans can be performed before processing them. While the scans are being viewed, detail enhancement can be obtained by (a) magnification of one-quarter of the picture to fill the whole screen (Plate IVA) and (b) altering (i) the window width, which selects the range of absorption values that can be demonstrated and (ii) the window level, which selects where the centre of the window shall be for a particular area of interest. This level has to be adjusted so that the window includes the appropriate EMI units of the tissue being investigated (Plate III). For example, when viewing a lung scan, different window levels must be selected to look specifically at pulmonary vessels, lung parenchyma and bony cage.

Localisation of level of cut. The exact level at which a scan has been taken is often difficult to determine, e.g. which particular vertebra has been demonstrated. It is also difficult to compare serial or repeat scans taken of the same patient on different occasions, even if only 24 hours apart. A routine method of identifying, recording and reproducing the level of cut is therefore essential, e.g.,

1. Scanography (Kreel, 1976), for which the patient lies on an X-ray table in the same position as for the scan. Markers are placed on the skin at pre-determined levels. A motorised tube—with a narrow transverse slit aperture—moves down the patient at a rate of about one metre in seven seconds and a scanogram is taken.

2. Referring scans numerically to surface markings. These markings usually include the infra-orbital line ($=A$), sternal notch ($=B$), xiphisternum ($=C$), iliac crests ($=D$) and symphysis pubis ($=E$). Measurements are made from these points in steps of 13 mm, this distance being the same as the thickness of the tomographic cut. Thus, $B3 = 26$ mm caudad from the sternal notch and $D2 = 13$ mm caudad from the iliac crests.

3. Placing markers on the skin at pre-determined levels and taking a radiograph before the scan is done. A grid made of lengths of radiopaque catheter—each piece of catheter 13 mm longer than the next—is taped on to the patient's skin and a radiograph is taken. The grid is left *in situ* for the scan and the image appears as a row of dots. These dots are counted and compared with the original radiograph (Sheldon *et al.*, 1977).

Preparation of the patient

1. When the abdomen or pelvis is to be examined, the patient should keep to a low residue diet for two days before the examination, to reduce intestinal gas which can cause artefacts on the scans.

2. If it is essential to avoid peristaltic movement, propantheline bromide (Probanthine) or hyoscine-N-butylbromide (Buscopan) can be given intravenously before the scan.

3. The patient should drink a glass of water immediately before the scan is done, to reduce the amount of gas in the stomach and so reduce artefacts.

Premedication. Usually none is required. Adequate basal narcosis is usually advisable for infants and small children.

Contrast medium enhancement. After the initial series of scans has been viewed, it may be necessary to obtain further information by repeating the sections following an intravenous injection of water-soluble contrast medium. Contrast medium increases the X-ray absorption in vascular organs and lesions and it can be used to improve the demonstration of lesions that are either more vascular or less vascular than the adjacent tissues.

When the area of interest is the head of the pancreas, a dilute solution of water-soluble contrast medium (e.g. Gastrografin) is given by mouth to outline the duodenum as well as to diminish artefacts caused by intestinal gas.

Positioning of the patient. For body scanning, the patient lies on the scanning couch, with the hands on the head to remove the arms from the area to be examined. Bags containing polystyrene beads are placed round the patient (secured by straps with 'Velcro' fastenings) to make as circular a shape (in section) as possible and to exclude as much air as possible from the scan.

Viewing of scans. For body scans the patient enters the aperture of the scanning unit fect first and for head scans head first. Thus, body scans are viewed from below upwards, so the right side of the patient appears on the left of the screen or photograph as in conventional radiography. Head scans are viewed from the top of the head downwards, so the right side of the patient appears on the right side of the screen or photograph.

Alternative scanning cycle. A 60-second scanning cycle is also available. By reducing noise this gives better detail in low contrast areas. The 20-second cycle is preferred for most examinations but the longer cycle can be used to advantage where extra detail is required, particularly in areas not affected by respiratory or peristaltic movement, e.g. the brain.

Image storage. Processed data are stored (*a*) on magnetic diskettes (6 scans per diskette) (*b*) on magnetic tape (240 scans per tape) (*c*) as a numerical print-out (*d*) photographically, using a polaroid camera, a bromide camera or a multi-image camera which uses X-ray type film which can be processed in an automatic film processor.

Radiation dose. At 140 kV, a series of eight scans gives a maximum skin dose of about 3 rads.

Uses. The value of C.T. scanning of the head has been established and its uses include:

1. *Intracranial structures*
   (*a*) Ventricles, to demonstrate size and position

(b) Brain, to detect haemorrhage
                tumour
                cyst
                oedema

2. *Extracranial structures*, to demonstrate presence and extent of tumours, e.g. in the orbits or sinuses.

3. *Skull*, particularly the base of the skull.

The investigation of other organs and structures of the body by C.T. scanning is still in its relatively early stages. The following uses have been described, but the full clinical importance has yet to be established.

4. *Thorax*,
   to demonstrate:
      Pulmonary lesions
      Pericardial and pleural effusions
      Mediastinal masses
      Rib metastases
      Lymph node enlargement, particularly in areas difficult to examine by conventional radiography, e.g. base of thymus

5. *Abdomen and pelvis* (Plate IVB),
   to demonstrate:
      Liver tumour
      Pancreatic tumour
      Aortic aneurysm
      Adrenal gland tumour
      Enlarged intra-abdominal glands
      Space-occupying lesions in the kidney;
   to determine cause of obstructive jaundice

6. *Musculo-skeletal system*,
   to demonstrate:
      Bone architecture
      Fracture, particularly spinal
      Extent of muscle masses
      Extent of soft tissue masses
      Size and shape of spinal canal

7. *Oncology*,
   to demonstrate:
      Extent of disease for staging
      Volume of tumour for radiotherapy field planning
      Densities of tissues for accurate dose calculations
      Response to treatment
      Recurrence of disease
   to indicate when chemotherapy should be stopped

12

Foreign bodies

Foreign bodies may be introduced into the body through any natural orifice or through a penetrating wound. The purpose of radiographic examination is firstly to establish the presence and identity of a foreign body, then to show its position relative to adjacent structures, to localise its position exactly if required and to assess any secondary or associated damage.

In the case of intra-ocular foreign bodies, geometric methods are used to give accurate localisation. In other parts of the body, localisation by precise relationship to known adjoining structures is usually all that is required. Complex geometric methods have been described for many years but are now seldom attempted and rarely necessary.

It is important to ensure that no artefact is present that could be misinterpreted, such as a fragment of metal or radiopaque glass in the hair, between layers of clothing, within the cassette or even in the Bucky tray.

To ascertain whether a foreign body is present, two views are taken at right angles to each other, with no movement of the patient between the two exposures and with no compression of the part under examination. A further radiograph is taken in one of these projections immediately afterwards to exclude misinterpretation from screen or film emulsion faults.

If the presence of a foreign body has been demonstrated, tangential views must also be taken to ascertain whether or not it is embedded in the tissues.

To assess associated trauma and secondary damage such as an abscess following a swallowed foreign body that has become impacted, or lung collapse after inhalation, basic views for the region in question are taken.

Absolute immobilisation of the region being examined and arrested respiration in the case of neck, thorax or abdomen, are essential to prevent small, low-density objects being blurred out of recognition.

If the nature of the foreign body is known, it may be useful to radiograph a similar object to see if it is radiopaque. This must be carried out with the object immersed in water to simulate soft tissues.

The area covered by the radiographs must be large enough to include any possible location of the foreign body and must not be restricted to the site of entry. This is particularly important if radiography is not carried out immediately after injury.

As foreign bodies can move considerable distances from the site of entry, particularly in muscle or in blood vessels, the best time to localise a foreign body is immediately before an incision is made to remove it. Thus radiography in the operating theatre, using a mobile machine, is often required.

The types of foreign bodies most commonly found are ingested, inhaled, inserted, embedded and those in the eye.

INGESTED

With adults, these are often fish bones or chicken bones, dentures or separate teeth and many other objects that may become lodged in the pharynx or oesophagus. With children, swallowed foreign bodies are often such things as coins, screws, small toys and other bizarre objects that may or may not be radiopaque. Radiographs may be required over a period of several days, with a final radiograph immediately before operation.

Basic views

CHILDREN

Antero-posterior. The whole alimentary tract must be shown. A 35 × 43 cm (17 × 14 in) cassette is used, with the lower border at the level of the symphysis pubis. A very short exposure time is used, to prevent movement blur.

Centre in the mid-line, at the level of the middle of the cassette.

ADULTS

Lateral view of neck. The patient stands in the lateral position against the cassette, with the chin raised and the shoulders lowered as much as possible. The upper border of the cassette is placed at the level of the top of the ear. The exposure is made on arrested inspiration. Fuller details are given on page 176.

Centre 5 cm (2 in) posterior to the anterior surface of the neck, at the level of the laryngeal prominence.

Left posterior oblique view of chest (for the oesophagus). The patient faces the X-ray tube and is rotated 45°, with the right side away from the cassette. The upper border of the cassette is adjusted to 2·5 cm (1 in) above the top of the shoulders. The exposure is made on arrested full inspiration. Fuller details are given on page 186.

Centre to the cassette.

Antero-posterior view of abdomen. The patient lies supine on the X-ray table. The lower border of a 35 × 43 cm (17 × 14 in) cassette is placed at the level of the symphysis pubis. The exposure is made on arrested expiration. Fuller details are given on page 195.

Centre to the cassette.

Supplementary view

Lateral view of the neck, with contrast medium. A further soft tissue lateral view is taken after the patient has swallowed either (*a*) a small quantity of barium which will outline the foreign body or (*b*) a piece of cotton wool soaked in barium or Dionosil which will usually adhere to the foreign body and make it more visible.

ADDITIONAL EXAMINATION
Barium swallow and meal (p. 256).

INHALED

With adults, these are usually single teeth, either from a denture or inhaled during dental extraction. With children, the most frequently inhaled foreign bodies are peanuts, but teeth and other small objects, which may or may not be radiopaque, fluids (e.g. household chemicals and poisons, or water following swimming accidents) are sometimes inhaled. Inhalation of a foreign body often results in collapse of part of a lung (Pochaczevsky *et al.*, 1975).

Postero-anterior (or antero-posterior) views of the chest are required on inspiration and on expiration, the latter to demonstrate areas of collapse or of greater radiolucency caused by the exit of air being blocked at the level of the obstruction.

For the radiographic views required, namely (*a*) postero-anterior (*b*) lateral (*c*) posterior oblique and (*d*) penetrated postero-anterior, see pages 184–187.

ADDITIONAL EXAMINATION
Bronchography (p. 360).

INSERTED

Objects may be found inserted into any natural orifice, i.e. nose, ears, urethra, vagina and rectum.

For the nose, basic occipito-mental and lateral views will be required (p. 95).

For the ear, basic skull views will be required (pp. 91 and 92). Tangential views may also be required. Sometimes a small amount of radiopaque oil is used to demonstrate a non-opaque foreign body.

For the urethra, vagina and rectum, an antero-posterior view of the pelvis is usually all that is required, as endoscopy is normally performed.

EMBEDDED

Embedded foreign bodies are usually objects such as glass fragments (which may or may not be radiopaque), lead shot and bullets. Trauma associated with the foreign body may present a more immediate problem than the localisation of the foreign body itself, e.g. in the abdomen.

For foreign bodies embedded in the limbs, antero-posterior, lateral and appropriate oblique views are required in order to demonstrate whether the foreign body is within the tissues and, if so, its position relative to important adjacent structures. For foreign bodies in the abdomen, antero-posterior and lateral views are required and it may also be necessary to opacify other structures, e.g. the alimentary or renal tract.

If available, xeroradiography (p. 77) is recommended for the detection of non-metallic foreign bodies in soft tissues (Woesner and Saunders, 1972).

FOREIGN BODIES IN THE EYE

The purpose of radiographic examination is to determine whether a radiopaque body is present and, if so, whether or not it is intra-ocular. If required, it can then be accurately localised.

Foreign bodies less than 0.25 mm in diameter are unlikely to be seen on postero-anterior views but should be visible on lateral views. Cassettes must be kept scrupulously clean to minimise the risk of artefacts on the intensifying screens being confused with minute foreign bodies in the eye. Non-screen film is often used in order to avoid this possibility but the increased exposure time entailed may cause blur due to movement and thus prevent a very small foreign body from being seen.

A head-band or other form of immobilisation must be used to prevent movement of the head.

Basic views

OCCIPITO-MENTAL
The patient sits facing the skull table, with the chin raised and the base line at 35° to the vertical, so that the floor of the orbits is horizontal. The patient is asked to look straight ahead at a point at eye-level. To differentiate between possible foreign bodies in the eye and screen artefacts, two radiographs are taken using different cassettes but without moving the patient's position between the two exposures.

Centre in the mid-line at the level of the lower orbital margin.

LATERAL
The head is turned into the lateral position, with the median sagittal plane parallel with the film, the interpupillary line at right angles to it and the base line horizontal. The patient is again asked to look straight ahead at a point at eye-level. Two exposures are made, using different cassettes. There must be no movement of the patient between the two exposures.

Centre to the outer canthus of the eye.

If either of these views demonstrates a possible foreign body, further occipito-mental views are taken with the patient looking upwards as far as possible for the first exposure and then downwards as far as possible for a further exposure. Lateral views are also taken with the patient looking first upwards and then downwards as far as possible. Care should be taken to ensure that the patient really does look in the direction requested and it is advisable to repeat the instruction immediately before the exposure is made.

If the images of the foreign body are widely separated when the patient looks in different directions, it may be assumed that the foreign body is intra-ocular. The radiographs described above will usually provide the ophthalmic surgeon with sufficient information as to the position of the foreign body to enable him to remove it but occasionally more accurate localisation is required. There are several methods of doing this but those most commonly used are the limbal ring method and the Bromley apparatus method (Sutton, 1975).

ADDITIONAL EXAMINATIONS

Shift subtraction (p. 45). Two radiographs are taken, identical except that in one view the patient looks up and in the other he looks down, as for the basic views. An intermediate positive film is made of the first radiograph and this is superimposed on the second, and subtracted. The image of the foreign body will appear as a light shadow in the first position and as a dark shadow in the second position.

Multi-section tomography. This has the advantage of avoiding both surgery and the placing of pointers and requires minimal patient co-operation (Lloyd, 1973). At least eleven non-screen films are placed in a suitable cassette (e.g. a multi-section cassette with the screens and spacers removed) or stacked on the Bucky tray. The patient lies with the head in the lateral position, the chin supported and the eyes looking straight ahead at a point at eye-level. The tube is centred to the outer canthus of the eye and the fulcrum of the tomographic unit is set at the level of the central axis of the cornea, measured from the table-top by a transparent double ruler. A set-square, with lead along its base and along its hypotenuse, is placed in front of the eye at right angles to the plane of the anterior surface of the cornea and with the edge of the lead base parallel with this plane.

The films are exposed, using one linear tomographic movement. An image of a cross will appear on each radiograph, due to the lead on the base and hypotenuse of the set-square. From the position of these crosses in relation to the foreign body, the latter can be accurately localised.

This method is very useful in the detection of multiple foreign bodies, for which other methods are not feasible.

13

Scintigraphy

Scintigraphy is a technique which depicts graphically the distribution of radioactivity within an organ or within the whole body. A suitable pharmaceutical compound labelled with an appropriate radionuclide is given to the patient, usually by intravenous injection, but occasionally by mouth. Although more properly called scintigraphy, because this term includes the use of the gamma camera which does not 'scan', the term radionuclide scanning (or radioisotope scanning) is often used.

The significance of the scintigraphic appearances is assessed in conjunction with radiographs of the same region.

Radionuclides employed. The choice of radionuclide for a particular investigation depends on several requirements:

1. It must emit gamma (γ) radiation of medium energy.

2. It must not emit alpha (α) particles (which are harmful) and should not emit beta (β) particles (which are not detected by conventional scanners or cameras and therefore increase the radiation dosage unnecessarily). Some radionuclides emit a β-particle at the same time as a γ-photon and this additional radiation is unavoidable.

3. It must be non-toxic.

4. It must have a suitable physical half-life, long enough not to make the time of examination too critical and to enable the examination to be completed, but otherwise as short as possible so as to avoid excessive radiation to the patient.

5. It should have a short biological half-life, i.e. it should not be retained in the body for any length of time after the images have been made.

6. It must be capable of labelling a pharmaceutical compound which will delineate the structure being investigated.

It is not always possible to satisfy all these requirements. Some radionuclides with high energy and long half-life (e.g. ^{75}Se) or coincidental beta emission (e.g. ^{131}I) are tolerated if there is no satisfactory alternative.

The radionuclide should be used with a pharmaceutical compound that is pharmacologically and chemically inert in the dosage used, i.e. it should have a suitable metabolic pathway.

One of the major disadvantages of radionuclides with a short half-life is that, because their activity declines rapidly, they have to be used immediately or soon after delivery. This has been overcome to some extent by using small generators which can provide enough radioactive material for several examinations to be carried out. Such generators may last for varying lengths of time, from one week to several months. The best known examples are a ^{99}molybdenum generator from which ^{99m}technetium can be eluted and a ^{113}tin generator from which ^{113m}indium can be eluted. The latter generator will last for several months before it is expended because ^{113}tin has a relatively long half-life.

In the case of very short-lived radionuclides the examinations must be done immediately after production. For example $^{87}Kr^m$, which is used for lung ventilation studies, has a half-life of 13 seconds.

^{99m}technetium can be incorporated into a large number of different compounds and so it can be used to investigate several different structures, for example:

Structure	Compound
Brain	Pertechnetate
Liver	Technetium sulphur colloid
Kidneys	Technetium chelates
Skeleton	Technetium phosphates
Placenta	Technetium labelled human serum albumin
Lungs	Technetium labelled microspheres

The most important of the other radiopharmaceutical compounds and the investigations for which they are used are:

Pancreas	^{75}selenium methionine
Kidneys (renogram)	^{131}I ortho-iodo hippurate
Abscesses and tumours	^{67}gallium citrate

Preparation of the patient. Usually no preparation is required and there is no need for restriction of food or fluid. Exceptions include the following cases:

1. When radionuclides are used that are taken up by the thyroid gland (e.g. iodine) the patient is given a preliminary dose of Lugol's iodide or sodium iodide the day before the examination to prevent this uptake and hence excessive irradiation of the thyroid, unless it is the thyroid itself that is being examined.

2. It is customary to give oral potassium perchlorate 1–2 hours before ^{99m}technetium pertechnetate brain scintigraphy, so as to decrease activity in the choroid plexus and salivary glands.

3. In pancreas scintigraphy, it is important to stimulate the formation of pancreatic juices and this can be achieved effectively and simply by the patient's fasting overnight and drinking one or two glasses of yoghurt (Butterman and Dressler, 1973) or a glass of milk and 'Complan' immediately before the examination.

Care of the patient. The examination can be performed on outpatients. No premedication is required and there are no after-effects. Although reactions of any kind are rare, appropriate resuscitative drugs and equipment (pp. 211 and 212) must be readily available.

Duration of the examination. The length of time the patient has to spend at the hospital varies and may often be several hours. Scintigraphy is commenced when the radionuclide reaches optimum activity in the part under examination. This varies according to the part under examination:

1. Liver and placenta—immediately after injection
2. Brain—1 to 2 hours
3. Kidneys—2 hours
4. Skeleton (using methylene diphosphate)—3 hours
5. Abscesses and tumours (using gallium citrate)—48 and 72 hours

Once scanning is begun, the time required to produce the image is considerably less when the gamma camera is used.

Apparatus. There are two types of instrument for radionuclide scintigraphy:

Linear scanner. This consists of three parts:

1. The detecting device containing the scintillation detector, collimator and photo-multiplier tube.
2. The amplifier and other electronic components.
3. The recording apparatus.

The scanner moves backwards and forwards mechanically across the area being scanned. Radioactivity is detected by a large scintillation crystal (of sodium iodide) which is shielded by lead. The crystal is situated in the scanner, above a lead collimator which prevents interference from radiation outside the area being scanned. The size of the area being scanned and the rate of the scan can be varied to suit the conditions of the examination.

Light flashes from the crystal are converted into voltage impulses in the photo-multiplier and then amplified. The recording device converts these impulses into a visible record, in the form of dots, either on paper or on X-ray film (Plate V). The dots on paper may be either black (the density of the dots per unit area being proportional to the number of impulses) or in a series of colours, each of which records a particular intensity of radiation.

The scanner has to be adjusted for each examination so that (*a*) it accepts only those impulses arising from the peak energy of the radionuclide being used and (*b*) the maximum activity from the area being examined is represented by the upper range of the photo-dot or colour scale.

By using a dual-headed scanner, anterior and posterior views or left and right lateral views can be done at the same time. Minification of the image enables a skeletal scan to be viewed on a single 35 × 43 cm film, which is a great advantage (Plate VIA and B). Usually a 5 : 1 minification is used for a whole body scan and 2 : 1 minification for a large organ (e.g. liver) scan.

Gamma camera. This has a static head which records radiation emitted from the whole of the area under examination at one time, instead of moving across it as does the scanner. It consists of a much larger sodium iodide scintillation crystal which is coupled to several photo-multiplier tubes. Several collimators are available and the choice for each examination depends mainly on the isotope being used. The diameter of the field covered is about 25 cm. The radiation registered is displayed on an oscilloscope and recorded by means of a polaroid camera. The exposure is allowed to continue until a predetermined number of scintillations has accumulated, e.g. 500,000 for a brain scintigram.

The main advantages in using the gamma camera are its silence and the speed with which the image is built up. The latter allows as many projections to be made as are needed for each examination and more examinations can be performed per day. A further advantage is the ability to record rapid fluctuations in radioactivity over the whole organ. These are the so-called 'dynamic' or rapid sequence studies which can be recorded either by a time lapse camera or on magnetic or video-tape which is replayed through the cathode-ray oscilloscope. This is a useful facility which has not yet been exploited fully. Where computer facilities are available, a number of useful procedures can be carried out, particularly in cardiac studies, renal studies and perfusion studies.

Radiation dose. The radiation dose to the area under examination is usually less than it is with equivalent radiological examinations. But with radionuclides (unlike X-radiation which apart from scattered radiation is confined to the area of the body actually radiographed) organs other than those being examined are involved. For example, technetium ($^{99}Tc^m$) used for brain scintigraphy is secreted into the stomach, ^{197}Hg (mercury) is excreted by the kidneys and radioactive iodine (^{131}I) is taken up by the thyroid.

Technique. The radionuclide is usually given by intravenous injection. After the length of time required for the radionuclide to reach optimum activity, the patient is positioned comfortably for the examination.

Unlike radiographs, the scintigraphy images merely record activity from one aspect of the organ. Thus, where one lateral radiograph of the skull may be adequate, two lateral scintigrams are necessary. When the patient faces the detection device, an *anterior* view is obtained; when the patient's position is reversed, a *posterior* view is obtained. When the patient's left side (or the left side of the skull) is towards the detection device, a left lateral view is obtained and conversely with the right.

Uses. The uses of scintigraphy include the examination of the following structures:

Brain (anterior, posterior and both lateral projections). Abnormality is shown by positive accumulation of the radionuclide. To demonstrate tumour, subdural haemorrhage.

Liver (anterior, posterior and right lateral projections). Abnormality is shown by absent activity. To demonstrate tumour, abscess, cyst.

Spleen (anterior, posterior and left lateral projections). Abnormality is shown by absent activity. To demonstrate size, cyst, reticulosis.

Pancreas (anterior projection with the scanning head tilted slightly cephalad to help separate the images of the pancreas and liver). Subtraction scintigraphy (p. 68) is used if possible, to make this separation more successful. Abnormality is shown by absent activity. To demonstrate tumour (particularly of the head of the pancreas), pancreatitis.

Kidneys (posterior projection. An anterior projection may also be helpful if there is a horse-shoe kidney or pelvic kidney). Abnormality is shown by absent activity. To demonstrate the kidneys in cases of acute renal failure, renal ischaemia, chronic pyelonephritis.

Skeleton. The whole skeleton should be viewed with either a gamma camera or a dual-headed scanner. Abnormality is shown by positive accumulation. To demonstrate primary and secondary bone tumours. Some non-malignant bone conditions have an increased radioactive accumulation and these should be recognised by taking the appropriate radiographs.

Lungs (anterior, posterior and both lateral projections). Abnormality is shown by absent activity. To demonstrate pulmonary embolus.

Abscesses or tumours (anterior and posterior projections). [67]gallium citrate is accumulated in macrophages and in some tumour cells. To locate occult abscesses and tumours and sometimes to assess the extent and activity of lymphomata. Abnormality is shown by positive accumulation.

Placenta (anterior projection, scanning from the symphysis cephalad and then the appropriate lateral projection). To demonstrate the position of the placenta, which is shown by positive accumulation.

Combination of scintigraphy and simple radiographic techniques often enhances the value of each and may avoid the need for complicated tests.

Some radionuclide tests have been superseded by other tests, e.g. ultrasonic scanning is now the method of choice for placental localisation, and C.T. scanning for most suspected brain lesions.

Subtraction scintigraphy

Subtraction scintigraphy is employed when another structure as well as the one being examined takes up the particular radionuclide used. The subtraction technique involves the electronic subtraction of two scintigrams taken using two different radionuclides. For example, in the demonstration of the pancreas, it is difficult to obtain an image of it free from the image of the liver. A radionuclide is injected which localises only in the liver and a scintigram is made. The second radionuclide is injected which is taken up by the pancreas *and* the liver and a second scintigram is made. The first is then subtracted from the second.

Some equipment performs this process simultaneously by means of dual analysers and electronic subtraction units (Butterman and Dressler, 1973).

RENOGRAPHY

Renography is a time-activity study of the renal areas following intravenous injection of a suitable radiopharmaceutical compound, usually ^{131}I-Hippuran. The results are recorded by a gamma camera, a curve for each renal area being obtained (Plate VII).

The curve consists of three phases: AB = a sharp rise during the first 30 seconds immediately after the injection, due mainly to rapid distribution of radioactivity in the circulation, BC = a slower rise, due mainly to renal accumulation, and CD = an exponential fall, due to ureteric drainage, which continues for about 15 to 20 minutes until all radioactivity has been eliminated from the renal areas.

Uses

1. *In testing for renal function.* An abnormal pattern on the renogram is produced by reduced renal blood flow, dehydration, impaired ureteric drainage or reduced function of the renal cells. But as several different clinical conditions can include one or more of these same abnormalities, the renogram can be interpreted accurately only in conjunction with other tests.

2. *Screening for renal ischaemia.* The curve of the renogram is characteristically low in renal artery stenosis because of diminished urine flow and prolonged renal transit due to poor perfusion. As renal function deteriorates further, the shape of the renogram curve becomes similar to that of a blood-clearance curve.

3. *Distinguishing between obstructive failure and parenchymal failure.* These two conditions produce different renogram curves.

4. *Demonstrating impaired drainage.* Impaired renal drainage, caused by hydronephrosis or by compression of the ureter by a tumour within the pelvis, is demonstrated by a very slow fall in the CD phase of the curve.

Serial renography is performed to follow up progress of known abnormalities, thus avoiding too frequent urography (see also p. 297).

14

Ultrasonography

Ultrasonography is a diagnostic procedure employing high frequency sound waves. The technique is frequently used as the examination of choice but may also be employed as a complement to other diagnostic procedures.

The frequency of the sound waves used in medical diagnosis may be between 1 and 15 MHz (1 MHz = 1 million cycles per second), 2 to 3·5 MHz being the most useful and practical frequencies.

Principles

Ultrasound is generated in pulses from a transducer consisting of a disc of lead zirconate titanate, which has piezo-electric properties (Wells, 1977).

When a voltage is placed across the disc, it creates a pulse of high frequency sound waves. The interfaces of different body tissues reflect the ultrasound as echoes. Ultrasound waves pass through the body in straight lines and they are reflected and refracted at the interfaces between the various structures of the body. Strong reflections (echoes) are obtained at the interfaces between substances with differing transmission (acoustic) properties. The echoes consist of mechanical vibrations which are returned to the transducer disc and converted by it into electrical impulses. These impulses are amplified and displayed on a cathode-ray oscilloscope and can then be photographed.

The transmission of the pulse and the detection of the echo take only a fraction of a thousandth of a second. Thus the process can be repeated many times per second and can be displayed on an oscilloscope so that the trace appears stationary.

During scanning, either the transducer is in direct contact with the patient's skin or there is an intervening water bath. To achieve satisfactory ultrasonic coupling when the transducer is in contact with the patient's skin, a thin layer of oil is first spread over the skin to act as a coupling medium. When a water bath is used, the part of the body being examined can be immersed in water, but usually the water is contained in a plastic bag or 'balloon' which is held in contact with the patient's skin. By this method it is more difficult to achieve satisfactory coupling because of the likelihood of trapping air between the patient and the flexible wall of the water bag.

Gases are not transonic. As a result, ultrasound is almost completely reflected at interfaces with gas. This introduces a restriction in the investigation of gas-containing structures. Such structures will also prevent the ultrasound reaching structures deep to them.

At present, it is not possible to distinguish between different fluids—e.g. blood, pus or ascitic fluid—by ultrasound. A solid tumour is less transonic and therefore more echogenic than a cystic mass. A vascular tumour may be more transonic than one that has low vascularity.

'A' scan

The returning echoes, as electrical impulses, are made to displace vertically the horizontal time-base on the cathode-ray screen. The amount of vertical displacement is proportional to the strength of the echoes from interfaces along the ultrasonic beam. The horizontal distances between the vertical displacements represent the distances between the various reflecting interfaces within the body.

The scale factor is often controlled by the operator, the scale usually being from about $\frac{1}{10}$th life-size to life-size itself where 1 cm on the screen represents 1 cm in tissue.

Uses of 'A' scan

1. To examine the mid-line structures of the brain (echo-encephalography) to determine whether they are shifted from their normal central position in the skull (Plate VIII). An automatic scanner performs this more efficiently because the echoes to be measured are selected automatically, thus removing the possibility of observer error.
2. To determine whether a structure is solid or cystic (usually combined with 'B' scan).
3. To examine the liver or kidneys (usually combined with 'B' scan).
4. To detect and localise foreign bodies in the eye.
5. To detect pleural effusions, ascites or pericardial effusions.
6. To guide the range and direction of biopsy or amniocentesis needles (usually combined with 'B' scan).

Compound 'B' scan

The returning echoes are displayed on the cathode-ray oscilloscope as dots instead of vertical deflections. The distance between the dots is a representation of the depth of the reflecting interface within the body.

The direction of the scan line corresponds with the orientation of the transducer. Maximum echo amplitude is detected when the transducer is at normal incidence to the tissue interfaces, because only then does the echo return directly to the transducer. Scans to emphasise organ boundaries must therefore be performed by oscillating the transducer as it is moved over the patient's skin. The transducer is usually rocked through an angle of 30° and moved both transversely and longitudinally.

By continuously recording the display while the transducer is moved across the organ, a record of the interfaces within that organ is obtained. The display can be recorded either photographically on film, or electronically on a storage cathode-ray tube or scan converter.

Early 'B' scanners produce a black and white display in which, whatever the strength of the returning echo, a similar dot is produced on the oscilloscope, the strength of the returning echo not being indicated. Tissue maps of a plane through the patient, showing organ boundaries, are produced.

Grey scale displays produced by more recent 'B' scanners, depict the amplitude of the returning echoes over a wide dynamic range. The strength of the returning echo is depicted in various shades of grey between black and white. Information can be obtained from the subtle echo variations which are produced by differing textures of organs or structures within the body. Scans to demonstrate organ texture are usually made with a single sweep of the transducer.

Uses of 'B' scan

1. Obstetric, to demonstrate:
   (a) Uterine size and to confirm pregnancy from about 6 weeks amenorrhoea
   (b) Foetal age
   (c) Number of foetuses and presentation
   (d) Foetal abnormality e.g. anencephaly
   (e) Position of placenta (Plate IX), or prior to amniocentesis
   (f) Hydramnios
   (g) Hydatidiform mole
   (h) Ectopic pregnancy

2. Gynaecological, to demonstrate:
   (a) Cysts
   (b) Tumours
   (c) Position of IUCD
       to differentiate between:
   (d) myofibromata and ovarian cysts
   (e) ovarian cysts and ascites in an elderly patient
3. Urological, to demonstrate:
   (a) Renal cysts
   (b) Renal tumours
   (c) Renal calculi
   (d) Hydronephrosis
   (e) Presence and structure of kidneys which are
       radiologically non-functioning
   (f) Bladder tumours
   (g) Site for renal puncture
4. Liver, to demonstrate:
   (a) Tumours
   (b) Cysts
   (c) Abscesses
   (d) Fatty degeneration
   (e) Cirrhosis
   (f) Volume
   (g) Biliary obstruction
   (h) Cholelithiasis
   (i) Gall-bladder function
5. Cardio-vascular system,
   (a) To demonstrate aortic aneurysms
   (b) To detect dissecting aneurysms and to follow them up
6. Breast, to demonstrate:
   (a) Cysts
   (b) Tumours
7. Abdomen, to demonstrate site for needle aspiration of ascites
8. Larynx, to demonstrate tumours
9. Ophthalmological, to demonstrate:
   (a) Retinal detachments
   (b) Tumours
   (c) Foreign bodies
10. Thyroid, to measure and to identify whether tissue is
    homogeneous, nodular or cystic
11. Pancreas, to differentiate between solid and cystic masses
12. Spleen, to demonstrate size

Döppler method

Any structure that pulsates or moves can be studied by this method as long as it is reasonably accessible. The movement of a reflecting surface alters the frequency of the returning echo. This change in frequency is usually in the audible range. The simplest Döppler machines play the change in frequency (obtained by subtracting the transmitted frequency from the received frequency) through a loud-speaker or earphones.

Uses

1. To detect foetal pulsations. It can be used (*a*) for early detection of pregnancy (from about 10–12 weeks) (*b*) to demonstrate whether or not a foetus is alive (*c*) to determine multiplicity and (*d*) to monitor the foetal heart beat, even during labour when conventional auscultation is difficult.

2. To demonstrate the presence or absence of pulsation in peripheral blood vessels and the characteristics of the pulsation. The transducer is scanned over the skin surfaces below which are the vessels to be investigated. Arterial and venous blood can be distinguished because of their different directions of flow and because of the strong pulsatile nature of arterial flow. Images of moving blood can be produced by new hybrid 'B' scanners and this technique may become an alternative to arteriography for cerebral and femoral artery investigations.

Echocardiography

Pulsed ultrasound from a small transducer is used and a continuous recording made of the movement of the echo from the selected portions of the heart.

Echoes are presented as bright dots along the time-base line. Moving objects are recorded either by photographing the screen while the time-base drifts slowly across or, more often, by means of a strip chart recorder which moves a continuous strip of either photographic film or ultraviolet-sensitive paper across the time-base line.

Uses

The principal use is in the examination of the mitral valve (Ross, 1975). It is possible to record the amplitude and rate of movement of the anterior cusp and thus to determine the presence of mitral stenosis and to grade its severity. Echocardiography is also used to investigate:

(*a*) aortic and tricuspid valve function

(b) left ventricular function
(c) congenital heart disease
(d) cardiac tumours such as myxomata
(e) hypertrophic obstructive cardiomyopathy

Real time scanners

The returning 'B' scan echoes are displayed in such a way that movement of the object being scanned is demonstrated. This is achieved either by mechanically moving a single transducer or electronically switching a row of transducer elements so that the ultrasonic beam sweeps rapidly through the plane being scanned. The electronically switched devices use either a 'linear' array of about 60 transducer elements or a 'phased' array of about 12 elements (Halliwell, 1978).

Mechanically moved transducers give better resolution and fewer artefacts than electronically switched transducers but they tend to be noisy and to vibrate. Sometimes a water bag is used to improve ultrasonic coupling.

The transducer is hand-held and not attached to the scanning gantry. This permits an easier and more rapid examination. Real time scans are often performed as an initial part of a conventional 'B' scan examination.

Uses

1. To observe and record foetal movements, e.g. cardiac cycle, kicking and thumb sucking.
2. To track veins and arteries in the abdomen and thus to help in their identification.

Patient care

Examination by ultrasonography causes little or no distress or discomfort to the patient. No ill-effects have yet been demonstrated from the use of ultrasound at routine diagnostic power levels. The risk of damage associated with its use is less than with ionising radiation and it is likely that there is a threshold intensity below which there are no cumulative effects.

For most examinations, no special preparation, premedication or after-care is required. In all pelvic investigations, e.g. early pregnancy and in localisation of the placenta in later pregnancy, it is important to scan through the urine-filled bladder which will displace the gas-containing intestine and thus permit the ultrasound beam to enter the pelvis.

Because gases are transonic, gas filling the transverse colon presents a major problem in ultrasonic examination of the abdomen, particularly in a non-ambulant patient. In such a case, the patient either has to be re-scanned a few days later when the gas may no longer be present or the gas has to be massaged out of the way.

In the investigation of a pregnant patient, an audible demonstration of the foetal heart usually has a reassuring effect on the patient.

15

Xeroradiography

Xeroradiography is a photo-electric process by which X-ray intensity transmitted by an object is recorded as a charge density pattern on the surface of a semi-conducting selenium plate. Thus the process differs from the photo-chemical process of conventional radiography which uses film as the recording medium.

The selenium layer is a good insulator in the dark and will retain a uniform superficial charge for some hours (Boag et al., 1972). The plates become electrically conducting when exposed to light or X-radiation, thus allowing the surface charge to leak away in the exposed areas and leave on the surface of the plate a 'charge image' of the incident radiation pattern. This charge image is then developed and transferred on to a plastic-coated paper and is viewed by reflected light.

The xeroradiographic image is of medium to low contrast but it displays very fine detail because of the so-called 'edge effect'. Any structure with a well-defined interface (e.g. blood vessels, bone, cyst, soft tissue, calcification) is clearly outlined because the field strength is greatest near any sharp discontinuity in the charge pattern, and an electro-static build-up of powder occurs on one side of the interface with a corresponding depletion on the other.

In xeroradiography there is a considerable latitude for exposure factors, particularly at high kilovoltage. In the examination of the breast, the kilovoltage used is 45–50 and a tube with a tungsten target can be used, one with a molybdenum anode being unnecessary. In the examination of denser structures such as the chest, or for antero-posterior views of the soft tissues of the neck, the use of higher kilovoltage with increased filtration reduces the incident skin dose and improves the image (Davis, 1977).

Xerograms have a wide image latitude and allow simultaneous demonstration of bone and soft tissue structures, with a high degree of detail (Ottoe et al., 1976). To demonstrate these by conventional radiography, several radiographs must be taken using different kilovoltage. Greater detail can be obtained by xerography because of its high resolution compared with conventional radiography, i.e. 15–50 lines per cm as against 8–16 lines per cm.

The part of the body being examined must not be covered, nor should a foam pad or mattress be used under it. A 'tunnel' is used to protect the plate from damage and pressure which would cause it to lose its charge. The part to be examined is placed directly on this tunnel.

Accurate marking of xerograms is essential because a mirror image is produced. Thus, the marker must be placed as for a postero-anterior radiograph and particular care taken to use the correct marker (Richardson, 1977).

Apparatus. The sequence of charging, processing, cleaning and relaxing the plates is now performed automatically (Rank Xerox System 125) and the apparatus consists of two units: (*a*) the conditioner and (*b*) the processor.

Conditioner. Charging, cleaning and relaxing of the plates takes place in this unit. Six plates, which are made of aluminium and coated on one side with selenium, are stored ready for use. When an empty cassette is inserted into the conditioner, a plate is taken from the storage magazine in the unit and the surface of the plate is charged uniformly to a positive potential of about 1,600 volts. The plate is then inserted into the cassette and is ready for use.

During exposure to radiation, a latent electro-static image is formed, corresponding to the various densities of the object being examined. After the exposure, the cassette is inserted into the processor.

Processor. The latent image is developed by means of electrically charged, finely divided plastic particles (blue in colour) which adhere to the discharge pattern of the latent image, thus rendering it visible. The image is then transferred on to a plastic-coated paper by bringing the plate and paper into contact with each other. This reverses the electro-static field and causes the powder to leave the plate and adhere to the paper. The paper is then heated to make the (blue) image permanent. The processing cycle takes 90 seconds.

The plates can be processed in either the positive or the negative mode. Positive xerograms provide better soft tissue demonstration but negative xerograms are of value when both bone and soft tissue detail need to be demonstrated. The negative mode image requires additional powder fixative.

After processing, the plate is put back into the conditioner where any residual powder is cleaned off and it is then 'relaxed' by heating it to remove any residual charge or the memory of a previous exposure. It is then stored ready for charging when next required.

Uses. The main uses of xeroradiography include:

1. Mammography (Plate X). Resolution of very fine detail is obtained in both the thicker and thinner parts of the breast, including minute specks of calcification not visible on film (Boag *et al.*, 1972; Gilbe, 1973).

2. Localisation of non-metallic foreign bodies, e.g. a fish bone in the throat or fabric in a wound (Richardson, 1977).

3. Demonstration of airways, from the nasopharynx to the carina, especially in children.

4. Demonstration of calcification in soft tissues.

5. Demonstration of soft tissue tumours (Ottoe *et al.*, 1976).

6. Investigation of peritendinitis of the shoulder joint (Reichmann *et al.*, 1975).

7. Demonstration of simultaneous bone detail and soft tissues of the face in orthodontic examinations.

8. Investigation of the skull, e.g. in facio-maxillary investigations or to demonstrate intracranial calcification.

9. Evaluation of extremity prostheses (Jing *et al.*, 1977).

10. Angiography. Xerox plates are, at present, much less sensitive than the film/screen combination used in conventional radiography and so their use in angiography is necessarily restricted to peripheral studies. Because of the 'edge effect' the quantity of contrast medium needed for the delineation of blood vessels is much less than with conventional radiographs and this has the advantage of less pain for the patient, greater safety and, in some cases, the avoidance of general anaesthesia because the examination is brought below the pain threshold (James *et al.*, 1973). Bone, soft tissues and contrast-filled vessels are each clearly demonstrated.

16

Thermography

In thermography the variations in the amount of heat being emitted by infra-red radiation from different structures or parts of the body are detected and recorded so as to produce a visual image.

Body heat is produced by cellular metabolism, is distributed by blood and lymph throughout the body and is lost by radiation (45%), evaporation (25%) and convection (30%). Heat lost by radiation in the infra-red part of the spectrum can be measured accurately (Lloyd Williams, 1960). Heat lost by evaporation and convection cannot easily be measured and the amount so lost (and hence the effect on the thermographic image) can be reduced by lowering the temperature of the part of the body being examined before thermography is carried out.

Malignant cells, because of their increased cellular metabolism, produce a rise in temperature in the overlying skin. An impaired blood supply causes a loss of temperature in the skin overlying the affected area due to retarded cellular metabolism; correspondingly, an increased blood supply produces a rise in temperature in the overlying skin (Ryan, 1969).

Equipment. A system of mirrors focuses the infra-red emission from the subject on to a sensitive detector (usually of indium antimonide). The detector converts the infra-red emission into an electronic impulse which is displayed on a cathode-ray tube as a thermal image of the area being scanned. On most equipment, areas of increased infra-red emission are displayed as white, and areas of lower infra-red emission as grey or black. Accurate measurements of temperature differences can be made by scanners which incorporate a quantitative facility. This may take the form of a single-line scan, a digital print-out of absolute temperature or a system of isotherms. Isothermal display selects a temperature range which is shown as a line, or an area of saturated white superimposed upon the regular display. Any one of these facilities will show differences in temperature between adjacent parts under examination, and the actual temperature can be measured.

Colour thermography is achieved by photographing the cathode-ray tube display with different coloured filters in front of the camera. For each filter used, a different isotherm is selected and the temperature patterns can be shown in colour. Some modern scanners incorporate their own colour facility. The display is recorded by photographing it using either a polaroid 35 mm film or electro-chemical paper.

Standardisation of equipment. Correct focus is of as much importance in thermography as in conventional photography. Detectors are liable to drift and their calibration should be checked against known 'black body' standards.

Preparation of the patient. Adequate cooling of the patient, for up to 20 minutes in a room temperature of 18°C, is recommended to avoid abnormal heat patterns from clothing, and to enhance the effect of radiation from deeper structures (Samuel, 1970).

Uses. The main uses of thermography are:

1. Early detection of malignant disease of the breast. Thermography has been found to detect the presence of very small lesions earlier than they can be detected by other means. The malignant area gives rise to increased infra-red emission (Plate XI). The examination is sometimes used as a screening technique as it can be carried out quickly, i.e. as many as twelve patients in one hour (Ryan, 1970).

2. Investigation of arterial disease. Thermographic findings can be correlated with arteriographic ones and may provide a useful method of following the course of disease and efficacy of treatment without further arteriography (Samuel, 1970). Thermography can be used to evaluate narrowing or obstruction of the carotid vessels (Wood, 1964). It is a useful method of determining the optimum site for amputation of a limb by allowing the vascularity of projected skin flaps to be assessed.

3. Investigation of incompetent valves in perforating veins (Patil et al., 1970). Incompetent valves allow blood to flow retrogressively from deep veins to superficial veins and because the temperature of blood in deep veins is higher than that of blood in superficial veins, this difference can be demonstrated by thermography and thus the incompetent valves can be accurately localised.

4. Demonstration of deep vein thrombosis before this is possible by clinical methods.

5. Assessment of burns, e.g. to distinguish between full thickness burns (which show decreased infra-red emission) and partial thickness burns (which show increased infra-red emission). Thermographic assessment makes earlier grafting possible, thus saving time

and reducing the risk of infection. It can also indicate whether a tube or pedicle graft is ready to move.

6. Assessment of the extent of pressure sores.

7. In metastatic malignant disease, e.g. superficial lymph gland or bone involvement, which can be demonstrated earlier by thermography than by radiography.

8. In some abdominal conditions. In some cases thermography can be useful in the investigation of conditions such as acute appendicitis, cholecystitis and subphrenic abscess; also in the investigation of the placenta.

Care of the patient. Thermography causes no distress or discomfort to the patient and because it detects and measures radiation emanating *from* the body and does not give radiation to the body, it has the advantage of being entirely non-destructive.

17

Forensic radiography

Forensic radiography is usually carried out in the mortuary or post-mortem examination room. Some hospitals or police departments have high-powered equipment but, as short exposure times are not needed, low-powered mobile equipment is adequate. A stationary grid, or a grid cassette, is used for examining the thicker parts of the body and non-screen film should be used for examining extremities to obtain optimum detail of bone and soft tissue.

Adequate radiation protection must be provided for the radiographer and any other persons present, by means of lead rubber aprons and mobile screens.

The main purposes of radiography in forensic examinations are: (a) identification (b) demonstration of missile or weapon tracks (c) location of foreign bodies (d) demonstration of injuries or disease (e) autoradiography and (f) research (Beeson, 1978).

Identification

Age. In the absence of any disease which might affect it, accurate assessment can be made of the bone age of a child by the appearance of the centres of ossification (p. 142) and of a young adult by the state of fusion of the epiphyses.

Matching of findings at post-mortem examination with previous radiographs or other records. Examples are:

1. Frontal sinuses. These are as individual as finger-prints.

2. Dentition. Radiographs taken post mortem can be compared with previous dental or skull radiographs.

3. Vertebral column. This may be helpful in cases where there has been a spinal fusion or laminectomy, where post-operative radiographs exist.

4. Chest. A chance finding such as a pericardial cyst or a calcified pleural plaque may be matched with a previous chest radiograph.

5. Old fractures or features resulting from orthopaedic operations (e.g. Smith Peterson pins, Kunschner nails, plating and screwing of

fractures, joint prostheses) especially when matched with previous post-operative radiographs (Graham, 1973).

Superimposition of radiograph and photograph. Radiographs of the skull after death can sometimes be matched with photographs of the face before death.

Demonstration of tracks. The tracks made by gun-shot wounds, stab wounds and bullet wounds, and their depth and proximity to vital organs can be demonstrated by contrast medium. The contrast medium must be introduced into the wound by gravity, and not injected, as pressure could form false channels (Graham and Butler, 1969).

Foreign bodies. The presence of objects such as bullets, fragments of glass, explosives or pieces of metal (e.g. broken needles in drug addicts) in the soft tissues can be demonstrated radiographically. The location of swallowed objects, e.g. teeth after a fight, or a small toy swallowed by a child, can assist in correlating time of death with possible cause of injury. In cases of shot-gun wounds, radiographs act as a record of the quantity, calibre, depth of penetration, spread and distribution of shot. In victims of bomb explosions, radiographs can demonstrate fragments of metal, including detonators, which may assist in identifying the bomb 'factory' (Beeson, 1978).

For low-density foreign bodies, e.g. glass, industrial non-screen films and low kilovoltage (about 35 kV) should be used.

Injuries or disease. Examples are:

1. Non-accidental injury in the young ('battered baby'). Radiographs of the whole skeleton, including the skull and long bones, are taken. Views of the extremities can give valuable information not only about recent injury but also about earlier and probably untreated fractures.

2. Age of fractures. This can be assessed by their state of union.

3. Assessment of laryngeal injuries in cases of strangulation. Radiographs must be taken before dissection.

4. Demonstration of Caisson disease (caused by too rapid decompression, e.g. in divers), by the presence of aseptic bone necrosis, usually in the heads of the femora or humeri, or both.

Autoradiography. This is the detection of radioactive substances, particularly those emitting α-particles, in the body, e.g. (*a*) remains of Thorotrast in a patient who has developed carcinoma many years after its administration or (*b*) plutonium particles inhaled or ingested by workers in nuclear energy establishments (McInroy *et al.*, 1976).

Research. The radiographer may be required to assist in any of the many fields of research that are often begun in the post-mortem room. These include the injection of contrast medium into arteries or veins (e.g. into the coronary arteries in the investigation of coronary heart disease) or into the pancreatic duct (in the study of the radiological anatomy of the pancreas, Sandin *et al.*, 1973).

Part II

REGIONAL RADIOGRAPHY

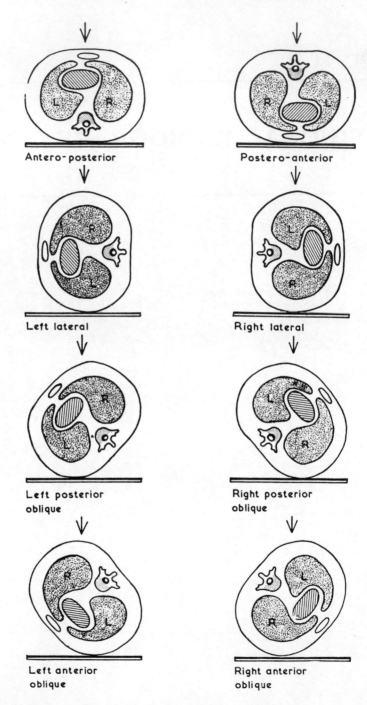

Antero-posterior

Postero-anterior

Left lateral

Right lateral

Left posterior
oblique

Right posterior
oblique

Left anterior
oblique

Right anterior
oblique

Fig. 2　Positioning for general radiographic views.

18

Skull

The skull is composed of 22 bones comprising the cranium (vault and base) and the facial bones. Except for the mandible, these are so closely connected that no movement between them is possible. The immovable joints between the bones have irregular, serrated edges and are called sutures.

The views required will vary according to the diagnostic problem. A complete examination requires several views for each region because of the anatomical complexity of the skull. To simplify radiographic description, three guide lines are referred to: (*a*) the radiographic base line* joining the outer canthus of the eye and the external auditory meatus (*b*) the interpupillary line joining the centre of the eyes when looking straight ahead and (*c*) the median sagittal plane dividing the skull in the mid-line from back to front.

Whenever possible a high-powered unit capable of giving a high milliamperage combined with a short exposure time should be used, preferably with a fine focus tube. When a mobile unit must be used for radiography of the skull in an accident department, intensive care unit or ward, exposure factors and film-screen speed should be adjusted to keep exposure times short enough to prevent blur due to movement by a patient unwilling or unable to co-operate.

Exposure factors should be selected to produce the highest possible detail with a wide range of contrast. High kilovoltage technique is not normally used in neurological radiography as minute specks of calcification, important for diagnosis, may not be shown. However, to demonstrate a fracture in an unco-operative patient, the use of high kilovoltage gives the advantage of a shorter exposure time.

In most departments where skull examinations are frequently carried out, a specialised unit (e.g. Schönander or Barizetti) forms part of the equipment and its use makes radiography of the skull

---

* The anthropological base line, i.e. the line joining the external auditory meatus and the lower orbital margin, is often now used instead but the radiographic base line is used throughout this chapter as it is more convenient in practice.

quicker and more accurate. These units have transparent tops, marked with central cross lines, beneath which is a grid that can be pulled out so that the patient can be observed either directly through the transparent top or via a mirror system. This enables a simple anterior centering point to be used for postero-anterior views of the skull. The X-ray tube is mounted on a curved cross-arm which is part of a circle the centre of which is also the centre of the table. Thus, in whatever way the tube is angled it is always centred to the table. By means of fine adjustments the tube may be off-centred when required.

The table, also, can be angled and this makes positioning for certain views, e.g. submento-vertical, easier and more comfortable for the patient.

In a general department, cassettes used for skull examinations should preferably not be used for other purposes, such as radiography of a limb in plaster of Paris, so as to avoid artefacts. Screens must be kept scrupulously clean and undamaged and a stationary grid should be reserved for skull examinations and carefully maintained to prevent damage leading to loss of definition.

A head-band or other form of immobilisation should always be used to reduce the risk of the patient moving or changing position during the exposure. Foam pads and sandbags, all preferably encased in polythene bags, should be available both for immobilisation and for the comfort of the patient.

To minimise the risk of cross-infection, the skull unit or X-ray table must be cleaned after use, particularly when a number of patients from an ear, nose and throat clinic are being examined (and in such circumstances the next patient will often feel reassured if this is done in his presence before his own radiograph is taken). For this purpose a supply of gauze swabs or tissues and antiseptic solution should be kept at hand.

To obtain optimum definition by reduction of scattered radiation, the smallest possible cone, or adjustment of the light beam diaphragm, must be used.

All clothing and radiopaque objects, e.g. spectacles, dentures, earrings, necklaces, hair pins and clips, must be removed from the head and neck. Collar studs and zip-fasteners at the back of the neck must also be removed because although they may not seem to be within the area under examination, they may nevertheless be projected within the skull on certain views, such as submento-vertical and Townes.

In the following sections of this chapter, anterior centering points are given for both antero-posterior and postero-anterior views. These centering points can be used both with a skull table and with a conventional X-ray table. It is much easier and more accurate to position the cassette, centre the X-ray tube and collimate the beam to the patient's facial landmarks (e.g. the lower border of the orbits, the nasion or the angle of the jaw) than to attempt to use centering points on the back of the head, as is conventionally quoted, as these may be difficult to locate accurately with a patient who has, for example, thick or blood-matted hair, or a tender head. When the patient is prone, with the forehead or chin on the X-ray table, the side of the face is always visible even if long hair may be slightly in the way sometimes.

CRANIUM

Anatomy. The cranium is composed of the frontal, occipital, sphenoid and ethmoid bones and the paired temporal and parietal bones. It forms the protective covering for the brain. The floor of the cranium is divided into anterior, middle and posterior cranial fossae.

Basic views

Occipito-frontal. The patient faces the skull table, with the forehead resting against it. The base line and median sagittal plane must be at right angles to the film.

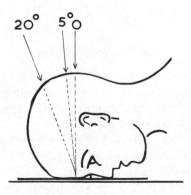

Fig. 3

Centre to the glabella, with the tube angled either 5° caudad to show the petrous bones within the orbits or 20° caudad to project the petrous bones below the level of the orbits (Fig. 3).

Lateral. The head is placed in the lateral position with the median sagittal plane parallel with the table, the interpupillary line at right angles to it and the base line horizontal.

Centre 5 cm (2 in) above the external auditory meatus.

Townes. The patient faces the X-ray tube, with the chin tucked in so that the base line is at right angles to the table. To achieve this, it may sometimes be necessary to place a pad under the occiput or to angle the table slightly. The median sagittal plane must be at right angles to the table.

Centre 5 cm (2 in) above the glabella, with the tube angled 30° caudad.

To ensure correct and easy centering, when using a skull unit, the patient or the table is adjusted initially so that the tube is centred to the tip of the nose. The tube is then angled 30° (Fig. 4).

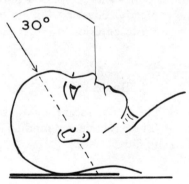

Fig. 4

Special circumstances

1. In all cases of trauma to the skull, the lateral view must be taken with a horizontal beam in order to show, for example, air in the ventricles, free fluid in the sphenoid sinuses (indicating possible fracture of the base of the skull) or an aerocoele.

2. In cases of serious injury, a lateral view of the cervical spine (using a horizontal beam) and an antero-posterior supine view of the chest are taken in addition to the routine skull views. The basic examination of a badly injured patient should include views of the cervical spine and chest, as the nursing of an unconscious patient requires

frequent turning, and it is essential therefore to know if there is injury to the neck or thorax (Lewin, 1966).

3. As an initial screening test for such conditions as headache, migraine or epilepsy (Bull and Zilkha, 1969) or as part of a skeletal survey, the examination may be restricted to a single lateral view.

Supplementary views

BASE OF SKULL

Submento-vertical. The patient faces the X-ray tube, with the chin and neck extended. If the patient is supine, the table is lowered gently and angled until the base line is parallel with the table. If the patient is sitting, the neck is extended as far as possible and the table is then angled until the base line is parallel with it (Fig. 5).

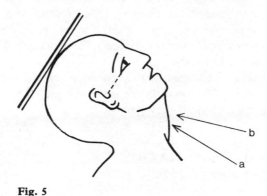

Fig. 5

Centre in the mid-line between the angles of the jaw, with the tube angled 5° towards the face (arrow a, Fig. 5).

Special circumstances

A submento-vertical view may be obtained on a patient who must remain lying on an X-ray table or on a stretcher, by placing the cassette at an angle behind the patient's head and raising the chin as much as possible, and placing foam pads under the neck and shoulders (Fig. 6).

Centre between the angles of the jaw, at right angles to the cassette.

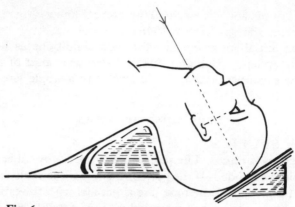

Fig. 6

JUGULAR FORAMINA

The jugular foramina lie at the posterior ends of the petro-occipital suture and they transmit the internal jugular veins and the glosso-pharyngeal, vagus and accessory (9, 10 and 11) cranial nerves.

Submento-vertical (under-tilted). The patient is positioned as for the base of skull view.

Centre between the angles of the jaw with the tube directed 70° to the base line, i.e. 20° towards the neck instead of 5° towards the face as in the base of skull view (arrow b, Fig. 5).

ADDITIONAL EXAMINATION

Jugular venography (p. 244).

PITUITARY FOSSA

The pituitary fossa is a mid-line structure and is situated in the middle cranial fossa. It is formed by the upper surface of the body of the sphenoid bone.

Lateral. The head is positioned as for the basic lateral view. A small aperture is used.

Centre 2·5 cm (1 in) above, and 2·5 cm (1 in) in front of, the external auditory meatus.

Postero-anterior. The head is positioned as for the basic occipito-frontal view. A small aperture is used.

Centre 5 cm (2 in) below the external occipital protuberance, with the tube angled 10° cephalad.

CRIBRIFORM PLATE OF ETHMOID BONE

Oblique. The patient sits facing the skull unit, with the chin raised so that the base line is at 35° to the horizontal. The head is rotated 45° towards the side under examination.

Centre through the orbit nearer the cassette, with the tube angled 10° caudad.

LOCALISED LESIONS INCLUDING DEPRESSED FRACTURES

Tangential views. From the lateral or occipito-frontal positions, the head is rotated so that the area in question, seen on the basic views, is in profile.

FACIAL BONES

Anatomy. The facial part of the skull is composed of the maxilla (upper jaw), the nasal, lachrimal, vomer, palatine and zygomatic bones and the mandible (lower jaw). The mandible is discussed separately.

Basic views

Occipito-mental. The patient faces the skull table, with the chin (and usually also the nose) in contact with it so that the base line is at 45° to the vertical.

Centre to the lower orbital margin.

30° Occipito-mental (over-tilted). The patient is positioned as last mentioned and the kV is increased by 8.

Centre to the lower orbital margin with the tube angled 30° caudad.

Lateral. The head is placed in the lateral position, with the median sagittal plane parallel with the table and the interpupillary line at right angles to it. The kilovoltage required is 10 less than for a lateral skull view.

Centre to the zygomatic bone.

Special circumstances

1. If the patient is unable to sit up or lie prone, 'reverse occipito-mental' views are taken. The patient lies supine with the chin raised and the neck extended as much as possible (Fig. 7).

2. Erect occipito-mental views of all patients with 'black eye'

should be taken in order to demonstrate orbital emphysema (usually associated with fracture into the ethmoid sinus) which is visible only on an erect film.

3. In all cases of trauma, the lateral view should be taken with a horizontal beam in order to show, for example, air in the ventricles, free fluid in the sphenoid sinuses (indicating possible fracture of the base of the skull) or an aerocoele.

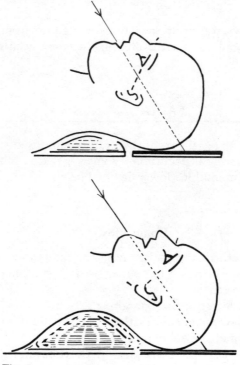

Fig. 7

Supplementary views

ZYGOMA

The zygoma is a 'quadrilateral' bone which articulates with the zygomatic processes of the maxilla, frontal and temporal bones. The zygomatic arch bows laterally from the posterior margin of the zygoma to just anterior to the external auditory meatus.

Fronto-occipital. The patient faces the X-ray tube, with the chin tucked in so that the base line is at right angles to the table. The median sagittal plane must also be at right angles to the table. The kilovoltage required is 10 less than for the basic Townes view.

Centre to the bridge of the nose, with the tube angled 30° caudad.

NASAL BONES
Lateral. A non-screen film and a small aperture are used.

Centre to the nasion.

Supero-inferior. The patient sits or lies with the chin raised and an occlusal film held gently between the teeth so that two-thirds of the film is outside the mouth. The frontal bone should be projected directly over the front teeth. The gonads must be protected, particularly if the patient is seated when it may be impossible to avoid directing the primary beam towards the gonads.

Centre through the frontal bone at right angles to the film.

Occipito-mental. To show deviation of the nasal septum. See p. 95.

MAXILLA
Oblique. The patient faces the X-ray table, with the forehead resting against it. The head is then rotated 40° towards the side under examination and the chin is raised so that the chin, cheek and nose are all in contact with the table.

Centre through the mastoid process remote from the film, with the tube angled 10° cephalad.

This view can also demonstrate retained roots of upper teeth.

ORBITS
These are formed by the roof of the antra, the floor of the anterior fossa and the lateral walls of the nose.

20° Occipito-frontal. The patient sits or lies with the head in the basic occipito-frontal position.

Centre to the nasion with the tube angled 20° caudad.

Occipito-mental (under-tilted). The patient is positioned in the basic position and the base line is then adjusted to 35° so that the floor of the orbits is at right angles to the film.

Centre to the lower border of the orbits.

Lateral. The patient is positioned as for the basic lateral view. A small aperture is used. The kilovoltage required is 10 less than for a lateral skull view.

Centre to the outer canthus of the eye.

OPTIC FORAMINA

These transmit the optic nerves and ophthalmic arteries. Views of both sides are taken for comparison.

Oblique. The patient faces the skull table with the eye under examination in the centre of the table. The head is then rotated 35° towards the side being examined so that the forehead, cheek, chin and nose are all touching the table. The base line should be at 35° to the horizontal (Fig. 8), i.e. 55° to the table.

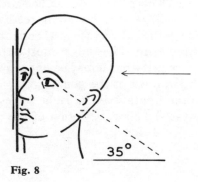

Fig. 8

Centre through the orbit nearer the film.

ADDITIONAL EXAMINATIONS

Tomography (p. 47), if possible with hypocycloidal movement. *Inclined plane axial tomography* (Lloyd, 1975). *Pan-oral tomography* (p. 171) (Canigiani and Wickenhauser, 1972).

TEMPORAL BONES

Anatomy. The temporal bones comprise the paired squamous, petrous, mastoid and tympanic parts and the styloid processes. The petrous part contains the organs of hearing and balance, i.e. the middle and inner ears and the internal auditory canals. It lies at 45° to the median sagittal plane.

Investigation may be required to demonstrate (*a*) fractures (*b*) pneumatisation of the mastoid cells (*c*) the middle and inner ear structures or (*d*) the internal auditory canals when disease of the facial or auditory nerves is suspected. The views required for the internal auditory canals and for the mastoid cells differ slightly and will be discussed separately.

Mastoid air cells

Basic views

Lateral oblique. The head is placed in the lateral position. Views of both sides must always be taken and a small cone or aperture is used.

Centre to the external auditory meatus nearer the film, with the tube angled 20° caudad.

Fronto-occipital. The patient faces the X-ray tube, with the chin tucked in so that the base line is at right angles to the table. A narrow slit aperture is used.

Centre to the glabella, with the tube angled 35° caudad, so that, when viewed from the side, the central ray passes through the external auditory meatus.

Submento-vertical. The patient faces the X-ray tube, with the neck extended. The skull table is adjusted until it is parallel with the base line. A narrow slit aperture is used.

Centre between the angles of the jaw so that, when viewed from the side, the central ray passes through the external auditory meatus.

Internal auditory canals

Basic views

Fronto-occipital. As for mastoid air cells (above).
Submento-vertical. As for mastoid air cells (above).
Occipito-frontal (per orbital). The patient sits or lies facing the skull table, with the base line at right angles to the table. A narrow slit aperture is used.

Centre to the centre of the orbits, with the tube angled 10° caudad.

Supplementary views

Modified 'Stenvers'. The patient faces the skull table, with the forehead resting against it and the base line at right angles to it. The table is adjusted so that the central cross-lines are just above the centre of the eyebrow of the side under examination (Fig. 9A). The head is then rotated 45° so that the side being examined is against the table (Fig. 9B). A small aperture is used. A view of each side must be taken.

Centre as just described, with the tube angled 12° cephalad.
Stockholm 'C'. This view is similar to a modified 'Stenvers' view

A

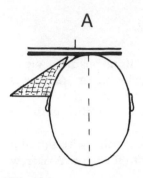

B

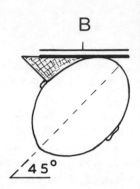

Fig. 9

but identical positioning of the two sides is more easily obtained. The head is placed in the lateral position. A small aperture is used.

Centre 1 cm ($\frac{1}{2}$ in) above, and 2·5 cm (1 in) in front of, the external auditory meatus, with the tube angled 12° cephalad and 30° occipito-frontally. The grid must be turned so that it is parallel with the central ray.

ADDITIONAL EXAMINATION
Tomography (p. 47), with hypocycloidal movement if possible. Tomography with hypocycloidal movement will determine whether a fracture of the petrous bone extends into the inner ear.

TEMPORO-MANDIBULAR JOINTS

Anatomy. The temporo-mandibular joint is a gliding synovial joint formed by the condyle of the mandible articulating with the mandibular fossa of the temporal bone. The joint has two cavities separated by a disc. When the mouth is opened, the head of the mandible glides forwards on to the condylar eminence. The joint is palpable and can be felt most easily when the mouth is opened slightly.

Basic views

Lateral oblique. A view of each side must always be taken for comparison. To demonstrate movement of the joint, views are taken firstly with the mouth closed and then with it open. The head is placed in the lateral position, with the median sagittal plane parallel with the skull table and the interpupillary line at right angles to the table. A small aperture is used. By means of lead letters the films are marked 'open' and 'closed' respectively.

Centre to the joint nearer the film, with the tube angled 25° caudad.

Fronto-occipital. The patient faces the X-ray tube, with the chin tucked in so that the base line is at right angles to the skull table. The mouth is opened as wide as possible.

Centre in the mid-line, with the tube angled 35° caudad so that, when viewed from the side, the central ray passes through the joint.

ADDITIONAL EXAMINATION
Tomography (p. 47).

MANDIBLE

Anatomy. The mandible is composed of a central, curved part called the body, and two ascending rami. In the centre of the body is the symphysis menti. The rami end in two processes, the coronoid and the condylar, separated by the mandibular notch. The condylar process consists of a head and a neck. The head forms part of the temporo-mandibular joint. The upper margin of the body is called the alveolar process and in it are sockets for the roots of the lower teeth.

In a lateral view, one half of the mandible obscures the other half and in a postero-anterior view the cervical vertebrae overshadow the symphysis menti. Therefore, oblique views are required to demonstrate the whole mandible.

Rami

Basic views

Occipito-frontal. The patient faces the X-ray table, with the forehead in contact with it. The base line and median sagittal plane must be at right angles to the table. The kilovoltage required is 10 less than for an occipito-frontal skull view.

Centre in the mid-line at the level of the angle of the jaw, making sure that the whole mandible is included on the radiograph.

Lateral oblique. The patient sits or lies with the head in the lateral position, with the side under examination nearer the cassette.

Centre 5 cm (2 in) below the angle of the jaw remote from the cassette, with the tube angled 30° cephalad.

Special circumstances

1. If the patient is unable to sit up or lie prone, a fronto-occipital view is taken. Oblique views can be taken with the cassette supported vertically by the side of the face, the X-ray tube being directed horizontally.

2. It is sometimes difficult to show the ramus of the mandible satisfactorily in patients who have short necks or thick shoulders. Such a patient should sit with the cassette held against the side of the face and should then bend towards that side, so that the median sagittal plane is at approximately 35° to the horizontal.

Centre 5 cm (2 in) below the angle of the jaw remote from the film, with the tube horizontal.

Supplementary view

Obliques. The patient faces the X-ray table, with the base line at right angles to it. Two views are taken, the head being rotated 10–15° to each side in turn.

Centre to the middle of the ramus nearer the cassette, with the tube angled 15° caudad.

Symphysis menti

Basic views

Postero-anterior oblique. The patient faces the X-ray table, with the forehead against it and the base line at right angles to it. Two views are taken, the head being rotated 20° to each side in turn.

Centre 5 cm (2 in) from the cervical spinous processes, directly through the symphysis menti.

Submento-vertical. The patient faces the X-ray tube, with the chin raised and the neck extended as much as possible. The skull table is then angled until it is parallel with the base line.

Centre between the angles of the jaw and at right angles to the cassette.

Infero-superior. The patient is positioned as for the submento-vertical view. An occlusal film is placed between the teeth. Two views are useful:

Centre (1) from below the chin, at right angles to the film (2) to the symphysis menti, at 45° to the film.

Special circumstances

A submento-vertical view may be obtained on a patient who must remain on a stretcher, as explained on p. 93 and Fig. 6.

ADDITIONAL EXAMINATION

Pan-oral tomography with the head rotated. If the head is rotated 25° the anterior mandible will be demonstrated without the cervical spine being superimposed (Esberg and Haverling, 1977).

Condyles

Basic views

Fronto-occipital. The patient faces the X-ray tube, with the chin tucked down so that the base line is at right angles to the film. The mouth is opened as wide as possible.

Centre in the mid-line, with the tube angled 35° caudad so that when viewed from the side the central ray passes through the joint.

Submento-vertical. As for symphysis menti (p. 102).

Lateral oblique. The patient sits or lies with the head in the lateral position. A view of each side is taken for comparison.

Centre to the temporo-mandibular joint nearer the cassette, with the tube angled 25° caudad.

Special circumstances

1. Following trauma, the whole mandible must be demonstrated because a blow to one side of the face, particularly near the angle of the jaw, can result in a fracture of the neck of the mandible on the other side, i.e. 'contre coup' injury.

2. When there are fractures of both sides of the mandible, there may also be a third fracture near the mid-line, causing the so-called magnification sign whereby the mandible appears too wide for the upper jaw (Trapnell, 1977). The mid-line fracture may be demonstrated on an occipito-frontal view (p. 101) but an intra-oral occlusal view may demonstrate a fracture not seen on other views. See infero-superior view (p. 102).

ADDITIONAL EXAMINATION

Pan-oral tomography (p. 171 and Plate XXI).

PARANASAL SINUSES

Anatomy. The paranasal sinuses consist of the maxillary antra and the frontal, ethmoid and sphenoid sinuses. They all communicate with the nasal cavity and are lined with mucous membrane continuous with that lining the nasal cavity.

Radiographs of the nasal sinuses must be taken with a horizontal beam to facilitate the demonstration of free fluid. The patient should be erect whenever possible. A small aperture, just sufficient to include the sinuses, is used (Lysholm, 1963).

The use of the air gap technique (p. 27) instead of a grid will reduce the radiation dose to the eyes (Crooks and Ardran, 1977).

Rare earth or very fast tungstate screens allow the more frequent use of the fine focus and shorter exposure times.

Basic views

Occipito-mental (to show antra and the frontal, anterior ethmoid and sphenoid sinuses). The patient sits facing the skull table, with the chin in contact with it so that the base line is at 45° to the vertical. The table may be angled 15° for easier positioning and to bring the cassette parallel with the long axis of the face. The mouth is opened wide so that the sphenoid sinuses are demonstrated (Fig. 10). (The petrous temporal bones must be projected below the antra; if they are superimposed on the lower part of the antra, the angle of the base line should be increased by raising the chin.)

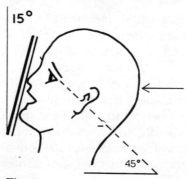

Fig. 10

Centre to the tip of the nose.

Occipito-frontal (to show the frontal and anterior ethmoid sinuses). The patient faces the skull table, with the chin raised slightly so that the base line is at 20° to the horizontal. The angle should be checked with a protractor. The skull table may be either vertical, or angled 20° so that it is parallel with the forehead (Fig. 11).

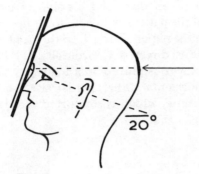

Fig. 11

Centre to the nasion.

Lateral (to show all the nasal sinuses, both sides superimposed). The head is placed in the lateral position, with the median sagittal plane parallel with the table and the interpupillary line at right angles to the table.

Centre 2·5 cm (1 in) from the outer canthus of the eye along the base line.

Submento-vertical (to show sphenoid and ethmoid sinuses). The patient sits facing the X-ray tube, with the chin raised and neck extended. The skull table is adjusted until it is parallel with the base line (Fig. 12).

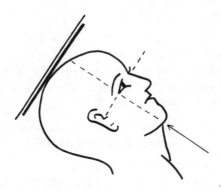

Fig. 12

Centre in the mid-line, 2·5 cm (1 in) behind the symphysis menti.

Special circumstances

1. To confirm the presence of a fluid level in the maxillary antrum, to differentiate between fluid and a polyp or cyst (Axelsson and Jensen, 1975) or if the patient is unable to sit up, an occipito-mental view is taken with the patient lying with the head in the lateral position and the tube is directed horizontally. The side of the head (affected side if known) is placed on a foam pad so that the median sagittal plane is horizontal. The chin is raised so that the base line is at 45° to the cassette, which is supported vertically in front of the patient's face (Fig. 13).

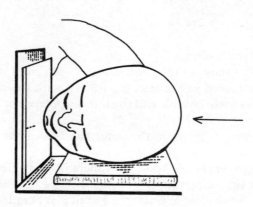

Fig. 13

Centre at the level of the tip of the nose and at right angles to the cassette, using a horizontal beam.

2. If fluid in the frontal sinuses is suspected, a 'brow-up' lateral view is taken to confirm its presence. The patient lies supine and the X-ray tube is directed horizontally.

Supplementary view

POSTERIOR ETHMOID SINUSES

Oblique. The patient faces the skull table, with the forehead resting against it. The head is rotated 40° and the chin raised so that the base line is at 30°. The nose, chin, cheek and eyebrow should all be in contact with the table.

Centre to the orbit nearer the film.

ADDITIONAL EXAMINATIONS

Tomography (p. 47). *Dacryocystography* (p. 350) (Lloyd *et al.*, 1974).

19

Vertebral column

The vertebral column consists of thirty-three vertebrae (seven cervical, twelve thoracic, five lumbar, five sacral and four coccygeal). The sacral segments are fused together to form the sacrum. The coccygeal segments (or in some cases only the lowest three of them) are fused together and form a small triangular bone.

A typical vertebra consists of a body and a neural arch together enclosing the vertebral foramen which transmits the spinal cord. The neural arch consists of paired pedicles and laminae, and bears several processes to which muscles and ligaments are attached. The articular facets are also paired and are situated on the superior and inferior surfaces of the arch. The superior processes face posteriorly and the inferior processes face anteriorly. These processes articulate with similar ones on the adjacent vertebrae, thus allowing flexion, extension and lateral flexion. In the thoracic region, rotation also occurs. Between the pedicles of adjacent vertebrae are intervertebral foramina which transmit the spinal nerves and vessels. Between the vertebrae are intervertebral discs which allow a small amount of movement between the adjacent vertebrae. These discs consist of a central nucleus pulposus enclosed by the fibro-cartilage of the annulus fibrosus.

The vertebrae in each region show variations from the basic pattern and full radiographic examination demands demonstration of all the integral parts. It may be required to demonstrate (a) local disease, requiring several coned views of the lesion, e.g. fractures, inflammation or neoplasm (b) spinal deformities, e.g. scoliosis, requiring views of the whole spine or (c) generalised or systemic disease, requiring a skeletal survey.

There must be no movement by the patient during the exposure but for most views it is not necessary for respiration to be arrested. The major difficulty to be overcome is presented by the overlying tissues.

Radiation protection. With the exception of the lumbo-sacral region and sacrum in female patients, it is always possible to protect the gonads from direct radiation, by accurate coning and lead rubber placed over the gonad area. Some radiation to the gonads resulting from internal scatter is inevitable but can be reduced by perfect technique.

Low backache is a common complaint in young adults and careful attention must be paid to gonad protection when radiographing the lumbar and sacral vertebrae. In antero-posterior views, when the patient's knees are flexed, lead rubber can be held by the patient so that it rests on the anterior surface of the thighs, the upper border being at the level of the anterior superior iliac spines. For lateral views of the lumbar spine, lead rubber is placed over the pelvis up to the level of the anterior superior iliac spines. In the male, gonad protection can be similarly applied for views of the sacral area.

Some diseases necessitate follow-up films over a number of years and young adults who have undergone surgery or an accident may require frequent radiography. The cumulative amount of radiation received by the gonads can be high if great care is not taken.

The 10-day rule (p. 19) should be observed if the degree of clinical urgency permits.

ADDITIONAL EXAMINATIONS
The vertebral column may be investigated by the following methods:

Tomography. To demonstrate conditions which may not be seen on plain films, e.g. osteolytic lesions in a vertebral body less than 1 cm in diameter (p. 47).

Myelography. To demonstrate encroachment on to the spinal canal, especially by non-opaque causes (p. 344).

Discography. To demonstrate herniation of a disc (p. 374).

Scintigraphy. To demonstrate primary and secondary tumours (p. 63).

Computed tomography. To demonstrate bone architecture and the size and shape of the spinal canal (p. 52).

Excretion urography, barium studies, etc. To investigate closely related structures.

CERVICAL VERTEBRAE

Anatomy. The cervical spine is convex forwards. The seven cervical vertebrae show marked differences from each other, particularly the first (atlas) which has an anterior arch instead of a vertebral body, into which fits the odontoid peg of the second cervical vertebra (axis). The spinous process of the seventh cervical vertebra is prominent, easily palpable and thus a useful surface landmark. The transverse processes each have a foramen transversarium for transmitting the vertebral artery.

In the antero-posterior view, the upper cervical vertebrae are obscured by the jaws and teeth. Although full extension of the neck will project the jaws upwards, the upper cervical vertebrae are then obscured by the occiput. But they can be demonstrated if this view is taken with the patient's mouth wide open. The vertebrae are then shown between the upper and lower jaws.

The intervertebral foramina face antero-laterally and thus oblique views are necessary to demonstrate them. The upper vertebral facets face antero-inferiorly and in a lateral view are therefore shown superimposed on the contra-lateral facet. Between the lateral margins of the vertebral bodies are synovial joints (the neuro-central joints) and therefore in a lateral view it is not possible to show the whole joint space as it is in other regions of the vertebral column.

The cervical spine is the most flexible part of the vertebral column and many positions are possible. In children, flexion and extension occur mainly in the upper cervical region but in adults movement occurs mostly in the lower part.

Basic views

Antero-posterior (CV1–3). The patient lies supine on the X-ray table or sits with his back to the skull table. The chin is tucked down so that the maxilla is superimposed on the lower border of the occiput. The mouth must be opened wide. Immobilisation of the head is important. A small aperture is used.

Centre to the middle of the open mouth.

Antero-posterior (CV3–7). The patient lies supine with the chin raised so that the mandible is superimposed on the occiput. The cassette is displaced cephalad in line with the central ray.

Centre in the mid-line at the level of the angle of the mandible, with the tube angled 15° cephalad.

Lateral. The patient sits or stands in the lateral position, with one shoulder against the cassette and with the shoulders lowered as much as possible. The chin is raised so that the angle of the mandible does not obscure the upper cervical vertebrae. For immobilisation a foam pad of appropriate thickness is placed between the side of the head and the cassette, the head being maintained in the lateral position. A long focus-film distance, 150 cm (60 in), is used to reduce magnification. The upper border of the cassette is placed at the level of the top of the pinna.

Centre behind the angle of the mandible.

Special circumstances

1. In some patients, particularly children, front teeth may obscure the upper vertebrae. Angulation of the tube 5° cephalad, or raising the chin, may enable the axis and atlas to be shown. If not, an antero-posterior view taken as follows may do so. For this view, the patient lies supine with the radiographic base line at right angles to the table. The head is immobilised. The patient is instructed in opening and closing the mouth rapidly and the exposure is made with the lowest possible milliamperage so as to allow a long exposure time, preferably at least 3 seconds.

Centre to the symphysis menti, with the mouth closed.

2. In cases of torticollis, where there is flexion and rotation, it is difficult to exclude a fracture or subluxation. It may be necessary to take three antero-posterior and three lateral views, at varying angles of patient and tube, to demonstrate all the cervical vertebrae completely.

3. When the odontoid peg or atlanto-axial joints are not clearly demonstrated on the basic views, tomography (p. 47) is invaluable.

4. A patient with a traumatic or destructive lesion of the cervical spine requires very careful treatment and should be moved as little as possible. He should be placed in position before any supporting collar is removed and he must not be moved further until it is replaced. A lateral view is taken with the cassette supported vertically, using a horizontal beam.

5. A patient with a suspected fracture or dislocation of the cervical spine must be examined on the casualty stretcher and should not be moved on to the X-ray table. Medical assistance should be obtained to apply traction to the arms so that a lateral view of the lower cervical vertebrae can be obtained. Such a view is taken with the cassette supported vertically, using a horizontal beam.

Supplementary views

INTERVERTEBRAL FORAMINA

Either anterior or posterior oblique views will demonstrate these foramina satisfactorily. Both sides are always examined. Correct labelling of the films is essential and this is best achieved by 'right posterior oblique' and 'right anterior oblique' lead markers.

In the right posterior oblique view, the left foramina are shown and in the left posterior oblique, the right foramina. In the left anterior oblique view, the left foramina are shown and in the right anterior oblique view, the right foramina.

Posterior obliques (Plate XII). The patient sits or stands with the back against the grid cassette or erect Bucky, and is then rotated 45° to each side in turn. The head is placed in the lateral position. A radiograph is taken in each position.

Centre in the mid-cervical region, to the side of the neck further from the cassette, with the tube angled 15° cephalad.

Anterior obliques. The patient lies in the half-prone position, with the head lateral and the neck at an angle of 45° to the table. The arm of the lower side is placed by the patient's side and the other arm is raised over the head. A radiograph is taken in each position.

Centre in the mid-cervical region, to the side of the neck nearer the cassette, with the tube angled 15° caudad.

ATLANTO-OCCIPITAL JOINTS
These are formed by the lateral masses of the atlas articulating superiorly with the convex atlantoid processes of the occiput.

Lateral. The patient is positioned with the head in the lateral position against the cassette.

Centre 2·5 cm (1 in) below the external auditory meatus.

Oblique. The head is placed in the antero-posterior position and then rotated 45° to each side in turn, a radiograph being taken in each position.

Centre to the middle of the orbit nearer the film.

POSTERIOR ARCH OF ATLAS
Lateral. The head is placed in the lateral position against the cassette. The tube is angled in order to separate the two sides of the arch.

Centre to the thyroid cartilage, with the tube angled 5° cephalad.

Special circumstances

1. With badly injured patients, when oblique views cannot be obtained by the conventional methods, but the patient can be rotated,

the articular facets and processes can be demonstrated by taking views in the following way (Lodge and Higginbottom, 1966):

Oblique I. The patient lies supine and the tube is directed horizontally at 120 cm (48 in) focus-film distance. The patient is then rotated 20° away from the tube. The cassette is supported vertically.

Centre to the fifth cervical vertebra, with the tube angled 5° cephalad.

Oblique II. The patient is then rotated 40° so that the side away from the tube is raised 20°.

Centre to the fifth cervical vertebra, with the tube angled 5° caudad.

Traction to the arms is applied at the wrists (and not the hands) in each case. Careful marking of the radiographs is essential as the two sides can be distinguished only by the markers. It is recommended that the right marker be put on the film when the right shoulder is downwards and the left marker when the left shoulder is downwards.

2. With badly injured patients who cannot be moved from the supine position for any of the previously described oblique views, the lower cervical vertebrae can be demonstrated by the following method:

Supine oblique. The patient lies supine and completely immobilised on the casualty stretcher (McCall *et al.*, 1973). The X-ray tube is rotated 45° and centred 5 cm (2 in) above and lateral to the sternal notch. The cassette is placed under the patient's neck so that the emergent beam passes through the centre of the cassette. Occasionally the tube has to be angled 10–15° cephalad when there is an exaggerated caudal obliquity of the lower intervertebral foramina, in which case the centering point is 5 cm (2 in) lateral to, and at the level of, the sternal notch. A grid cannot be used when there is double angulation of the tube.

MOBILITY AND STABILITY

Lateral views in flexion and extension. The patient is positioned as for the basic lateral view and two radiographs are taken, one with the neck flexed as much as possible so that the chin rests on the chest and the other with the neck extended and the chin raised as much as possible. For the flexion view, the cassette should be placed transversely, so that all the cervical vertebrae are included.

Centre to the mid-cervical region.

CERVICO-THORACIC VERTEBRAE

Fractures and dislocations of the upper spine frequently occur in the cervico-thoracic region. It is important that radiographs are obtained as soon as possible after injury and without moving the patient from the position, usually supine, in which he presents for X-ray examination. The most useful view is usually the lateral, which is always taken first, processed and scrutinised before any attempt is made to take an antero-posterior view which, unless a special trolley with a radiolucent top is used, usually necessitates sliding a cassette under the patient's neck and shoulders.

The upper thoracic vertebrae are usually obscured in the lateral view by the shoulders. In large patients, or those who 'hunch' their shoulders, the lower cervical vertebrae may also be obscured by the shoulders. This region, therefore, presents particular problems.

Traction applied to the arms is often successful in lowering the shoulders sufficiently to demonstrate C7 and T1 on the basic lateral view but it must only be attempted under medical supervision. When traction is applied, the assistant, wearing a lead coat, should stand at the end of the stretcher or X-ray table and apply traction by holding the patient by the forearms or above the elbows, and not just by the hands or wrists.

A patient with a traumatic or destructive lesion of the cervical or thoracic spine should be placed in position before any supporting collar is removed and he must not be moved further until it is replaced.

Experience shows that no single method of obtaining the lateral view is always successful in demonstrating this region adequately on every patient and it may be necessary sometimes to attempt several of the views described below.

Because of the thickness of tissue present at the shoulders, it is usually necessary to use a grid for all views.

Basic views

I. For the patient who can stand:

Lateral. The patient stands in the lateral position with one shoulder against the cassette which is placed vertically. The shoulders should be lowered as much as possible. If the condition of the patient allows, he should hold a sandbag in each hand to pull the shoulders downwards. A 24 × 30 cm (10 × 12 in) cassette is used, with its upper border at the level of the top of the pinna. A long focus-film distance, usually 150 cm (60 in), is used. The kilovoltage required is 5–10 more than for the lateral view of the cervical spine.

Centre behind the angle of the mandible.

Lateral (with one arm raised). The patient stands in the lateral position with the arm nearer the cassette raised above the head. The other shoulder is lowered as much as possible (Fig. 14).

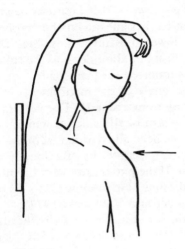

Fig. 14

Centre just above the shoulder further from the cassette.

Antero-posterior. The patient lies supine on the X-ray table, with the chin raised slightly. The kilovoltage required is 5–10 more than for the antero-posterior view of the cervical spine.

Centre to the sternal notch.

Supplementary views

Lateral (to show the spinous processes). The patient stands in the lateral position, with the neck flexed as much as possible so that the chin rests on the chest. The arm nearer the cassette is brought forward and curved round the waist and the other arm is held in front of the body. A cassette containing two sets of screens can be used (see Multiple Radiography, p. 35) and will give an additional view of the spinous processes which otherwise may be over-exposed, even if high kilovoltage is used to reduce differences in density between the vertebral bodies and the spinous processes.

Centre behind the shoulders, at the level of the head of the humerus.

Lateral oblique (Plate XIII). From the lateral position, the patient is rotated about 20° by placing the arm further from the cassette behind his back. The other arm is brought forward. The shoulders are thus no longer superimposed.

Centre to the middle of the clavicle further from the cassette.

II. For the patient who cannot stand but can be moved:

Lateral. The patient lies supine on the X-ray table or stretcher, with the shoulders lowered as far as possible. The cassette is supported vertically against one shoulder and the tube directed horizontally. The head is supported on foam pads.

Centre behind the angle of the mandible.

Lateral (with one arm raised). The patient is turned into the lateral position. The arm of the side on which he is lying is raised above the head and the head allowed to rest on it. The other shoulder is lowered as much as possible, by traction, if appropriate, under medical supervision. If the patient has very broad shoulders, caudad angulation of the tube may help to show C7 to T2 between the images of the shoulders (Scher and Vambeck, 1977).

Centre: either to the acromium process further from the table, with the tube vertical, *or* to the spinous process of C7 with the tube angled 15° caudad.

Lateral oblique. From the lateral position, the patient is rotated about 20° by placing the arm further from the cassette behind his back. The other arm is brought forward. The shoulders are thus no longer superimposed.

Centre to the middle of the clavicle further from the cassette.

Antero-posterior. The patient lies supine on the X-ray table. The kilovoltage required is 5–10 more than for the antero-posterior view of the cervical spine.

Centre to the sternal notch.

III. For the patient who must not be moved:

Lateral. The cassette is supported vertically by the side of one shoulder, with its upper border at the level of the pinna of the ear. The shoulders are lowered as much as possible, by traction under medical supervision. A long focus-film distance, usually 150 cm (60 in) is used and the tube is directed horizontally.

Centre behind the angle of the mandible.

This radiograph should include the whole cervical spine to exclude injury higher up. It should be scrutinised before any other view is taken.

Lateral (with one arm raised). One arm is carefully raised above the head and the cassette is supported vertically against the axilla. The other shoulder is lowered as far as possible, by traction under medical supervision. If the patient has very broad shoulders, caudad angulation of the tube may help to show C7 to T2 between the images of the shoulders.

Centre to the acromium process further from the cassette.

Antero-posterior. The casette is placed under the patient's neck and shoulders, care being taken not to move him.

Centre to the sternal notch.

Supine oblique (see p. 113). This view will demonstrate which side a fracture is on, but is less good for demonstrating fracture or dislocation.

ADDITIONAL EXAMINATION
Tomography (p. 47).

THORACIC VERTEBRAE

Anatomy. The thoracic spine is concave forwards. The 12 thoracic vertebrae show a gradual transition, the upper vertebrae resembling the cervical and the lower vertebrae resembling the lumbar vertebrae. The bodies of the vertebrae increase in size from the upper to the lower parts of the region. The body of each thoracic vertebra and the transverse processes of all but the last two vertebrae, have facets for articulating with the heads and tubercles of the ribs.

The apophyseal joints are nearly vertical, their superior articular processes facing backwards and their inferior processes facing forwards. The intervertebral foramina are deep and are clearly demonstrated on a lateral view. The spinous processes extend downwards and backwards as far as the level of the body of the vertebra two below. The spinous processes of the lowest three thoracic vertebrae are shorter, thicker and more nearly horizontal than the others.

In the antero-posterior view, the upper four thoracic vertebrae are overshadowed by the translucency of the air-filled trachea and the lower vertebrae are obscured by the denser shadows of the heart, mediastinum and sub-diaphragmatic structures. Thus, demonstration of all the thoracic vertebrae on one exposure is difficult.

In the lateral view, the upper two (sometimes three) vertebrae are obscured by the dense shoulder structures and the other vertebrae may be obscured by lung vascular shadows, particularly if the exposure is made on arrested respiration.

Centering. The centering points given for the views that follow are based on the fact that the spinous process of the seventh cervical vertebra is easily palpable. The conventional centering points are usually measured from the sternal angle and when this is used by students and inexperienced radiographers, the cervico-thoracic junction (which must be included on the radiograph) is often not demonstrated. Sometimes even the first thoracic vertebra is not demonstrated. Furthermore, the sternal angle is not always easy to locate and palpation of the sternum may be painful for some patients, e.g. following mastectomy or radiotherapy. In practice it is therefore more satisfactory for the cassette to be placed so that its upper border is 4 cm (1½ in) cephalad to the spinous process of the seventh cervical vertebra.

Basic views

Antero-posterior. The patient lies supine on the X-ray table, with the knees flexed over a small pillow for comfort. Either a 17 × 7 in or 30 × 40 cm (15 × 12 in) cassette is used, with the upper border 4 cm (1½ in) above the spinous process of the seventh cervical vertebra. A narrow aperture should be used but if there is a possibility that the patient has a kyphosis or scoliosis, the aperture must be widened.

Centre in the mid-line, at the level of the middle of the cassette.

Lateral. The patient lies on his side, with the knees flexed to assist balance. The arm nearer the table is placed in front of the patient and the other arm is placed above the head. The shoulders are thus no longer superimposed. Foam pads must be placed under the body to maintain the spine parallel with the table. A long exposure time is used and the patient is encouraged to breathe gently throughout the exposure so as to blur out lung and rib shadows. Immobilisation is essential. A 30 × 40 cm (15 × 12 in) or 35 × 43 cm (17 × 14 in) cassette is used, with the upper border at the level of the seventh cervical spinous process.

Centre through the axilla to the centre of the cassette.

Special circumstances

For a patient with kyphosis (p. 125) more exposure (usually mA.s as well as kV) is required than for a normal patient and more for the antero-posterior view than for the lateral view of the same patient. It may be painful for the patient to lie on his back and so soft pads should be suitably placed to relieve pressure. An erect antero-posterior view may be more comfortable for such a patient. More information is usually obtained from the lateral than from the antero-posterior view. When severe curvature is present, the light beam diaphragm must not be closed to the usual narrow aperture.

Supplementary views

Antero-posterior and lateral, weight-bearing. The patient sits or stands in front of the erect Bucky or vertically-placed grid cassette. The positioning and centering are the same as for the basic horizontal views.

Obliques. From the supine position the patient is rotated 45° to each side in turn. Foam pads and sandbags are used to support the patient. A radiograph is taken in each position.

Centre in the mid-clavicular line of the raised side, 5 cm (2 in) below the sternal angle.

THORACO-LUMBAR VERTEBRAE

In the antero-posterior view, the thoraco-lumbar region is over-shadowed by the denser mediastinal and sub-diaphragmatic structures. In the lateral view, the diaphragm is superimposed on the thoraco-lumbar region, thus producing great differences in density between the air-containing thoracic cavity and the denser sub-diaphragmatic area. The lateral view of the thoraco-lumbar region must therefore be taken on full arrested expiration because the diaphragm is then at its highest level and the maximum amount of the vertebral column is demonstrated below the diaphragm.

Basic views

Antero-posterior. The patient lies supine, with knees and hips flexed, and the soles of the feet on the table.

Centre in the mid-line, at the level of the twelfth thoracic vertebra, about 10 cm (4 in) superior to the lower costal margin.

Lateral. The patient lies on the side, with the knees flexed. Small pads are placed under the waist, hip or shoulder to maintain the spine parallel with the table. The exposure is made on full arrested expiration.

Centre 7·5 cm (3 in) anterior to the spinous process at the same level as for the antero-posterior view.

Special circumstances

In investigations for suspected ankylosing spondylitis, localised views of the thoraco-lumbar junction and a view of the sacro-iliac joints are required.

LUMBAR VERTEBRAE

Anatomy. The lumbar spine is convex forwards. The lumbar are the largest and strongest of the vertebrae. Their spinous processes are broad and directed horizontally. The posterior intervertebral joints are oblique in direction, the inferior facets facing forwards and laterally, the superior facets facing backwards and medially.

Owing to the angle between the lower border of the fifth lumbar vertebra and the first sacral segment, the lumbo-sacral junction is not clearly demonstrated on an antero-posterior view of the lumbar spine. Angulation of the tube is necessary so that the central ray passes through the joint space. The lumbo-sacral angle varies from patient to patient, being between 15° and 25°. The larger angle is found in women.

The pars interarticularis is the portion of bone joining the superior and inferior articular facets and is best demonstrated in posterior oblique views.

The 10-day rule should be observed if the degree of clinical urgency permits.

Basic views

Antero-posterior. The patient lies supine with the knees and hips flexed, and with the soles of the feet on the table to reduce the lumbar lordosis. The light beam diaphragm should be restricted to a narrow aperture just large enough to include the lumbar spine and sacro-iliac joints.

Centre in the mid-line, at the level of the lower costal margin.

Lateral. The patient lies on his side, with the knees flexed and the hands placed on the pillow. Usually two pillows under the head and a pad under the waist are required to maintain the spine parallel with the table. For male patients with broad shoulders and narrow hips, a pad may be required under the hips.

An aluminium wedge filter can be used to avoid over-exposure of the spinous processes in the lateral views, particularly for a very slim patient. The filter increases in thickness from 0 to 1 cm, thus allowing the full exposure to the vertebral bodies while reducing the exposure to the spinous processes.

Centre 7·5 cm (3 in) anterior to the spinous process, at the level of the lower costal margin.

Lateral of the lumbo-sacral junction. The patient remains in the last-mentioned position. The light beam diaphragm is restricted to a small aperture sufficient to cover an area of about 15 × 15 cm on the radiograph.

Centre 5 cm (2 in) below the iliac crest, 7·5 cm (3 in) anterior to the spinous process of the fifth lumbar vertebra.

Special circumstances

If the patient has been in bed for some time, there may be a large quantity of intestinal gas present, making demonstration of the lumbar vertebrae difficult. Therefore, a patient who is to have a lumbar spine examination should be ambulant for some hours beforehand, if possible. If this is not possible, gas shadows may be blurred out by using a long exposure time, with the patient breathing gently throughout the exposure.

Supplementary views

LUMBO-SACRAL JUNCTION

Antero-posterior. The patient is positioned as for the basic antero-posterior view. A small aperture is used and the cassette should be displaced cephalad in line with the central ray.

Centre in the mid-line, at the level of the anterior superior iliac spines, with the tube angled 15° to 25° cephalad. (The exact tube angulation may be measured from a lateral view of the lumbo-sacral spine.)

Lateral. See above.

PARS INTERARTICULARIS

Posterior obliques. From the antero-posterior position, the patient is rotated 45° to each side in turn, the raised side being supported with foam pads and sandbags. The knee of the side nearer the film is flexed and should rest on a sandbag for support. A radiograph is taken in each position.

Centre in the mid-clavicular line of the raised side, at the level of the lower costal margin.

SPONDYLOLISTHESIS

(Anterior displacement of one vertebral body on another, usually at the lumbo-sacral junction but occasionally between the fourth and fifth lumbar vertebrae.)

Posterior obliques. The patient is positioned as for the oblique views of the lumbar spine (p. 121). A small aperture is used. A radiograph is taken in each position.

Centre 5 cm (2 in) medially from the anterior superior iliac spine of the raised side.

POSTERIOR VERTEBRAL ARCHES

Semi-axial view (Abel and Smith, 1977). The patient lies supine with the knees flexed and the soles of the feet on the table.

Centre in the mid-line, at the level of the lower sternum with the tube angled 45° caudad so that the emergent beam is at the level of the spinous process of the third lumbar vertebra.

SACRUM

Anatomy. The sacrum is roughly triangular in both antero-posterior and lateral projections and the body is concave forwards. The anterior margin forms the sacral promontory. The upper part of the sacrum is directed posteriorly at an angle varying from patient to patient and may be almost horizontal. Paired intervertebral foramina open on to the anterior and posterior surfaces.

The 10-day rule should be observed if the degree of clinical urgency permits. For female patients, the gonad dose is less if postero-anterior instead of antero-posterior views are taken.

Basic views

Either **antero-posterior.** The patient lies supine on the X-ray table, the knees flexed over a small pillow. An 18 × 24 cm (10 × 8 in) cassette, placed transversely, is displaced cephalad so that its upper border is at the level of the iliac crests.

Centre in the mid-line, 5 cm (2 in) below the anterior superior iliac spines, with the tube angled 10° to 25° cephalad. If the lateral view is taken first and processed, the exact angle may be measured from it, but male patients usually require 10° to 15° and female patients 20° to 25°.

Or **postero-anterior.** The patient lies prone with the pelvis positioned symmetrically. The cassette is displaced caudad in line with the central ray.

Centre in the mid-line at the level of the posterior iliac spines, with the tube angled 15° caudad.

Lateral. The patient lies on the side, with the knees flexed. The upper border of the cassette should be at the level of the anterior superior iliac spines and should be large enough, e.g. 24 × 30 cm (12 × 10 in) to include the sacrum and coccyx.

Centre 5 cm (2 in) anterior to, and at the level of, the posterior iliac spines, which are easily palpable.

Special circumstances

Radiographic demonstration of the sacrum and coccyx is often hampered by intestinal gas and faecal shadows. If possible the patient should take a suitable aperient on each of the two nights before the examination. If this is not possible, tomography (p. 47) is of advantage.

Supplementary views

Stereoscopic antero-posterior. The patient is positioned as for the basic antero-posterior view. The tube is moved 3 cm (1¼ in) from the mid-line for each exposure (Stereography, p. 36).

COCCYX

Anatomy. The coccyx is an extremely variable structure. It usually points forwards and downwards but it may be at a pronounced angle to the sacrum. Unlike the sacrum, it is of small and delicate proportions.

The 10-day rule should be observed if the degree of clinical urgency permits.

Basic views

Antero-posterior. The patient lies supine, the knees flexed over a small pillow. The cassette is displaced caudad in line with the central ray.

Centre in the mid-line 5 cm (2 in) below the anterior superior iliac spines, with the tube angled 15° caudad.

Lateral. The patient lies on the side, with the knees flexed.

Centre to the coccyx, which is easily palpable.

Special circumstances

When it is impossible for the patient to lie in the supine position (e.g. after trauma or if suffering from coccydynia) a postero-anterior view is taken with the tube angled 15° cephalad.

SACRO-ILIAC JOINTS

Anatomy. The sacro-iliac joints are atypical synovial joints between the lateral margins of the sacrum and the ilium. The articular surfaces interlock and restrict movement to a minimum. The joints are of a complex shape, S-shaped in cross-section with the sacral articular surface directed postero-inferiorly. Thus tube angulation is required in the antero-posterior view and oblique views also are required for complete demonstration of the joints.

The 10-day rule should be observed if the degree of clinical urgency permits. For female patients, the gonad dose is less if postero-anterior rather than antero-posterior views are taken.

Basic views

Either **antero-posterior.** The patient lies supine, with the pelvis positioned symmetrically and the knees flexed over a small pillow. A 24 × 30 cm (12 × 10 in) cassette is used transversely with its upper border at the level of the iliac crests.

Centre in the mid-line 5 cm (2 in) below the anterior superior iliac spines, with the tube angled 20° cephalad.

Or **postero-anterior.** The patient lies prone with the pelvis positioned symmetrically. The cassette is displaced caudad in line with the central ray.

Centre in the mid-line at the level of the posterior iliac spines, with the tube angled 15° caudad.

Obliques. From the supine position the patient is rotated 25° to each side in turn. The knee nearer the table is flexed and the pelvis is supported by foam pads and sandbags. A radiograph is taken in each position. A narrow slit aperture is used so that a view of both joints is obtained.

Centre 4 cm (1½ in) medially to the anterior superior iliac spine and directly through the joint on the raised side.

Supplementary views

SUBLUXATION

To demonstrate subluxation of the sacro-iliac joints which can occur following pregnancy, erect antero-posterior views are taken. The patient stands with her back against the erect Bucky or vertically-placed grid cassette. The cassette is displaced cephalad as for the basic view. Two radiographs are taken, with the patient standing with all her weight on each leg in turn.

Centre 5 cm (2 in) below the anterior superior iliac spines, with the tube angled 20° cephalad.

ADDITIONAL EXAMINATIONS
Stereography (p. 36). *Tomography* (p. 47).

SPINAL DEFORMITIES

Scoliosis is lateral curvature of the spine, with rotation. The whole spine from the occiput to the sacrum must be included on the radiographs. The patient is radiographed in the erect antero-posterior position. The epiphyses of the iliac crests must be included. During correction of the condition, follow-up films are required. Either a long, 90×35 cm (36×14 in), cassette is used, with one exposure, or two overlapping 35×43 cm (17×14 in) cassettes are used, with two exposures.

Kyphosis is antero-posterior curvature of the spine. Collapse of the vertebral bodies occurs eventually, giving acute angulation and a 'hunch-back' appearance. An antero-posterior view, centred to the apex of the curve, and coned views of collapsed vertebrae are usually required. The lateral view usually gives more information than the antero-posterior and it is also less uncomfortable for the patient. An antero-posterior view requires more exposure than a lateral view of the same patient. Soft pads must be used for the patient's comfort, particularly in the supine position which may be very painful to adopt.

20

Shoulder girdle

The bones of the shoulder (pectoral) girdle comprise two scapulae and two clavicles. The lateral ends of the clavicles articulate with the scapulae at the acromio-clavicular joints; the medial ends of the clavicles articulate with the sternum at the sterno-clavicular joints. Posteriorly, there is no bony attachment, position being maintained by the tone of the muscles of the shoulder girdle. The head of the humerus articulates with the glenoid fossa of the scapula to form the shoulder joint.

For radiographic examination of the shoulder girdle, all radio-paque objects must be removed from the neck, shoulders and arms and usually the patient is asked to undress down to the waist and to wear a suitable gown. After an injury (e.g. fracture or dislocation) the patient will be unable to do this and it will be necessary to ensure that the region is free from radiopaque objects, without causing the patient further distress by undressing.

Films. Screen film is used, with or without a grid depending on the physique of the patient. Either a grid or an air gap is necessary in the case of patients with well-developed deltoid muscles, to improve contrast by reducing the amount of scattered radiation and also, usually, for the sterno-clavicular joints and for a lateral view of the scapula. A curved cassette is very useful in obtaining an axial view of the shoulder. When an infero-superior view of the shoulder is taken, a method of supporting the cassette horizontally is required.

Non-screen film and a grid can be used (Stripp, 1964). This technique produces extremely good detail but results in greatly increased radiation dose. The technique is probably best employed as a supplementary, rather than a routine, method.

Radiation protection. With accurate coning and positioning, radiography of the shoulder girdle should be a low dose examination, but lead shielding of the gonads is essential. This is particularly important for the supero-inferior axial view of the shoulder, when the gonads may be in the direct X-ray beam.

SHOULDER JOINT

Anatomy. The gleno-humeral joint is a ball and socket synovial joint formed by the hemispherical head of the humerus articulating with the glenoid fossa of the scapula. The greater tuberosity of the humerus has three facets for the insertion of the spinati and teres minor muscles. Between the greater and lesser tuberosities lies the bicipital groove through which passes the tendon of the long head of the biceps muscle. About 2·5 cm (1 in) distal to the tuberosities is the surgical neck of the humerus, frequently the site of fractures.

When the arm is hanging by the side, the head of the humerus is directed medially, upwards and backwards and the glenoid fossa faces forwards and laterally. Thus in the antero-posterior view of the shoulder, the joint space is not shown clearly unless the patient is rotated into a posterior oblique position.

The shoulder joint is protected superiorly by the coraco-acromion ligament which is attached to the coracoid and acromion processes, both of which are easily palpable and form useful surface landmarks.

A wide range of movements is possible because the capsule of the joint is very loose, especially inferiorly, and because the glenoid fossa is shallow. These movements are abduction, adduction, flexion, extension and rotation. All these together permit circumduction.

Basic views

Antero-posterior. The patient, either erect facing the tube, or

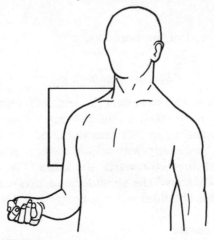

Fig. 15

supine, is rotated approximately 30° until the scapula of the side under examination is parallel with the film. The elbow is flexed and the forearm is directed forwards (Fig. 15). The shoulder should be relaxed and not elevated ('hunched') as this can give a distorted view of the joint and may even simulate subluxation.

Centre to the coracoid process.

Axial (supero-inferior) (Plate XIV). The patient sits beside the X-ray table, with the arm abducted and the elbow flexed at right angles. A curved cassette is placed under the axilla and the patient leans over it so that the shoulder region is as flat as possible (Fig. 16). If the arm is not sufficiently abducted, distortion of the joint will occur. Depending on the height of the patient it may be necessary either to raise him on pillows or to raise the cassette.

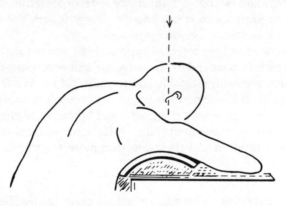

Fig. 16

Centre to the head of the humerus.

Special circumstances

1. If the patient is unable to abduct the arm sufficiently for a supero-inferior axial view to be taken, an infero-superior view may be taken, with the patient standing and the arm abducted as much as possible. The X-ray tube, preferably with a long cone, is placed at the side of the patient and directed towards the axilla. The cassette is supported horizontally above the shoulder and pressed firmly against the neck so that the shoulder will not be projected off the film (Fig. 17).

Centre to the cassette.

2. If the arm cannot be abducted because it is in a sling, or is too

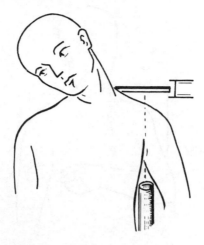

Fig. 17

painful to be moved, the patient faces the cassette and is then rotated until the spine of the scapula of the side being examined is at right angles to the cassette.

Centre to the head of the humerus.

Supplementary views

MUSCLE CALCIFICATION
Internal and external rotation. (These views are also essential to obtain further information concerning any lesion shown on the basic views.) Two radiographs are taken. For one view, the patient is positioned as for the basic antero-posterior view. The elbow remains flexed and the forearm is placed either across the chest (Fig. 18A) or behind the back, to produce full internal rotation of the shoulder joint. For the other view, the patient is re-positioned in the antero-posterior position, with the elbow flexed. The arm is then externally rotated as far as possible (Fig. 18B).

Centre to the coracoid process, for each view.

RECURRENT SUBLUXATION
'Stryker's' view. The patient lies supine, with the palm of the hand on top of the head and with the elbow directed forwards.

Centre to the coracoid process, with the tube angled 10° cephalad.

SUB-ACROMIAL CALCIFICATION
25° Antero-posterior. The patient lies supine with the elbow

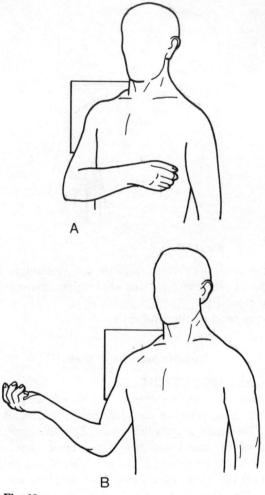

A

B

Fig. 18

flexed. The upper border of the cassette is placed level with the top of the shoulder.

Centre to the acromion process, with the tube angled 25° caudad.

BICIPITAL GROOVE
The patient stands, bending slightly forwards, with the arm against the side and the palm of the hand against the thigh. The tube is directed cephalad at the same angle as the humerus, to silhouette the groove.

Centre to the groove, which is palpable between the tuberosities.

SCAPULA

Anatomy. The scapula is a large, flat, triangular bone, situated one on each side of the postero-lateral aspect of the thorax. It has a costal and a dorsal surface. The dorsal surface is divided into a smaller supraspinous fossa and a larger infraspinous fossa by the spine of the scapula which widens laterally and forms the acromion process. The acromion process projects over the shoulder joint, giving it some protection, and also articulates with the lateral border of the clavicle at the acromio-clavicular joint. The coracoid process projects from the upper border of the scapula and serves as an attachment for various muscles, including the biceps. The large, flat surfaces of the scapula also serve for muscle attachment to strengthen the shoulder joint.

Basic views

Antero-posterior. The patient faces the X-ray tube and is rotated about 30° to bring the plane of the scapula parallel with the cassette. A long exposure time is used, with the patient breathing gently. This helps to blur out lung and rib shadows to give a clearer view of the scapula.

Centre to the head of the humerus.

Lateral. The patient faces the cassette, with the elbow of the side being examined flexed and the arm slightly abducted. The patient is rotated about 60–75° with the side under examination towards the cassette, until the plane of the scapula is at right angles to the cassette.

Centre to the medial border of the scapula.

Special circumstances

1. If the arm is in a sling and adducted across the body, the lateral view can still be taken but the degree of rotation usually has to be reduced to about 30°.

2. If the patient is in a wheel-chair or on a stretcher, the lateral view is taken with the patient facing the X-ray tube, the hand of the side under examination being placed on the opposite shoulder. The patient is rotated about 25° with the side under examination away from the cassette, until the plane of the scapula can be felt separated from the thorax.

Centre to the head of the humerus.

Supplementary views

CORACOID PROCESS

Antero-posterior. The patient faces the X-ray tube and is rotated about 30° to bring the plane of the scapula parallel with the cassette. The arm is raised over the head.

Centre to the lateral border of the scapula.

SUPRASPINOUS FOSSA

The patient stands facing the X-ray tube and bending forwards so that the spine of the scapula is vertical and thus parallel with the vertically-placed cassette. Because of the large object-film distance, the focus-film distance is increased to at least 180 cm (72 in) (Stripp, 1963).

Centre just medial to the acromio-clavicular joint.

ACROMIO-CLAVICULAR JOINT

Anatomy. This is a gliding synovial joint between the acromial end of the clavicle and the medial margin of the acromion process of the scapula. It allows a little gliding movement in conjunction with movements of the scapula.

Basic view

Antero-posterior. A view of each joint is always taken, either separately or both on the same radiograph. The patient stands facing the X-ray tube and, if his condition allows it, equal weights are held in each hand so as to increase the effect of gravity and open up the joint spaces.

For a view of both sides on the same radiograph, the patient remains facing the X-ray tube.

Centre in the mid-line at the level of the joints and using a slit aperture.

For a view of one side only, the patient is rotated slightly so that this side is nearer the film.

Centre to the joint (which is easily palpable) using a small aperture.

CLAVICLE

Anatomy. The clavicle is a curved bone, the medial part being convex forward and the lateral part being concave forward. At its medial end it articulates with the sternum at the sterno-clavicular joint. At its lateral end it articulates with the acromion process at the acromio-clavicular joint. It is the first bone to ossify, between the fifth and sixth weeks of intrauterine life.

Basic views

Postero-anterior. The patient faces the cassette and is rotated slightly so that the long axis of the clavicle is parallel with it. The cassette is placed transversely and adjusted so that the clavicle is in the mid-line of the cassette. A narrow transverse aperture is used.

Centre to the middle of the clavicle.

Infero-superior. The patient faces the X-ray tube, and is rotated slightly so that the clavicle is parallel with the cassette. The cassette is placed transversely with its upper border 7·5 cm (3 in) above the level of the top of the shoulder, in line with the central ray.

Centre to the lower border of the clavicle, with the tube angled 30° cephalad.

Special circumstances

1. For an injured patient, positioning for an antero-posterior view is often easier. He sits or lies facing the X-ray tube and is rotated slightly until the clavicle under examination is parallel with the cassette. A small pad is placed under the other shoulder for support and the head is turned towards the injured side.

Centre to the middle of the clavicle.

2. For a child, a view of both clavicles is usually taken. He lies supine with the shoulders on the cassette which must be wide enough to include both shoulders. The beam is collimated to a narrow transverse aperture.

Centre in the mid-line at the level of the clavicles.

21

Upper limb

The upper limb consists of the arm, forearm and hand. The term 'arm' in medical terminology refers to that part of the upper limb between the shoulder and the elbow and not to the whole limb as in common parlance. The bones of the upper limb comprise the humerus, radius, ulna, carpals, metacarpals and phalanges.

For radiographic examination of the upper humerus, the shoulder and arm must be free from radiopaque objects and usually the patient is required to undress down to the waist and to wear a suitable gown. For the rest of the limb, it is usually possible for the sleeve to be pushed up sufficiently high. Objects such as watches, bracelets and rings must be removed from the area being examined but it is often necessary to allow a patient to keep on a wedding ring.

Films. The thickness of the soft tissues varies throughout the length of the limb. For the humerus, screen film is used, with or without a grid according to the physique of the patient. Non-screen film is used for the rest of the limb, unless the part being examined is in plaster of Paris.

Radiation protection. The upper limb should be a low radiation dose area and the major hazard during its examination is the inadvertent directing of the X-ray beam towards the gonad region. Protection against irradiation must always be used, either by a lead rubber apron or by a lead rubber screen, adjustable in height. When radiographs of the forearm or hand are being taken, the patient must never sit with the knees under the X-ray table.

HUMERUS

Anatomy. The humerus is the largest bone of the upper limb. The proximal end is described in the section on the shoulder (p. 127) and the distal end in the section on the elbow (p. 136). The shaft is cylindrical and about half-way along it, on the lateral aspect, is the deltoid tuberosity for attachment of the deltoid muscle.

In radiography of the humerus, it is important to note that the position of the hand does not determine the position of the humerus, because of the rotation that is possible between the arm and the forearm at the elbow joint.

The soft tissues of the arm are much thicker at the proximal end than at the distal end, particularly in muscular men. It is therefore often difficult to obtain an optimum exposure for radiographs of the arm as a whole. For examinations of the proximal and distal ends of the humerus, reference should be made to the techniques for the shoulder (p. 127) and elbow (p. 136). Following injury to the arm, the limb is often held across the body, usually in a sling, and radiography may have to be carried out with the limb in this position so as to avoid distress or further injury to the patient.

Investigation of the humerus is most commonly required after recent injury, to show the presence and extent of any fracture and the exact position of the fragments. The most frequent sites for fractures of the humerus are the surgical neck and the supracondylar region.

Basic views

Antero-posterior. The patient faces the X-ray tube and may be examined either erect or supine. The upper border of the cassette is placed 2·5 cm (1 in) above the top of the shoulder and should be large enough to include both the shoulder joint and the elbow joint. The elbow is extended, with the palm of the hand facing forwards. The epicondyles must be equidistant from the cassette.

Centre to the mid-shaft of the humerus at the level of the middle of the cassette.

Lateral. The patient faces the cassette, the arm is abducted, the elbow flexed and the hand placed on the abdomen. The patient is then rotated away from the side being examined until the humerus is against the cassette. The epicondyles must be superimposed. The upper border of the cassette is adjusted to 2·5 cm (1 in) above the top of the shoulder.

Centre to the mid-shaft of the humerus at the level of the middle of the cassette.

Special circumstances

1. For a lateral view, if the arm is strapped to the side, the patient faces the cassette and is rotated away from the side under examination

until the plane of the scapula is at right angles to the cassette. The upper border of the cassette is placed 2·5 cm (1 in) above the top of the shoulder and the cassette may need to be supported obliquely.

Centre to the mid-shaft of the humerus.

2. For a lateral view to show bone alignment or the position of fragments in a mid-shaft fracture, when the patient cannot be positioned as in either of the above methods, a trans-thoracic lateral view may be taken. The patient stands or sits with the side being examined against a grid cassette, the other arm over the head and the body bending slightly towards the side being examined so that the two shoulders are not superimposed.

Centre through the axilla further from the cassette.

ELBOW

Anatomy. The articulation at the elbow is a complex one. It comprises the hinge joint between the arm and the forearm (allowing flexion and extension) and the proximal radio-ulnar pivot joint (allowing pronation and supination—rolling movements of the radius and hand around the ulna, which remains still).

The elbow joint is formed by the trochlea of the humerus articulating with the trochlear notch of the ulna, and the capitulum articulating with the head of the radius. Proximal to the trochlea and capitulum, the shaft of the humerus expands to form the medial and lateral epicondyles, the medial being easily palpable and more prominent than the lateral.

On the posterior surface of the lower end of the humerus, between the medial surface of the trochlea and the medial epicondyle, is the ulnar groove for the passage of the ulnar nerve.

The elbow has multiple centres of ossification, secondary centres appearing between the ages of 2 and 12 years; comparative views of the other elbow are often required in children.

Basic views

Lateral. This view is usually taken first as the position is easier for the patient. The patient sits beside the X-ray table, with the elbow flexed at right angles and the hand in the lateral position. The arm and forearm must be in the same plane, so either the patient sits on a low stool or the film is raised on a firm support until it is at the correct height. If a skull unit is available, positioning is simplified as the elbow is placed on the skull table which is then gently raised until the arm and forearm are at the same level. The epicondyles must be superimposed. A sandbag is placed on each side of the forearm for immobilisation and support.

Centre to the lateral epicondyle.

Antero-posterior. From the lateral position, the elbow is extended and the arm outstretched with the back of the hand on the table or resting on a foam pad. The epicondyles must be equidistant from the film. For immobilisation, a sandbag is placed gently on the hand.

Centre between, and 2·5 cm (1 in) distal to, the epicondyles.

Special circumstances

1. If the patient is unable to extend the elbow, two antero-posterior views are taken, one with the arm on the film and the other with the forearm on the film, the elbow being extended as much as possible in each case. The tube is directed at right angles to the film.

2. If the elbow is in extreme flexion, the arm should be placed on the film and the hand supported or placed on the shoulder. The kilovoltage required is 10 to 15 more than for the basic antero-posterior view.

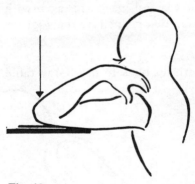

Fig. 19

Centre 5 cm (2 in) distal to the olecranon process through both arm and forearm (Fig. 19 and Plate XV).

3. If the patient must remain supine (e.g. in cases of severe illness or multiple injuries) an antero-posterior view may be taken by supporting the film under the elbow at the height at which the arm and forearm are in the same plane. If the arm is across the chest, a lateral view may be taken by placing the film between the elbow and chest.

Special attention must be paid to radiation protection of the gonads. The patient is asked to arrest respiration whilst the film is exposed.

Supplementary views

HEAD OF RADIUS
Antero-posterior with the forearm in mid-pronation. The palm of the hand is on the table.

Lateral. The forearm is fully pronated so that the radial aspect of the hand is on the table.

Antero-posterior with the elbow flexed. The elbow is flexed at right angles, with the arm and forearm equidistant from the film. The X-ray tube is directed at right angles to the film.

SUPRACONDYLAR FRACTURE
There should be no movement of the elbow. Antero-posterior and lateral views are taken in whatever degree of flexion is present, the antero-posterior view usually being taken as shown in Figure 19. The lateral view may have to be taken with the film placed between the elbow and the chest.

After reduction of the fracture, the limb will be in a 'collar and cuff', or other means of support, and must not be removed from it. Antero-posterior and lateral views are taken with the elbow maintained in the position determined by the support.

ULNAR GROOVE
The patient sits with his back to the X-ray table. The shoulder is

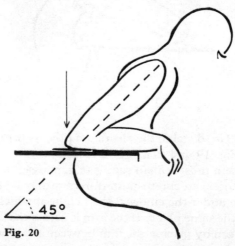

Fig. 20

extended, the elbow flexed and the forearm placed on the film. The arm is adjusted so that it is at an angle of 45° to the film (Fig. 20).

Centre to the groove, which is easily palpable, on the medial side of the elbow.

FOREARM

Anatomy. The bones of the forearm are the radius and the ulna, which articulate with each other at the proximal and distal radio-ulnar joints. They articulate with the humerus at the elbow joint and with the proximal row of carpal bones at the wrist. The head of the radius is at the elbow and the head of the ulna is at the wrist.

Supination and pronation involve rotation of the radius and hand about the ulna which remains still. On full supination, the radius and ulna lie approximately parallel with one another, when the patient is in the anatomical position. On pronation, the distal end of the radius rotates medially around the anterior surface of the head of the ulna so as to bring the radius obliquely across in front of the ulna, with the dorsal surface of the radius facing anteriorly. Therefore, to obtain a true antero-posterior view of the forearm, the elbow must be extended and the palm of the hand must face upwards.

Basic views

Antero-posterior. The patient sits beside the X-ray table, with the elbow extended. The back of the hand should rest on the table and a sandbag is placed gently on the fingers for immobilisation. The humeral epicondyles should be equidistant from the film. The film should be long enough to include both the elbow and the wrist joints.

Centre to the middle of the forearm.

Lateral. From the antero-posterior position, the elbow is flexed at right angles and the hand is placed in the lateral position with the thumb uppermost. A sandbag is placed against the palm of the hand for immobilisation. The film should be long enough to include both joints.

Centre to the middle of the forearm.

Special circumstances

If the elbow cannot be extended, the antero-posterior view is taken with the limb in the same position as for the lateral view but supported on foam pads or a pillow. The film is supported vertically by the side of the forearm. A horizontal beam is used.

WRIST JOINT AND CARPUS

Anatomy. The wrist joint is a condyloid joint between the fore-arm and the proximal row of carpal bones. The proximal articular surface is formed by the distal end of the radius and the triangular cartilage. The latter is attached to the medial side of the distal end of the radius and to the ulnar styloid process. The distal articular surface is formed by the proximal surface of the scaphoid, lunate and triquetral bones of the carpus.

The carpus consists of two rows of carpal bones. The proximal row consists of the scaphoid, lunate, triquetral and pisiform. The distal row consists of the trapezium, trapezoid, capitate and hamate. The pisiform is a sesamoid bone lying in the tendon of the flexor carpi ulnaris muscle and it articulates with the triquetral. The carpus has a transverse concavity on the palmar aspect, which is roofed by the flexor retinaculum ligament to form the carpal tunnel through which pass the flexor tendons and the median nerve.

Movements of the wrist are flexion, extension, abduction and adduction. Adduction, usually termed ulnar deviation, is used in radiography of the scaphoid to open up the joint space and to show the whole length of the bone.

Basic views

Postero-anterior. The patient sits beside the X-ray table, with the elbow flexed and the forearm and hand placed palm down, with the styloid processes equidistant from the film. Sandbags are placed gently on either side of the forearm for immobilisation.

Centre between the styloid processes.

Lateral. From the antero-posterior position, the hand and fore-arm are rotated 90° so that the ulnar aspect of the wrist is in contact with the film. The wrist is then rotated a further 5° so that the styloid processes are superimposed.

Centre to the radial styloid process.

Special circumstances

1. A true lateral view of the wrist may be difficult to obtain after

reduction of a Colles' fracture when plaster obscures the surface land-marks. Two or more views with slight variation in positioning may be necessary to obtain a true lateral view. It is sometimes of advantage to mark the centering point (when established) on the plaster in case further views are required.

2. If, because of pain, the patient is unable to adopt the position for one of the basic views, the film is supported vertically and a horizontal beam is used.

Supplementary views

CARPAL BONES

Oblique I. From the basic postero-anterior position, the hand and forearm are rotated 45° with the thumb raised from the film. A pad is placed under the palm of the hand for support. A small aperture is used.

Centre to the ulnar styloid process.

Oblique II. From the basic lateral position, the hand and forearm are rotated 45° backwards (i.e. 90° from the Oblique I position). A pad is placed under the back of the hand for support.

Centre to the ulnar styloid process.

Antero-posterior. (This view demonstrates well the carpal joint spaces but may be too uncomfortable for an injured patient). The elbow is extended and the back of the hand is placed on the table. The radial and ulnar styloid processes must be equidistant from the film.

Centre midway between the radial and ulnar styloid processes.

SCAPHOID

Postero-anterior with ulnar deviation. The patient is positioned as for the basic view of the wrist. Keeping the forearm still, the hand is then deviated laterally (adducted). The patient must be shown what to do but the wrist must never be forced into this position.

Centre between the styloid processes.

Obliques. From the postero-anterior position, the radial side of the hand is raised 30°, then 60°. A radiograph is taken in each of these two positions. A small aperture is used.

Centre to the scaphoid.

Lateral. As for the basic lateral view of the wrist (p. 140).

CARPAL TUNNEL

The patient stands with his back to the X-ray table, with the palm of the hand resting on the table. The patient leans away from the table so that the palm is raised about 7·5 cm (3 in) from it (Fig. 21). The forearm should be at an angle of about 45° to the table.

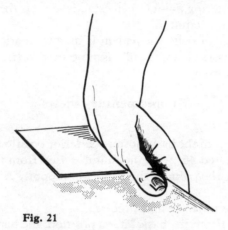

Fig. 21

Centre to the apex of the curve of the carpal bones.

BONE AGE
To assess radiographically the skeletal age of a patient, a dorsi-palmar (postero-anterior) view of the left hand and wrist is taken. The assessment is made from a skeletal atlas (Greulich and Pyle, 1959; Tanner *et al.*, 1975).

ADDITIONAL EXAMINATIONS
Macroradiography (p. 38). *Arthrography* (p. 366).

HAND

Anatomy. The digits of the hand are referred to as the thumb, and the index, middle, ring and little fingers.

The hand is composed of three sets of bones, the carpal and meta-carpal bones and the phalanges. The thumb has two phalanges and each of the fingers has three. When the hand is placed palm down, the thumb is oblique in direction; when the hand is lateral, the thumb rests in a postero-anterior position. Thus, separate views are required for the thumb and the rest of the hand. In the postero-anterior (dorsi-palmar) view, the bases of the metacarpals overshadow each other and to separate them an oblique view is required.

The hand, particularly the heads of the metacarpals, is one of the earliest sites of rheumatoid arthritis.

Basic views

Dorsi-palmar. The patient sits beside the X-ray table, with the elbow flexed and the palm of the hand on the film. The fingers should be separated slightly.

Centre over the head of the third metacarpal bone.

Oblique. From the dorsi-palmar position, the palm of the hand is raised to an angle of 45° and the thumb supported on a foam pad.

Centre to the head of the fifth metacarpal bone.

Supplementary views

FOREIGN BODIES

To demonstrate the presence and position of a foreign body, a dorsi-palmar view and a lateral view are taken. For the lateral view, the hand is placed in the lateral position so that the palm is at right angles to the film. The thumb is allowed to rest on a foam pad.

Centre to the head of the second metacarpal bone.

HYPERPARATHYROIDISM

To demonstrate the presence of subperiosteal bone resorption of cortical bone (usually in the middle phalanges) a dorsi-palmar view of both hands is taken (Doyle, 1972). There must be excellent soft tissue detail, so non-screen film and low kV (40 to 50) are advised. To avoid movement blur, the patient must be immobilised, for which elaborate methods will be necessary as the patient may be twitching. For the same reason a very short exposure time is essential.

METACARPO-PHALANGEAL JOINT SPACES

1. **Oblique.** The hands are 'cupped', as for catching a large ball (Fig. 22) and are immobilised in this position with foam pads and sandbags.

Centre between the hands at the level of the heads of the fifth metacarpal bones.

2. To demonstrate peripheral cysts near the attachment of the capsule of the joint to the bone (usually the earliest site of rheumatoid arthritis) the following view is taken (Brewerton, 1967). The back of the hand is placed on the film. The hand is then adjusted so that the dorsal aspect of the fingers remain on the film and the metacarpo-phalangeal joints are flexed at an angle of 65°. The thumb is extended.

Centre to the metacarpo-phalangeal joints, with the tube angled 12° to the ulnar side of the hand.

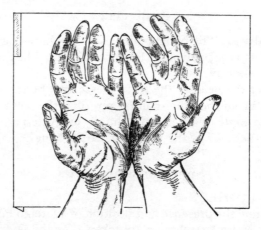

Fig. 22

FINGERS
Postero-anterior. The hand is positioned as for the basic view for the hand, but a smaller film and aperture are used. The film should include the finger (if any) on each side of the one being examined.

Centre to the head of the metacarpal bone of the finger under examination.

Lateral. For the index finger or middle finger, the hand is turned on to the radial side and the finger being examined is extended as far as possible and held in position by a foam pad and sandbag. For the ring finger or little finger, the hand is turned into the lateral position. The finger being examined is extended and supported and the other fingers are held out of the way.

Centre to the metacarpo-phalangeal joint of the finger being examined.

THUMB
Lateral. The hand is placed palm downwards and the ulnar aspect is raised on a foam pad so that the thumb is in the lateral position. The base of the first metacarpal must be included as this is frequently the site of a fracture (Bennett's fracture).

Centre to the first metacarpo-phalangeal joint.

Antero-posterior. The arm is extended along the X-ray table, with the palm downwards. The hand is then rotated until the posterior aspect of the thumb is in contact with the film. The fingers are supported out of the way of the X-ray beam.

Centre to the first metacarpo-phalangeal joint.

22

Pelvic girdle

The pelvic girdle is composed of two innominate bones and the sacrum and coccyx. The innominate bones, each composed of the ischial, iliac and pubic bones, articulate anteriorly with each other at the symphysis pubis and posteriorly with the lateral border of the sacrum at the sacro-iliac joints. The head of the femur articulates with the acetabulum of the innominate bone to form the hip joint.

The pelvis forms a complete ring. In the child, the ilium, ischium and pubis are separated by the Y-shaped cartilage which ossifies soon after puberty. The size and shape of the pelvis vary between male and female subjects, the female pelvis being wider and shallower, allowing passage of the foetal head during parturition.

Radiographically, the most important anatomical features of the pelvis are the iliac crests, the anterior and posterior iliac spines and the symphysis pubis, all of which are easily palpable and are used as centering points.

A view of the pelvis must be included in the initial examination following trauma to the femur.

All radiopaque objects must be removed from beneath and above the patient, even if, as is often the case with accident patients, he is not completely undressed. The patient's hands should be placed on the chest so that they do not obscure any part of the pelvis.

Radiation protection. For male patients, gonad protection must be employed whenever possible. For female patients, the gonads are in the direct beam and cannot be protected by lead shielding. Zealous attention must therefore be paid to careful radiographic technique. For the examination of the hip joints in female patients, protection of the gonads can be carried out by lead rubber, suitably placed, care being taken that no part of the hip joint is obscured by it. The 10-day rule (p. 19) should be observed if the degree of clinical urgency permits.

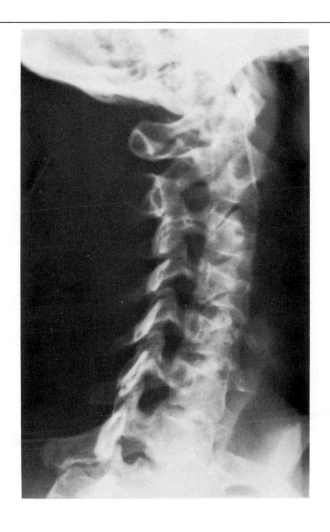

PLATE XII. Cervical spine, left posterior oblique view (p. 112).

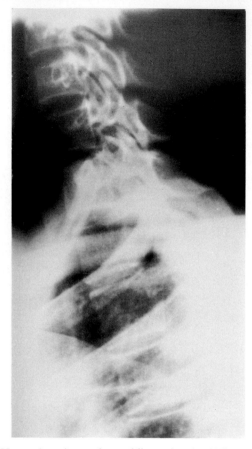

PLATE XIII. Upper thoracic vertebrae, oblique view (p. 116).

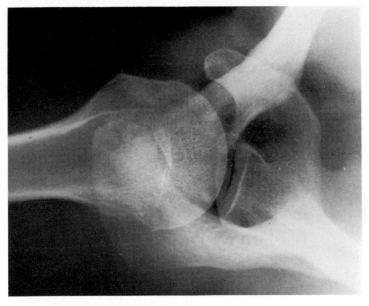

PLATE XIV. Shoulder, axial view (p. 128).

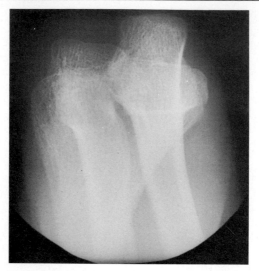

PLATE XV. Elbow, view in flexion (p. 137).

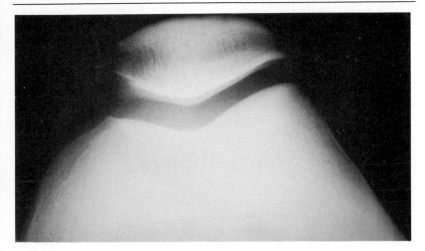

PLATE XVI. Patella, 'skyline' view (p. 157).

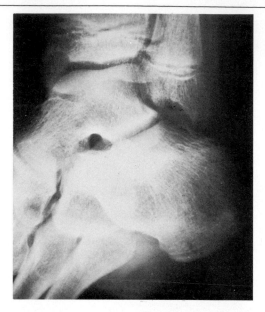

PLATE XVII. Sub-talar joints, medial axial oblique view (p. 163).

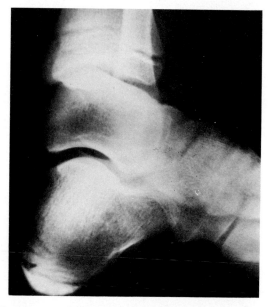

PLATE XVIII. Sub-talar joints, lateral axial oblique view (p. 163).

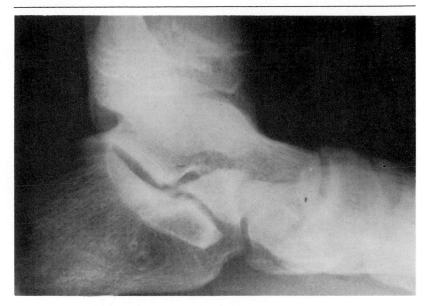

PLATE XIX. Sub-talar joints, 'Anthonsen's' view (p. 163).

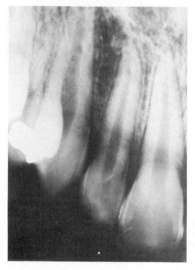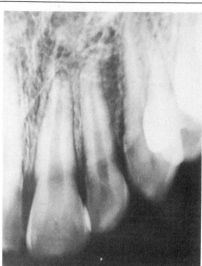

PLATE XX. Intra-oral views (p. 166).

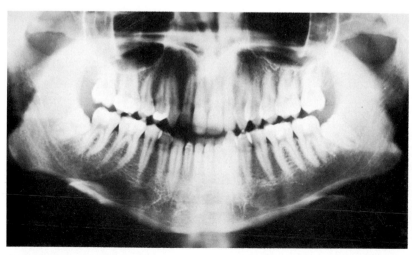

PLATE XXI. Pan-oral tomogram (p. 171).

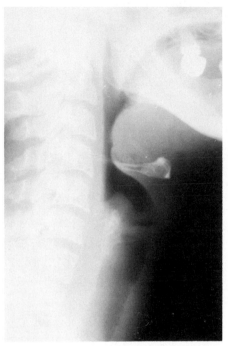

PLATE XXII. Neck, lateral soft tissue view (p. 176).

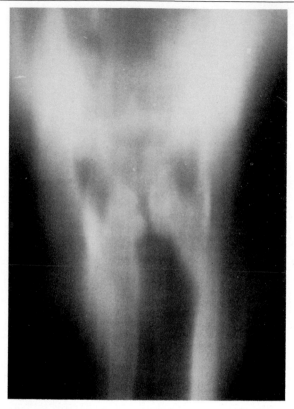

PLATE XXIII. Larynx (p. 176). Tomogram showing swelling of the left chord extending below the glottis.

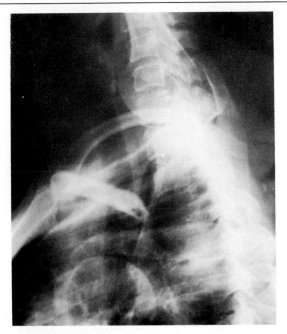

PLATE XXIV. Thoracic inlet, lateral view (p. 178).

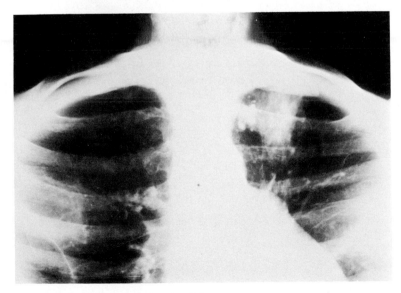

PLATE XXV. Chest, apical view (p. 186).

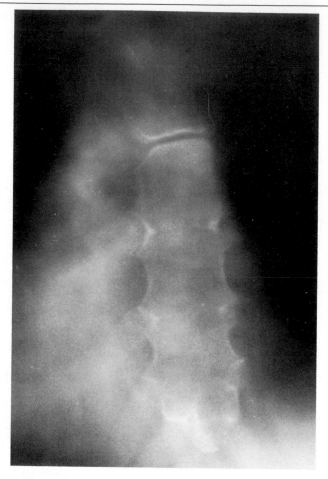

PLATE XXVI. Sternum, inclined plane tomogram (p. 49 and p. 191).

PELVIS

Basic view

Antero-posterior. The patient lies supine with the legs extended. The pelvis must be positioned symmetrically, with the anterior superior iliac spines equidistant from the cassette. If necessary, small foam pads are placed under the patient to achieve this. The feet are separated slightly and, if possible, internally rotated. A 35 × 43 cm (17 × 14 in) cassette, placed transversely, is used.

Centre in the mid-line, 5 cm (2 in) below the anterior superior iliac spines.

Special circumstances

An emaciated (usually elderly) patient presents difficulties in the selection of exposure factors because the lateral margins of the pelvis are often grossly over-exposed if reasonable penetration of the denser medial area is obtained. The use of higher kV (100 kV or more) decreases the radiographic contrast between the two areas (see p. 30).

Supplementary views

Lateral. For a lateral view of the whole pelvic girdle, the patient lies in the lateral position, with the legs extended and a small pad between the knees to keep the pelvis lateral. Alternatively, this view may be taken with the patient standing. If the patient's condition precludes either of these positions, it may be taken with the patient supine, using a horizontal beam.

Centre to the upper border of the femoral head.

ILIUM
Posterior oblique. If the condition of the patient allows, he is rotated 35° towards the side being examined. The knee of that side is flexed and the limb rotated outwards and supported.

Centre to the iliac fossa.

SYMPHYSIS PUBIS
Antero-posterior. Positioning is as for the basic view. A small aperture is used.

Centre to the symphysis pubis.

Antero-posterior erect (to investigate subluxation following pregnancy). The patient stands with her back against the erect Bucky or vertically-supported grid cassette. Two radiographs are taken, with the weight on alternate feet.

Centre to the symphysis pubis.

SACRUM AND COCCYX
See under vertebral column (pp. 122 and 123).

SACRO-ILIAC JOINTS
See under vertebral column (p. 124).

HIP JOINT
See under hip joint (below).

ADDITIONAL EXAMINATIONS
Stereography (p. 36). *Tomography* (p. 47).

HIP JOINT

Anatomy. The hip joint is a ball and socket synovial joint formed by the femoral head, which is two-thirds of a sphere, articulating with the acetabulum. The acetabulum is a deep depression on the lateral surface of the innominate bone and faces downwards for weight-bearing. Anteriorly, the hip joint is closely related to the femoral artery.

A small depression, the fovea, can be seen radiographically as a small translucent area on the medial border of the femoral head. To the fovea is attached the ligamentum teres.

The capsule of the hip joint is very strong. Anteriorly it covers the neck of the femur and extends to the inter-trochanteric line but posteriorly it does not cover the whole of the femoral neck. The epiphysis of the femoral head is entirely intra-capsular.

The femoral neck is directed postero-inferiorly. In the antero-posterior view, with the feet medially rotated 30°, it is clearly demonstrated. If the limb is allowed to adopt its natural position and become slightly laterally rotated, the neck of the femur is foreshortened. After injury to the neck of the femur, any attempt to rotate the limb is likely to cause considerable pain and the hip will have to be radiographed with the limb in the presenting position.

Movements of the hip joint are flexion, extension, adduction, abduction and rotation.

Basic views

Antero-posterior. An antero-posterior view demonstrating both hips is routinely taken after trauma and for the investigation of congenital abnormalities and arthritis. The patient lies supine with the feet separated slightly. If possible, the lower limbs are internally rotated 30° and immobilised in this position by means of sandbags placed on the lateral sides of the ankles. The pelvis must be positioned symmetrically, with the anterior superior iliac spines equidistant from the table.

Centre in the mid-line, 2·5 cm (1 in) above the symphysis pubis.

Lateral. From the antero-posterior position, the patient is rotated towards the side being examined, the knee is flexed and the leg is abducted and allowed to rest on the table, or is supported.

Centre to the femoral pulse, which is easily palpable in the groin.

Special circumstances

1. After total hip arthroplasty, the basic antero-posterior view of both hips can give an inaccurate assessment of acetabular anteversion because that view is not centred to the hip (Georgen and Resnick, 1975). Therefore an antero-posterior view of the affected hip should be taken, with the patient positioned as for the basic antero-posterior view.

Centre to the femoral pulse of the side under examination.

2. After surgery, or in any other follow-up investigation involving a single hip, the antero-posterior view need be of that hip only.

3. After internal fixation, the whole of the pin (or plate) must be shown on follow-up films.

Supplementary views

NECK OF FEMUR

Lateral (often known as 'true lateral'). The patient lies supine with the pelvis raised on foam pads and the injured limb extended. The foot should be medially rotated if possible, so that the femoral neck is not foreshortened. The other knee is flexed and the foot placed on a stool or other means of support, so that the limb is raised above the level of the injured one. The cassette is supported vertically against the injured hip, pushed against the waist and adjusted so that it is parallel with the neck of the femur. The X-ray tube, preferably with a long cone to reduce scatter, is directed horizontally at right angles to the cassette (Fig. 23).

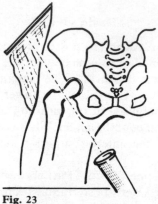

Fig. 23

Centre to the groin.

Lateral (with the patient sitting). For some patients, positioning for this view may be easier than for the view last described. It is useful for follow-up examination but is not performed for an initial examination following trauma. The patient sits on a thick foam pad, at the edge of the X-ray table or chair, with his legs separated, knees flexed and feet supported. A grid cassette is supported vertically at the posterior aspect of the buttock and thigh and is placed parallel with the neck of the femur. The X-ray tube is directed horizontally at right angles to the cassette.

Centre to the medial aspect of the thigh, at the level of the femoral pulse.

CONGENITAL DISLOCATION OF THE HIP
(HIP DYSPLASIA)

'Von Rosen'. The child lies supine with each leg abducted 45° (producing a mutual angle of 90°) and internally rotated (Von Rosen,

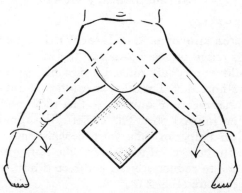

Fig. 24

1962; Fig. 24). A template with a right-angled corner is used as a guide for the positioning of the legs which should be held firmly in this position, either by a member of the medical staff, or by a perspex jig (Smith and Robinson, 1969).

Centre in the mid-line at the level of the femoral pulse.

Antero-posterior with hyperextended hips. The child lies supine with the legs fully extended. The knees are pushed down on to the X-ray table (Grech, 1972).

Centre in the mid-line at the level of the femoral pulse.

EPIPHYSES
'Frog'. The child lies supine with the knees flexed and the hips abducted. The soles of the feet are placed together and the hips externally rotated, the thighs resting symmetrically on equal-sized foam pads (Fig. 25). Sandbags are placed against the foam pads and against the feet for immobilisation.

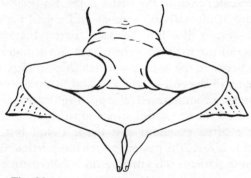

Fig. 25

Centre in the mid-line at the level of the femoral pulse.

ADDITIONAL EXAMINATIONS
Tomography (p. 47). *Arthrography* (p. 368).

23

Lower limb

The lower limb consists of the thigh, leg and foot. The term 'leg' in medical terminology refers to that part of the lower limb between the knee and the ankle, and not to the whole limb as in common parlance. The bones of the lower limb include the femur, patella, tibia, fibula, tarsus, metatarsus and phalanges.

The thickness of the soft tissue in the proximal parts of the limb is very much greater than in the distal parts. Radiography therefore requires the use of intensifying screens and a grid for the proximal parts and non-screen film for the distal parts. Intermediate parts require the use of intensifying screens but not usually a grid. The dividing lines between the areas for which these different techniques are appropriate will depend on the size and physique of the patient.

It is sometimes recommended (Stripp, 1966) that non-screen film and a grid be used for all examinations of the knee and lower thigh. This technique gives excellent soft tissue detail but involves increased radiation dose to the patient which it is particularly important to avoid in young patients who may require follow-up examinations. The technique is probably better employed as a supplementary than as a routine method.

When the part being examined is encased in plaster of Paris, screen film is usually necessary.

For radiographic examination of the thigh, the patient should undress from the waist down and wear a suitable gown. For examination of the knee, if the patient is wearing trousers it should be ascertained, before the patient gets on to the X-ray table, whether the trousers are wide enough to be pushed up well above the knee. If not, they must be removed. Turn-ups or folds of thick fabric may appear as radiopaque shadows and obscure important detail in the lower end of the femur. Stockings must be removed and this can usually be done in the X-ray room but tights are more difficult to remove and a cubicle is usually required.

Gonad protection is particularly important in radiography of the hip and thigh because of the proximity of the gonads and therefore zealous attention must be paid to the prevention of unnecessary radiation, both direct and scattered (p. 17). Examination of the knee, leg and foot should involve virtually no gonad irradiation when correct radiographic technique is practised. A lead apron should be worn by the patient, particularly for intercondylar views of the knee and for weight-bearing views of the feet.

FEMUR

Anatomy. The femur consists of a shaft, an upper extremity (bearing a head, neck and two trochanters) and a lower extremity (bearing medial and lateral condyles which are separated by an intercondylar notch). The femur is the longest and most massive bone in the body. It is oblique in direction, the obliquity varying in different subjects but usually being greater in women than in men because of the greater width of the pelvis.

Radiographic examination for trauma or pathology of the upper half of the femur must include the hip joint (p. 148) and the lower half must include the knee (p. 154).

Basic views

Antero-posterior (from the hip downwards). The limb should be extended and medially rotated so that the patella is parallel with the table. Sandbags are placed at each side of the leg for support. The upper border of a 35 × 43 cm (17 × 14 in) cassette is placed at the level of the anterior superior iliac spines, so that the hip joint is included on the radiograph. The beam is collimated to the width of the thigh.

Centre to the shaft of the femur at the level of the middle of the cassette.

Lateral (from the knee upwards). If possible, the patient is rotated towards the side being examined, with the knee flexed and the leg allowed to rest on the table. A pad is placed under the ankle so that the femoral condyles are superimposed and the knee is lateral. The lower border of a 35 × 43 cm (17 × 14 in) cassette is placed at the level of the tibial condyles so that the knee joint is included on the radiograph. The beam is collimated to the width of the thigh.

Centre to the shaft of the femur at the level of the middle of the cassette.

Special circumstances

1. For the lateral view, if the patient is unable to turn towards the side being examined, a horizontal beam is used. The opposite limb is raised above the level of the one being examined and supported. A grid cassette is supported vertically on the lateral aspect of the affected limb.

2. If views of the whole femur are required at an initial examination, an antero-posterior view of the lower femur and a lateral view of the upper femur are taken as well as the two basic views.

3. Following trauma to the femur, a view of the whole pelvis must be included in the initial examination (p. 147).

Supplementary views

Localised antero-posterior, lateral and two or more oblique views of any lesion may be required.

ADDITIONAL EXAMINATIONS
Tomography (p. 47). *Arteriography* (p. 219).

KNEE

Anatomy. The articulation at the knee is a complex synovial joint formed by the articular surfaces of the condyles of the femur, the upper end of the tibia and the posterior surface of the patella. The condyles of the femur are separated posteriorly by the deep inter-condylar notch. Between the condyles of the tibia is a non-articular area comprising the tibial spines (intercondylar tibial tubercles) to which are attached the anterior and posterior horns of the semi-lunar cartilages.

The patella is the largest sesamoid bone in the body and is situated in the tendon of the quadriceps femoris muscle. To the inferior part of the apex of the patella is attached the ligamentum patellae which is inserted into the tibial tubercle on the anterior aspect of the tibia just distal to the condyles.

The stability of the knee joint depends partly on strong collateral ligaments and if these are ruptured stress views will demonstrate separation of the joint surfaces.

Movements of the knee are flexion and extension, with slight rotation in extension. When completely extended, the knee is said to be 'locked' as it will then support the weight of the body without muscular effort.

Basic views

Antero-posterior. The patient sits or lies with the knee extended and the limb in slight medial rotation so that the patella is parallel with the cassette. Sandbags are placed against the malleoli to immobilise the limb in this position.

Centre 1 cm ($\frac{1}{2}$ in) distal to the apex of the patella.

Lateral. The patient is turned towards the side being examined, the knee flexed, with the heel resting on a pad or on the opposite ankle. The position of the knee is adjusted until the patella is at right angles to the cassette and the femoral condyles are superimposed.

Centre to the medial tibial condyle.

Special circumstances

1. If the patient has severe injuries, or is arthritic or obese, the positioning for the basic lateral view may be painful or difficult to maintain. In such cases, the patient should remain in the supine position, with the knee resting on a foam pad to raise it from the table. The cassette is supported vertically between the knees and the tube is directed horizontally and centred to the lateral condyle. When the investigation is for suspected lipo-haemarthrosis, the above view (because a horizontal beam is used) is preferable to the basic lateral view.

2. If the patient has fat or very muscular knees, or has increased bone density (e.g. in Paget's disease), improved image detail is obtained if the air gap technique (p. 27) or a grid is used.

Supplementary views

Obliques. The knee is extended and the limb rotated 45° medially and laterally in turn. Either the supine or the prone position may be used. Two radiographs are taken.

Centre to the joint.

Intercondylar (to demonstrate loose bodies and conditions such as osteochondritis dissecans). The patient sits or lies with the knee flexed over a curved cassette. The angle at the knee should be approximately 135°. The upper border of the curved cassette is placed well up under the thigh to compensate for angulation of the tube. Sandbags are placed on each side of the ankle to immobilise the leg in slight medial rotation.

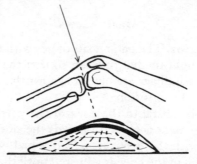

Fig. 26

Centre to the upper border of the tibia, with the tube at right angles to the shaft and parallel with the tibial plateau (Fig. 26).

PATELLA

Postero-anterior. The patient lies prone with a small pad placed under the ankles for comfort. The kilovoltage required is 5 more than for the antero-posterior view.

Centre to the crease of the knee.

Obliques. The patient lies prone with the knee extended and the foot over the end of the table. Two radiographs are taken, one with the foot internally rotated slightly and the patella pushed medially, the other with the foot externally rotated slightly and the patella pushed laterally. The kilovoltage required is 10 less than for the antero-posterior view (Stripp, 1966).

Centre to the crease of the knee.

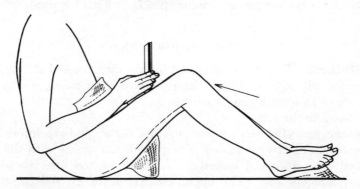

Fig. 27

Infero-superior or 'Skyline' (Plate XVI). There are several satisfactory methods of obtaining this view. The simplest is for the patient to sit with the knee flexed at about 135° and the foot resting on a sandbag. The cassette is supported vertically about 15 cm (6 in) proximal to the femoral condyle. The tube is placed at the level of the foot and is directed upwards at an angle of about 10° (Fig. 27). If a light beam diaphragm is used, the tube is adjusted until a silhouette of the knee is seen on the cassette. The gonads must be protected.

Centre to the inferior surface of the patella.

LIGAMENTS
Antero-posterior in forced abduction and adduction. These stress views are taken to demonstrate torn ligaments. The patient is positioned as for the basic antero-posterior view. The knee is then forcibly abducted and then adducted by the orthopaedic surgeon and held in each position whilst the exposure is made.

ALIGNMENT
Antero-posterior, weight-bearing. To show the angle of the femur to the tibia in conditions such as genu valgus, genu varus or Blount's disease, a weight-bearing antero-posterior view is taken. A 35 × 43 cm (17 × 14 in) cassette is used so that as much as possible of both limbs is included.

Centre between the patellae.

TIBIAL TUBERCLES
Lateral. To demonstrate osteochondritis of the tibial tubercles (Osgood-Schlatter's disease), lateral views of both knees are taken. Soft tissue detail must be visible. A small aperture is used. The kilovoltage required is 5 less than for the basic lateral view.

Centre to the tubercle, which is easily palpable on the anterior surface of the tibia.

ADDITIONAL EXAMINATIONS
Tomography (p. 47). *Arthrography* (p. 370).

TIBIA AND FIBULA

Anatomy. The bones of the leg are the tibia and fibula which articulate with each other at the proximal and distal tibio-fibular joints, with the femur at the knee joint and with the talus at the ankle joint. The tibia is the weight-bearing bone of the leg and its anterior surface is subcutaneous along its whole length, forming the shin.

Basic views

Antero-posterior. The knee is extended and the leg medially rotated slightly so that the malleoli are equidistant from the cassette which should be long enough (usually either 20 × 40 cm or 17 × 7 in for adults) to include both the knee joint and the ankle. If this is not possible, the joint nearer the site of injury should be included. The beam should be collimated to the width of the leg.

Centre to the mid-shaft of the tibia.

Lateral. From the antero-posterior position, the knee is flexed and the leg laterally rotated until the malleoli are superimposed and the patella is at right angles to the film. The beam should be collimated to the width of the leg.

Centre to the mid-shaft of the tibia.

Special circumstances

1. With a tall patient, it may be impossible to include the whole tibia on one film and additional views of either the ankle or the knee are taken.

2. If the patient is unable to rotate the leg into the basic lateral position, a lateral view is taken using a horizontal beam.

Supplementary views

LOCALISED VIEWS
Antero-posterior, lateral and two or more oblique views of any lesion may be required.

PROXIMAL TIBIO-FIBULAR JOINT
Oblique. The leg is extended and medially rotated slightly (about 10°).

Centre to the head of the fibula, which is easily palpable.

ADDITIONAL EXAMINATIONS
Tomography (p. 47). *Arteriography* (p. 219).

ANKLE

Anatomy. The ankle joint is a hinge synovial joint formed by the lower ends of the tibia and fibula fitting over the trochlea of the talus. The lateral malleolus is longer than the medial malleolus and both are easily palpable. Between the lower ends of the tibia and fibula is the inferior tibio-fibular joint which is a fibrous syndesmosis joint.

The stability of the ankle joint depends on strong collateral ligaments and, if these are ruptured, stress views will demonstrate separation of the joint surfaces.

Movements at the ankle joint are mainly flexion and extension, usually referred to as dorsi-flexion and plantar-flexion. When the toes are pointed downwards, slight abduction and adduction are possible.

Basic views

Antero-posterior. The patient sits or lies with the limb extended and immobilised in slight medial rotation so that the malleoli are equidistant from the film. The lower border of the film should be 2·5 cm (1 in) distal to the malleoli.

Centre between the malleoli.

Lateral. The patient is turned towards the side being examined, with the knee flexed. The position of the ankle is adjusted until the malleoli are superimposed. The lower border of the film should be 2·5 cm (1 in) distal to the lower border of the malleoli.

Centre to the medial malleolus.

Special circumstances

If the patient is unable to turn on to the side being examined, the lateral view is taken using a horizontal beam.

Supplementary views

LIGAMENTS

Antero-posterior in forced eversion or inversion. These stress views are taken to demonstrate torn medial and lateral ligaments. The patient is positioned as for the basic antero-posterior view. The ankle is then forcibly inverted or everted by the orthopaedic surgeon and held in that position while the exposure is made. The ankle may be held by the surgeon (wearing a lead rubber apron and gloves) or by some mechanical means such as a suction head-clamp (Sandin, 1966).

ADDITIONAL EXAMINATIONS
Tomography (p. 47). *Arthrography* (p. 366).

FOOT

Anatomy. The foot is composed of three sets of bones, the tarsal and metatarsal bones and the phalanges. It is arched transversely and longitudinally. Alteration of these natural arches may require radiographic examination.

The bones of the tarsus are the talus, calcaneum, navicular and cuboid, and the medial, intermediate and lateral cuneiforms. There are five metatarsal bones, the first being much thicker and slightly shorter than the others. The phalanges are small, there being two in the first toe and three in each of the other toes. On the plantar (posterior) aspect of the head of the first metatarsal bone are two sesamoid bones.

The thickness of the mid-foot is much greater than that of the toes and therefore in radiographs of the whole foot the toes are usually slightly over-exposed. Neither the joint spaces between the tarsal bones, nor those between the bases of the metatarsals, are clearly seen on a dorsi-plantar view as the bones overlap and oblique views are therefore necessary to demonstrate them clearly.

Basic views

Dorsi-plantar. The patient sits with the sole of the foot on the film and with the leg at an angle of approximately 45°.
Centre to the navicular, with the tube angled 25° towards the ankle.
Dorsi-plantar oblique. From the dorsi-plantar position, the leg is allowed to lean medially until the sole of the foot is at an angle of 45° to the film. The leg is immobilised in this position, either by supporting it on the other knee or by means of foam pads and sandbags.
Centre to the medial border of the foot, at the level of the navicular.

Special circumstances

If the patient is in a wheel-chair, satisfactory views may be obtained by allowing the patient to remain in it, with the foot positioned on the film which is placed on the floor.

Supplementary views

Dorsi-plantar, weight-bearing (to demonstrate hallux valgus). The patient stands with both feet on the film, which is placed on the floor. The weight should be equally distributed and both feet are included on the film.

Centre between the feet, at the level of the navicular, with the tube angled 25° towards the ankles.

Lateral, weight-bearing (to demonstrate pes planus). The patient stands on a small platform, with the film supported vertically between the feet and with its lower edge 2·5 cm (1 in) below the level of the soles of the feet. The tube is directed horizontally at the level of the soles of the feet and the platform must therefore be high enough for this to be achieved. A view of each foot is taken in turn.

Centre to the sole of the foot at the level of the navicular.

Lateral (to demonstrate foreign bodies). The patient sits on the X-ray table, with the knee flexed and the leg rotated outwards so that the plantar aspect of the foot is at right angles to the table.

Centre to the middle of the foot or to the site of entry of a foreign body.

CALCANEUM

Lateral. The foot is placed in the lateral position. A small aperture is used.

Centre to the calcaneum.

Axial. If the patient is able to stand, the following method is recommended because the X-ray beam is not directed towards the gonads. The patient stands with the heel or heels being examined on the cassette, with the posterior border about 2·5 cm (1 in) from the edge of the cassette. The patient bends the knees slightly and leans forwards, with a chair in front of him for support (Fig. 28).

Centre to the heel, or mid-way between the heels if both are being examined, at the level of the upper border of the calcaneum, with the tube angled 30° towards the toes.

Special circumstances

If the patient is unable to stand or is unsteady, he is examined in the sitting position with the legs extended and the foot dorsi-flexed

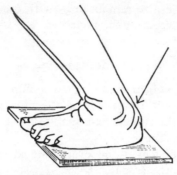

Fig. 28

as much as possible. The toes are pulled back by a bandage round them, held by the patient.

Centre to the plantar aspect of the calcaneum, with the tube angled 30° cephalad.

CALCANEAL SPUR
This condition is often bilateral and lateral views of both calcanei are required.

Centre to the calcaneum.

TOES
Dorsi-plantar. The sole of the foot is placed on the table. (The toe being examined can usually be separated from neighbouring ones by a pad of cotton wool.) A small aperture is used and the kilovoltage required is about 8 less than that for a view of the whole foot.

Centre to the toe being examined.

Lateral. For a lateral view of the first (great), second or third toes, the foot is placed on its side, with the medial aspect in contact with the film. The fourth and fifth toes are held out of the way, either by the patient's finger or with a bandage. For the fourth or fifth toes, the foot is placed on its side, with the lateral aspect in contact with the film. The other toes are held out of the way as much as possible.

Centre to the toe being examined.

Oblique. If the toes cannot be separated easily, an oblique view is taken. The foot is rotated medially 45° and supported.

Centre to the great toe.

OS TRIGONUM
This is a centre of ossification of the posterior tubercle of the talus, which occasionally ossifies as a separate bone.

Lateral. The foot is placed in the lateral position. A small aperture is used. A separate view of each foot is taken.

Centre 2·5 cm (1 in) posteriorly to the medial malleolus.

SUB-TALAR JOINT

Anatomy. The sub-talar joint consists of two articulations, the talo-calcaneal and the talo-calcaneal-navicular. Eversion and inversion of the foot occur at the sub-talar joints, movements being limited by strong inter-osseous ligaments.

There are three parts to the joint: anterior, middle and posterior. The groove between the middle and posterior articular facets is called the sulcus tarsi. Several views are needed to demonstrate the joint completely (Isherwood, 1961).

Basic views

Dorsi-plantar oblique. The patient sits on the X-ray table, with the knee flexed and the sole of the foot on the film. The limb is then rotated medially so that the sole of the foot is at 45° to the film.

Centre to the medial side of the foot, at the level of the navicular.

Medial axial oblique (Plate XVII). To show the sulcus tarsi. The patient sits with the limb extended and the foot dorsi-flexed. The position of the foot is maintained by means of a bandage which is held by the patient. The limb is then rotated 60° medially and the foot is supported on a foam pad.

Centre 2·5 cm (1 in) distal to the lateral malleolus, with the tube angled 15° cephalad.

Lateral axial oblique (Plate XVIII). To show the posterior part of the joint. The patient sits with the limb extended and the foot dorsi-flexed, the position again being maintained by a bandage held by the patient. The limb is then rotated 60° laterally and the foot is supported on a foam pad.

Centre 2·5 cm (1 in) distal to the medial malleolus, with the tube angled 15° cephalad.

'Anthonsen' (Plate XIX). The patient sits on the X-ray table, with the knee flexed and the lateral aspect of the foot resting on the film. The focus-film distance is adjusted to 30 to 35 cm (12 to 14 in).

Centre just below the medial malleolus, with the tube angled 25° caudad and 30° towards the toes (Anthonsen, 1943).

Supplementary view

Axial view of the calcaneum (to demonstrate talo-calcaneal 'bar'). The positioning is the same as for the basic axial view for the calcaneum (p. 161 and Fig. 28) but about 8 kV more is required.

ADDITIONAL EXAMINATION
Arthrography (p. 366).

LENGTH MEASUREMENTS

Accurate measurements of the bones of the lower limb are required as part of the initial investigation before children undergo leg-equalising treatment by surgical correction (such treatment being carried out usually by producing premature fusion of the epiphysis in the longer bone at a time calculated to allow the remaining growth of the epiphysis of the shorter bone to produce equality in length). These measurements are also required to assess progress of the treatment over a period of several years.

The principal requirements of the examination are that the measurements must be accurate and the method of obtaining them must be simple and easily reproduced.

The bones (or just the ends of them) are recorded radiographically together with a suitable measuring device, either a long ruler or a grid. Use is made of the vertical central ray (the beam being restricted to a narrow aperture) centred over each of the joints, so as to avoid magnification of the bones relative to the measuring device.

There are two main methods in common use:

Method I. In the simplest method, a ruler with radiopaque markings is placed along the mid-line of the X-ray table and slots into an angled board against which the patient's feet rest. This device is adjustable to allow the feet to be placed as symmetrically as possible, even when there is gross discrepancy between the lengths of the two limbs. The patient lies on the ruler, with the pelvis positioned symmetrically so that the anterior superior iliac spines are equidistant from the table, or as nearly so as possible. The feet are adjusted so that the malleoli are equidistant from the table.

Using a narrow transverse slit aperture, views of both hips, both knees and both ankles are taken on successive thirds of a 35 × 43 cm (17 × 14 in) cassette. The Bucky is used for each view. The X-ray tube is centred first to the level of the upper border of the femora, in the mid-line just proximal to the level of the femoral pulse. The upper third of the cassette is used, the middle and lower thirds being covered by lead rubber. The tube is then centred to the lower border of the femoral condyles, just distal to the apex of the patellae. The cassette is adjusted so that the middle third is in line with the central ray and the upper and lower thirds of the cassette are covered with lead rubber. The tube is then centred to the lower borders of the medial malleoli. The lower third of the cassette is placed in line with the central ray and the upper and middle thirds of the cassette are covered with lead rubber.

This method is accurate enough for clinical management of a patient, but it is not absolutely accurate when gross disparity is present between the length of the limbs, because then the tube cannot be centred directly over each joint.

Method II. This method (usually termed 'scanography') ensures that the images of all the joints are produced by the central ray and therefore whatever the disparity of the limbs there is no geometric distortion.

A measuring grid or ruler and a narrow slit aperture are again employed. But, in this method the X-ray tube is moved down the length of the limbs during a long exposure of about 6 seconds. The entire length of the limbs is thus radiographed, the central ray being at right angles to the limbs all the time. A 3 mm aperture and a 35×90 cm $(14 \times 36$ in) cassette are normally used. The tube may be hand-propelled or preferably motorised and usually the X-ray unit is equipped with a variable milliamperage control so that the mA can be decreased as the tube moves down the length of the limbs.

In each method, measurements of each limb are made from the top of the femoral head to the lower border of the medial condyle, and from the top of the medial spine of the tibia to the lower border of the medial malleolus.

24

Mouth and neck

The most important structures that will be described in this chapter are the teeth, salivary glands, pharynx, larynx, trachea and neck. Most of these are soft tissue structures, only the teeth and calcified laryngeal cartilages having a high inherent density. For the mandible see p. 101.

TEETH

Radiographic examination of the teeth is normally undertaken in a specialist department but sometimes it has to be done in a general department. Examinations using intra-oral and occlusal films are usually required. Radiography of the lower jaw using extra-oral film is described elsewhere (p. 101). Specialised equipment for pan-oral radiography is becoming more widely available and is finding increased application.

With conventional radiography it is not possible to show all the teeth on one film, because of the curved shape (roughly a parabola) of the jaws. Several teeth can usually be seen on each view but only two, or sometimes three, teeth are demonstrated clearly without distortion or superimposition (Plate XX). To demonstrate all the teeth multiple exposures are therefore required.

Anatomy. There are two sets of teeth: the deciduous ('milk') teeth, which erupt during the first two years, and the permanent teeth, which erupt between the sixth and twenty-fifth years and replace the milk teeth. The deciduous teeth comprise four incisor, two canine and four molar teeth in each jaw. The permanent teeth comprise four incisor, two canine, four premolar and six molar teeth in each jaw.

Each tooth consists of three parts: the crown, the neck and the root. Within the tooth is a pulp cavity containing sensitive tissue (pulp) and at the apex of the root is a small foramen for passage of nerves and vessels. Radiographically, the main part of the tooth appears as a dense, homogeneous structure with the root canal and pulp cavity as radiolucent areas in the centre and the denser enamel covering the crown. The periodontal membrane joins the root to the alveolar margin and the tooth socket is lined by lamina dura.

The teeth are numbered according to established dental formulae. Conventionally, those of the upper and lower jaws of each side are numbered from 1 to 8 for permanent teeth and from *a* to *e* for deciduous teeth. Thus:

R $\dfrac{8\ 7\ 6\ 5\ 4\ 3\ 2\ 1\ |\ 1\ 2\ 3\ 4\ 5\ 6\ 7\ 8}{8\ 7\ 6\ 5\ 4\ 3\ 2\ 1\ |\ 1\ 2\ 3\ 4\ 5\ 6\ 7\ 8}$ L   R $\dfrac{e\ d\ c\ b\ a\ |\ a\ b\ c\ d\ e}{e\ d\ c\ b\ a\ |\ a\ b\ c\ d\ e}$ L

Adult teeth   Deciduous teeth

By this formula, individual teeth are indicated thus: $\overline{8|}$ for adult right lower third molar, $\underline{|3}$ for adult left upper canine, $\overline{|c}$ for deciduous left lower canine.

In 1971, the Fédération Dentaire Internationale instituted a two-digit dental recording system, which is easier to write or type and which, unlike the conventional formula, can be relayed by Telex because it dispenses with the quadrant sign. Thus:

R $\dfrac{18\ 17\ 16\ 15\ 14\ 13\ 12\ 11\ |\ 21\ 22\ 23\ 24\ 25\ 26\ 27\ 28}{48\ 47\ 46\ 45\ 44\ 43\ 42\ 41\ |\ 31\ 32\ 33\ 34\ 35\ 36\ 37\ 38}$ L

Adult teeth

R $\dfrac{55\ 54\ 53\ 52\ 51\ |\ 61\ 62\ 63\ 64\ 65}{85\ 84\ 83\ 82\ 81\ |\ 71\ 72\ 73\ 74\ 75}$ L

Deciduous teeth

In this formula, the first digit indicates the quandrant and also distinguishes between adult and deciduous teeth. For example, individual teeth are indicated thus: 48 for adult right lower third molar, 23 for adult left upper canine, 73 for deciduous left lower canine.

Radiation protection. Relatively high skin doses are received during dental radiography because (*a*) only low kilovoltage (55–60 kV) is available on most dental units and (*b*) a short focus-film distance is used.

The total tube filtration must be equivalent to not less than 1·5 mm of aluminium up to 70 kV (Code of Practice, 1972, 3.14). A field-defining spacer cone, with a diameter at the end of the cone of not more than 6 cm should be used. It must provide a minimum focus-skin distance of not less than 20 cm for equipment operating above 60 kV and not less than 10 cm at lower kV. Open-ended cylindrical or divergent cones, affording the same protection as the tube housing, should be used in preference to the so-called 'pointer' cones, although in practice the former may prove difficult to use and there is some preference for pointer cones which have been modified so as to collimate the beam satisfactorily.

The cable should be long enough to enable the operator to stand at least one metre away from an X-ray tube operating at up to 70 kV, and 1·5 m at higher kV.

A lead apron should always be worn by the patient. This is particularly important when upper occlusal views are being taken. The X-ray beam should be directed away from the body whenever possible. The dental film should be held in place by a special holder but if this is not available the patient supports the film with a finger or thumb. Neither the radiographer nor any member of the staff must hold dental films in position whilst exposures are made.

Films. Intra-oral and occlusal films are non-screen type and they have a water-proof wrapping. They are often backed with lead foil to absorb radiation. Both intra-oral and occlusal films are pliable and thus can be bent slightly when being placed in the mouth but they must not be bent once in position as otherwise the teeth will appear distorted on the radiograph. Intra-oral films are 31×41 mm ($1\frac{1}{4} \times 1\frac{5}{8}$ in) or 22×35 mm ($\frac{7}{8} \times 1\frac{3}{8}$ in) and occlusal films are 57×76 mm ($2\frac{1}{4} \times 3$ in). As these sizes are too small for lead markers, each film has an embossed spot on the 'tube-side' and a routine should be followed for placing the film so that the embossed spot always appears on the occlusal surface so as not to obscure important detail.

Positioning of the patient. The patient may be examined either sitting or lying down, the sitting position being the more usual. The head must be supported and if a dental chair is not available, the patient should be seated in front of an erect cassette-stand, or skull table, with the head resting on a foam pad.

There are two methods of positioning the patient, film and X-ray tube for obtaining intra-oral periapical views:

1. *Bisecting-angle method.* This is the conventional method and more often used. Precise tube angulation and positioning of the patient's head are needed. Two positioning lines are used.

The upper positioning line extends from the ala of the nose to the tragus of the ear. The lower positioning line extends from the angle of the mouth to the tragus.

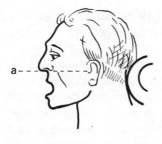
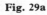
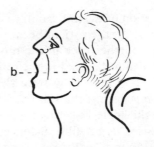

Fig. 29a   **Fig. 29b**

When the patient is examined in the erect position, the appropriate positioning line must be horizontal. Thus, if the upper teeth are being examined the chin is tucked in very slightly (Fig. 29a) and if the lower teeth are being examined the chin is raised (Fig. 29b). Foam pads should be placed behind the neck to support the head in the correct position.

The film must be placed sufficiently high or low in the mouth to ensure that the whole tooth is shown. For the incisors and canines the film is placed vertically in relation to the teeth and for all other teeth transversely. The film is placed in the mouth to lie in contact with the teeth and soft tissues. The film is therefore in close contact with the crowns of the teeth but some way from the apices because of the shape of the gums and palate and so it is at an angle to the long axis of the tooth. To reduce distortion, the X-ray tube is directed at right angles to an imaginary line bisecting this angle. The required angle will therefore depend on the individual patient but, as a general rule, angulation of the tube to the positioning lines, and the centering points are:

Upper Jaw	Average angle	Centre
Incisors	+55°	Tip of nose
Canines	+50°	Ala of nose
Premolars	+30°	Just below mid-point of orbit
Molars	+20°	Just below zygoma

Lower Jaw	Average angle	Centre
Incisors	−20°	Symphysis menti
Canines	−20°	Just lateral to symphysis menti
Premolars	−10°	In line with mid-point of orbit
Molars	− 5°	In line with outer canthus

2. *Paralleling method.* With this method a true orientation of the teeth with their supporting structures can be obtained with minimum

distortion or magnification (Tolman, 1975) but it is often less comfortable for the patient because the apical edge of the film has to be placed further back in the mouth.

The film is placed in the mouth, parallel with the long axis of the teeth. It is held away from the crowns of the teeth, with the edge which is against the soft tissues in approximately the same position as in the angle-bisecting method. To avoid magnification due to the increased object-film distance, the focus-film distance is increased to 40–50 cm (16–20 in). A long, cylindrical cone and very fast dental films are used. The narrower dental films are used more frequently in this method than in the angle-bisecting method, particularly for the anterior maxillary teeth.

Various methods of holding the films in place are used in different departments. These range from specially designed holders incorporating bite blocks and locating rings, to a simple haemostat. If none of these is available, a cotton roll can be placed between the film and the lingual surface of the crowns of the teeth and the film held in place by the patient's finger. The tube is directed at right angles to the film.

Occlusal views. These are taken to obtain a plan view of the teeth or to demonstrate cysts or other pathology in the alveolar process of the jaws. The occlusal film is placed horizontally in the mouth and is held gently between the teeth.

1. For the upper incisor teeth, the X-ray tube is centred to the bridge of the nose and directed at an angle of 65° to the film (nasal occlusal view).

2. For a plan view of the upper teeth, the tube is centred to the vertex of the skull and directed at right angles to the film (vertex occlusal view). This view should only be used when an occlusal cassette is available, because of the radiation dose to the eyes.

3. For the lower teeth, the chin is raised and the head positioned as for the submento-vertical view of the skull (p. 93).

4. For the lower incisor teeth, the tube is centred to the symphysis menti and directed at 40° to the film.

5. For a plan view of the lower teeth, the tube is centred under the mandible and directed at right angles to the film.

'Bite-wing' views. To demonstrate the crowns of the teeth, particularly at the points of contact between the teeth, usually in the investigation of caries, views are taken of the upper and lower teeth at the same time. On these views, the roots of the teeth are not shown. A special holder for the film is used, which allows the film to be held against the lingual aspect of the upper and lower teeth. A bite-block is incorporated in the device enabling the film to be held firmly in position. Alternatively a self-adhesive paper tab can be used.

The X-ray tube is centred to the occlusal plane and directed at right angles to the film. Both upper and lower crowns are demonstrated on one film but a second film for the premolar region may be necessary in large jaws or when the dental arch is very curved.

Exposures. With a dental unit, a focus-film distance of about 23 cm (9 in) is used and exposure times of between $\frac{1}{4}$ and $\frac{1}{2}$ second are required. With a general unit, a focus-film distance of 50 to 62 cm (20 to 25 in) is used and the kilovoltage is usually increased to about 75 kV.

With a general unit, the fine focus should be used so as to obtain maximum detail on the films.

Pan-oral tomography (Plate XXI). Several machines have been designed to obtain tomographs of the whole of both dental arches on one film. They are used to (a) investigate the jaws at a first orthodontic visit (b) demonstrate impacted teeth (c) demonstrate fractures of the mandible (d) demonstrate the temporo-mandibular joints and (e) demonstrate changes due to gross pathology in the maxilla.

Examples of such machines are the Orthopantomograph and the Panorex. They consist of an X-ray tube, with a slit diaphragm, linked to a film holder. As in most forms of tomography, the tube and film move in opposite directions. The film rotates during the exposure and the narrow beam of radiation from the slit diaphragm traverses its whole length.

The patient's head is carefully positioned in a modified craniostat and is adjusted so that the upper and lower arches are kept in focus during the exposure.

With the Orthopantomograph, the tomograph changes its axis of rotation twice during the exposure so as to remain at right angles to the curved shape of the dental arches.

With the Panorex, when one side of the jaws has been tomographed and the X-ray beam approaches the cervical vertebrae, the radiation is automatically switched off, the chair with the patient in it moves laterally and the other side of the jaws is tomographed. In the resulting radiograph, there is a blank space down the middle of the film but there are two separate and different views of the central teeth. With other pan-oral machines, these teeth are usually obscured partially by the image of the cervical vertebrae.

Reference should be made to specialised works (e.g. Manson-Hing, 1976) for further details of this form of tomography.

Cephalometry. This is used mainly in the investigation and follow-up of cases of malocclusion or asymmetry. Internationally recognised criteria ensure that radiographs taken for these purposes are always comparable. For details of this technique, reference should be made to specialised works (e.g. White *et al.*, 1967; Stafne and Gibilisco, 1975).

ADDITIONAL EXAMINATION

Xeroradiography (p. 77) for orthodontic examinations where demonstration of teeth, jaws and soft tissues are all required.

SALIVARY GLANDS

Anatomy. There are three pairs of salivary glands: parotid, submandibular and sublingual.

Parotid. These are the largest of the salivary glands and extend from the zygoma to the angle of the mandible. Each envelops the ascending ramus from behind and projects forward towards the masseter. A small part (the accessory) lies separately between the zygomatic arch and the parotid (Stenson's) duct. This duct is about 5 cm (2 in) long and is of a uniform, relatively narrow, calibre throughout. It leaves the anterior border of the gland and opens into the mouth at an orifice in the cheek opposite the second upper molar tooth.

Submandibular. These glands are each about the size of a walnut and are situated below and medial to the body of the mandible, extending from the angle of the mandible to the first molar teeth. Each gland is made up of a larger superficial part and a smaller deep part. It is separated from the parotid gland by the stylo-hyoid ligament. Wharton's duct, which is about 5 cm (2 in) long, leads from the gland and opens into the mouth at a papilla at the side of the frenulum of the tongue. The duct is wider than Stenson's duct except at its orifice where it is much narrower. The main part of the gland lies in the soft floor of the mouth, at the level of the body of the mandible.

Sublingual. These glands are situated beneath the mucous membrane of the mouth and are separated from the submandibular glands by the stylo-hyoid muscle. Several sublingual ducts open separately into the floor of the mouth; some may open into Wharton's duct.

Radiographic examination of the salivary glands and ducts is usually required to demonstrate calculi, these being most common in the submandibular and occasionally found in the parotid. Of the salivary glands, the parotid is the most frequent site of neoplasm. Soft tissue exposures are required in radiography of the salivary glands.

Parotid

Basic views

Antero-posterior. The patient sits or lies facing the X-ray tube, with the base line at right angles to the table. The head is then rotated 5° so that the side being examined is in profile.
Centre mid-way between the angles of the mandible.
Lateral. The head is placed in the lateral position with the median sagittal plane parallel with the table and the interpupillary line at right angles to it.
Centre to the angle of the mandible.
Lateral oblique. The head remains in the lateral position.
Centre to the angle of the mandible with the tube angled 15° to 20° cephalad.

Submandibular

Basic views

Lateral. The head is placed in the lateral position as above. To project below the level of the mandible a possible calculus in the duct, the floor of the mouth is depressed by a wooden spatula, or by a pad of swabs, held by the patient. The chin must be raised.
Centre 2·5 cm (1 in) anterior to the angle of the mandible.
Infero-superior. The patient sits with the head in the submento-vertical position, with the chin well raised. An occlusal film is placed diagonally well back in the mouth, so that the greatest amount of the side under examination is shown. The patient should close the teeth gently to steady the film.
Centre from below the angle of the mandible, at right angles to the film.

Sublingual

Basic views

Radiographic examination is seldom required.
Lateral. As for submandibular gland and duct (above).
Infero-superior. Because the sublingual glands are anterior to

the submandibular, the film need not be placed so far back in the mouth.

ADDITIONAL EXAMINATION

Sialography (p. 353).

PHARYNX

Anatomy. The pharynx extends from the base of the skull to the cricoid cartilage and is situated behind the nose, mouth and upper part of the throat. It is divided into three parts (*a*) the nasopharynx, which lies behind the nose and above the soft palate; it communicates with the middle ears via the eustachian tubes (*b*) the oropharynx, which lies behind the mouth and extends from the soft palate to the epiglottis; it is common to both respiratory and alimentary tracts and (*c*) the laryngopharynx, which extends from the upper border of the epiglottis to the lower border of the cricoid cartilage, where it becomes continuous with the oesophagus.

Radiographic examination of the pharynx is carried out to demonstrate tumour, abscess or the presence of a foreign body. Enlargement of the adenoid lymphoid tissue may be shown in radiographs of children. The air within the pharynx provides excellent contrast.

Basic views

Lateral ('Post-nasal space'). The patient sits or stands lateral to the cassette. The head is placed in the lateral position, with the chin raised, and immobilised. A long focus-film distance, usually 150 cm (60 in), is used. A small aperture is used, large enough to cover an 18 × 24 cm (10 × 8 in) cassette. The upper border of the cassette is placed at the level of the glabella. Soft tissue technique is employed and the exposure is made on arrested inspiration.

Centre to the lower border of the zygoma.

Submento-vertical. Whenever possible, a skull unit is used. The patient sits facing the X-ray tube, with the chin raised. The table is angled until it is parallel with the base line (Fig. 5, p. 93).

Centre between the angles of the jaw, at right angles to the base line.

Occipito-mental (to demonstrate lateral displacement of the coronoid process and extra-pharyngeal extension of a lesion in the nasopharynx) (Gupta *et al.*, 1973). The patient faces the skull table, with the chin (and usually also the tip of the nose) in contact with it so that the base line is at 45° to the vertical. The patient should open the mouth as wide as possible (Fig. 10, p. 104).

Centre to the lower orbital margin.

Palatography

The production of the correct sounds in speech is controlled by the positions of the tongue and soft palate and the closure between the oropharynx and the nasopharynx.

Palatography is the radiographic demonstration of these features and is of value to plastic surgeons and speech therapists in the management of anatomical abnormalities of the palate, such as cleft palate, palatal disproportion and related pharyngeal malformations (Kamdar and Oza, 1973).

Lateral soft tissue views of the nasopharynx are taken as for the basic view (p. 174) (*a*) with the palate at rest (*b*) with the patient phonating 'nnn'—when the palate is depressed against the back of the tongue and (*c*) phonating 'eee'—when the palate is fully elevated and the nasopharynx closed (Pitt and Ingram, 1975).

Short exposure times are essential to minimise blur due to movement of the palate. Very fast intensifying screens should be used. High kilovoltage also is sometimes recommended. The head must be immobilised and if palatography is carried out frequently, a cephalostat should be available. If not, an erect chest stand and head-clamps are used. When a child is being examined, the assistance of a parent or nurse may be needed to hold the child firmly by the chin and the top of the head.

Sometimes a thin strip of barium paste is placed along the centre of the tongue before the radiograph is taken, to show the position of the tip and bulk of the tongue. The placing of the paste is most easily carried out by using a drawing-up cannula attached to a syringe of paste and drawing a line along the length of the tongue (Pitt and Ingram, 1975). But this may be difficult with an unco-operative child.

ADDITIONAL EXAMINATIONS

Tomography (p. 47), lateral, antero-posterior and submento-vertical views may all be required for a full assessment. *Nasopharyngography* (p. 356). *Barium swallow* (p. 256) to demonstrate cricopharyngeal spasm or pharyngeal web or pouch. *Xeroradiography* (p. 77). *Nasopharyngoscopy* (Pigott and Makepeace, 1975).

LARYNX

Anatomy. The larynx is made up of a ring of cartilaginous structures, the most important of which are the thyroid, cricoid and arytenoid cartilages. The upper opening of the larynx is in the floor of the pharynx and the lower end is continuous with the trachea. The main function of the larynx is to act as a valvular sphincter guarding the entry into the pulmonary air tract; the production of sound is a secondary feature (Lederman, 1971).

Radiographic examination of the larynx is carried out to demonstrate paresis, oedema or fibrosis but most often in the investigation of malignancy. The most useful view is a soft tissue lateral view (Fig. 30 and Plate XXII) because in the antero-posterior view the midline structures are obscured by the much denser cervical vertebrae. Tomography (Plate XXIII) is essential for a complete examination.

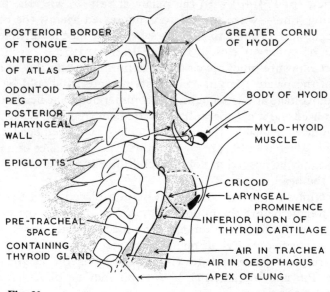

POSTERIOR BORDER OF TONGUE
ANTERIOR ARCH OF ATLAS
ODONTOID PEG
POSTERIOR PHARYNGEAL WALL
EPIGLOTTIS
PRE-TRACHEAL SPACE
CONTAINING THYROID GLAND

GREATER CORNU OF HYOID
BODY OF HYOID
MYLO-HYOID MUSCLE
CRICOID
LARYNGEAL PROMINENCE
INFERIOR HORN OF THYROID CARTILAGE
AIR IN TRACHEA
AIR IN OESOPHAGUS
APEX OF LUNG

Fig. 30

Basic view

Lateral (Plate XXII). The patient stands or sits with one shoulder against the cassette and with the head in the lateral position. The chin is raised and the shoulders are lowered as much as possible. A 24 × 30 cm (12 × 10 in) cassette is used, with its upper border at the level of the top of the pinna. A long focus-film distance, 150 cm (60 in), is used. The exposure is made on arrested deep inspiration or with the patient performing the Valsalva manœuvre (forced expiration against a closed glottis, p. 178).

Centre 5 cm (2 in) posterior to the anterior surface of the neck at the level of the laryngeal prominence.

Supplementary views

Further soft tissue lateral views taken with the patient (*a*) breathing gently (*b*) phonating 'eee' and (*c*) bearing down ('straining'), may be needed for a full assessment of the larynx (Ardran and Kemp, 1975).

Post-laryngectomy patients

Soft tissue radiographs of the neck are sometimes taken to demonstrate the pattern of air trapping when a patient who has undergone laryngectomy attempts speech. Such a patient who speaks well will show a large collection of air in the oesophagus and behind the base of the tongue, and muscular bands may be visible in the oesophagus which help to control speech and increase volume. A post-laryngectomy patient who does not speak well, shows no ability to reproduce a controllable air collection (Ryan, 1970).

ADDITIONAL EXAMINATIONS

Tomography (p. 47) in the antero-posterior position, to show the extent of neoplasm below the level of the vocal chords, or to show movement of the chords (the patient phonating 'eeeee'), or to show the presence of a polyp (the patient breathing gently). *Laryngography* (p. 358). *Barium swallow* (p. 256) before laryngectomy (even if the patient is complaining of dysphonia and not dysphagia) to demonstrate the extent of the tumour and thus the extent and nature of the operation (Lederman, 1971). *Cine-fluorography barium swallow*, to demonstrate extrinsic involvement of the vocal folds (Ardran and Kemp, 1975). *Thermography* (p. 80) to demonstrate gland metastases in the neck (Ryan, 1970). *Subtraction* (p. 41) between radiographs taken on quiet respiration and phonation (Hemmingsson, 1972). *Xeroradiography* (p. 77).

THORACIC INLET

Anatomy. The thoracic inlet is bounded posteriorly by the first thoracic vertebra, anteriorly by the manubrium sterni and laterally by the first ribs. Through it pass the trachea, oesophagus, vessels and nerves.

The most common reason for radiographic examination is in the assessment of thyroid enlargement.

Basic views

Antero-posterior. The patient lies supine on the X-ray table, with the chin raised. The exposure may be made either on arrested full inspiration or, preferably, with the patient performing the Valsalva manœuvre. For this, the patient is asked to take in a deep breath and then to breathe out hard whilst keeping the mouth closed and pinching the nose.

Centre to the sternal notch.

Lateral (Plate XXIV). The patient stands in the lateral position, with the chin raised and the arm nearer the cassette raised over the head (Fig. 14, p. 115). The exposure is made on full arrested inspiration. The focus-film distance used is 100 cm (48 in). High kilovoltage is used.

Centre just above the head of the humerus remote from the cassette.

Supplementary views

Lateral. The patient stands lateral to the cassette, with one shoulder against it, the hands behind the back and the shoulders forced back. The chin should be raised. This is a difficult position to maintain and immediately before the exposure is made the patient should be encouraged again to pull the shoulders right back. The upper border of the cassette is placed at the level of the angle of the jaw.

To reduce the contrast between the upper and lower parts of the trachea, high kilovoltage technique is employed or a wedge filter may be used. The use of a multilayer cassette is of advantage to show with one exposure both the dense retrosternal area and the less dense upper part of the trachea (p. 35). The exposure is made on arrested full inspiration or, preferably, with the patient performing the Valsalva manœuvre.

Centre to the sternal notch.

Lateral soft tissue view of neck. If the upper trachea is over-exposed on the basic lateral view, a further lateral view is taken as for the larynx (p. 176).

TRACHEA

Anatomy. The trachea is an extensile tube strengthened by U-shaped cartilages between 16 and 20 in number. It extends from the lower border of the larynx to its bifurcation into the left and right bronchi at the level of the fifth thoracic vertebra.

Basic views

Antero-posterior. As for thoracic inlet (p. 178).
Lateral. As for thoracic inlet (p. 178).

ADDITIONAL EXAMINATIONS
Tomography (p. 47) and *inclined hilar tomography* (Mayall, 1965; p. 49 and Plate IB). *Xeroradiography* (p. 77).

25

Chest

In a general department, radiography of the chest is the examination most frequently performed. Most cases are routine, to exclude radiographically demonstrable disease, to demonstrate possible pleural or pulmonary pathology and to follow the progress of such lesions. The next largest group of cases are patients with cardiac disease who require a somewhat different radiographic examination. Radiography of the chest is also required for investigation of the mediastinum, diaphragm and chest wall. The views required in all these cases will vary with the presenting clinical problem.

Care should be taken to ensure that no radiopaque objects are left on under the cotton gown, if worn, and that waistbands, belts, etc., are low enough not to obscure the lung bases. Even though a patient is asked to undress to the waist, it is possible to overlook some radiopaque objects and a hand placed on the patient's back during positioning will detect anything worn under the gown and avoid the necessity for repeat radiographs. Long hair must be pinned up out of the way. Occasionally, a patient may wear a medallion on a chain that cannot be unfastened. If so, the medallion should be placed between the patient's teeth, together with as much of the chain as is necessary to prevent it obscuring the lungs.

Radiation protection. The gonads must always be protected either by a lead apron, worn at the back and fastened round the patient's waist, by a lead screen (adjustable in height) or, for an infant, by a piece of lead rubber placed over the abdomen and pelvis. The upper border of the lead should be as high as possible without obscuring the costo-phrenic angles; in practice, the upper border of the protection is placed just above the iliac crests.

LUNG FIELDS AND HEART

An erect view should be taken whenever possible, but occasionally, when a patient has multiple injuries or has had a recent operation, it may be necessary to take a radiograph with the patient supine.

Respiration. To avoid blur caused by respiratory movement, radiographs of the chest must always be taken on arrested respiration. The lungs are best demonstrated when they are well aerated and therefore radiographs are usually taken on full inspiration, as the diaphragm is then at its lowest level and the largest expanse of lung is visible. Cardiac pulsation can produce blur even when respiration has been arrested and so the shortest possible exposure time must be used.

Positioning of the patient. Care must be taken in positioning, to ensure that there is no rotation of the patient, as abnormal projection of the heart or mediastinum may simulate pathology. If the medial ends of the clavicles appear on the radiograph, as equidistant from the spinous processes of the vertebrae, this shows that the patient is correctly positioned.

In the normal standing position, a large proportion of the lungs is obscured by the scapulae. To move the scapulae away from the thorax, the elbows are flexed, the backs of the hands are placed on the hips and the elbows are pushed gently forwards. When doing this, the shoulders must not be raised, so that the apices of the lungs are not obscured by the clavicles. The position required is awkward for the patient and the field of vision is restricted. Clear instructions regarding position, breathing and swallowing should be given in advance and ample time must be allowed for the patient to carry them out.

Small pleural effusions produce no radiological changes on a postero-anterior view except for obliteration of the costo-phrenic angles which must therefore be clearly demonstrated. In the erect position, the apices of the lungs are higher than might be expected and the upper border of the cassette should be placed 5 cm (2 in) above the level of the shoulders to ensure that the apices are included.

Infants and children. Small children are usually happier in the antero-posterior position (rather than in the postero-anterior position) because they can see what is happening around them, and therefore more accurately positioned films are usually obtainable in the antero-posterior position. The radiographer can also watch the child breathing and so take the radiograph on full inspiration if the child is too young to co-operate in breathing.

With a child under 5 years, better diagnostic radiographs can be obtained in the supine than the erect position and there may be little advantage in trying to obtain an erect view if the child is unco-operative (Hunter *et al*., 1973). But with encouragement and patience, even a small child can usually be examined in the erect sitting position if an antero-posterior rather than a postero-anterior view is attempted.

With a small child, the apparent size and shape of the heart may be altered if he leans backwards slightly, in a semi-lordotic position, and care should be taken to avoid this.

A baby's chest is wider than it is long, so for the antero-posterior view, the cassette—usually 18×24 cm (8×10 in)—is placed transversely. For the lateral view the cassette is placed lengthways because the posterior part of a baby's chest can be as much as twice as deep as the anterior part. The top of the cassette should be at the level of the nose because a baby has a very short neck and if the cassette is placed as it would be for an adult, the apices are not included. For the same reason, the name space on the cassette should be put at the bottom, to avoid obliterating the apices with it.

The positioning of infants for radiography of the chest should be such as to ensure minimum disturbance. Thus antero-posterior supine views are recommended unless it is important to demonstrate air-fluid levels (Gordon and Ross, 1977).

Centering. The conventionally quoted centering point is the fourth or fifth thoracic vertebra. In practice, this is too vague and will vary with every radiographer; a 'high' centering point usually becomes the aim and when such a point is used the whole head is likely to be irradiated unnecessarily. Instead, *before* the patient is positioned, the light beam diaphragm should be adjusted to within the limits of the cassette being used. The patient is then positioned and the beam centred to the cassette, the aperture being then further decreased if necessary. By this method, only the part being examined is irradiated and the centering is more accurate than with the conventional method. This is particularly important for follow-up cases.

Focus-film distance. To minimise cardiac magnification, a long focus-film distance is used. This distance, either 150 or 180 cm (5 or 6 ft), is kept constant for all erect chest radiographs in the same department. When it is necessary to take a supine view in the department, the focus-film distance is almost always less than 150 cm and depends on the tube column or suspension. In practice, 120 cm (48 in) is usually the longest focus-film distance possible and this is kept constant for all supine views. When there is any variation from this focus-film distance, it should be noted on the radiograph for the radiologist's information.

When using mobile equipment, it may sometimes be impossible

to obtain the required distance above the level of the bed for a supine view, and in such cases the longest focus-film distance obtainable should be used.

Air gap technique. If the patient is positioned a little distance, e.g. 15 to 25 cm (6 to 10 in), away from the cassette, the resulting air gap avoids the necessity for using a grid to reduce scattered radiation when high kilovoltage is used. The use of an air gap instead of a grid enables the exposure and hence the radiation dose to the patient, to be reduced by nealy 50 per cent (Ardran and Crooks, 1976).

To avoid magnification, the focus-film distance has to be increased. A focus-film distance of 350 cm (12 ft) and a patient-film distance of 15 cm (6 in) produce the same magnification as with the usual technique for chest radiography where the focus-film distance is 180 cm (6 ft) and the patient is in contact with the cassette.

A device (e.g. a rigid plastic frame fixed to the cassette stand) is needed for positioning and maintaining the patient at the desired distance from the cassette.

Contrast and definition are improved because very little scattered radiation reaches the film, and grid lines are avoided.

The quality of chest radiographs can be improved also by additional filtration (0·1 mm copper and 0·1 mm aluminium) fitted close to the tube window, with an additional differential filter in the case of well-developed female patients.

Film quality. The precise quality required for a radiograph of the chest is always decided by the radiologist, as personal preferences in chest radiography vary greatly. High or low kilovoltage technique may be used but as a general rule the contrast should be just sufficient to reveal detail throughout both dense and translucent areas, the lung vascular shadows should be clearly visible and bone detail in the ribs should be clear. Penetration should be such that the intervertebral disc spaces are just visible behind the heart but detail of the thoracic spine should not be seen clearly.

The choice of exposure factors is most satisfactorily determined by using a photo-timer or, if this is not available, a method of thickness/weight calculation is an advantage (Dawson et al., 1966. See also Exposures, p. 23).

Lateral view. In the postero-anterior view, one-third of the lungs is obscured by the heart and diaphragm. Some authorities hold that a lateral view should always be taken, particularly at an initial examination, but in some departments for reasons of economy a lateral view is taken only if a lesion is suspected from the postero-anterior view. The lateral view will reveal lesions that may be obscured by the heart or diaphragm and, if a lesion is shown on the postero-anterior view, will localise the lesion and demonstrate any character-istic outline such as effusion or collapse. It will also confirm anatomi-cal abnormalities, such as a depressed sternum, which may have produced a confusing view of the heart on the postero-anterior view.

Basic views

Postero-anterior. The patient faces the cassette, with the chin raised and placed on top, and in the mid-line, of the cassette. The top of the cassette should be 5 cm (2 in) above the level of the shoulders. The elbows are flexed, the backs of the hands placed on the hips and the elbows pushed forwards. For fuller details see page 181.

Centre to the cassette.

Lateral. From the postero-anterior position, the patient is rotated 90° so that the side under examination is against the cassette. The arms are folded over the head and the axilla is placed against the cassette (Fig. 31). The elbows must be raised, as otherwise the soft tissues of the arms, and sometimes even the humeri, may obscure the lung apices.

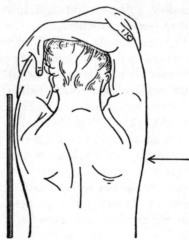

Fig. 31

Centre to the axilla at the same level as for the postero-anterior view.

Special circumstances

If the presence of pleural effusion, haemothorax or pneumothorax is suspected in a patient who is too ill to sit up, a view must be taken with the tube directed horizontally to demonstrate fluid—which lies posteriorly, or air—which collects uppermost. Therefore a lateral decubitus view is taken (see under Supplementary Views). To demonstrate a pneumothorax, the patient lies with the affected side uppermost and the exposure is made on full expiration. To demonstrate a haemothorax or a pleural effusion, the patient lies on the affected side, raised on foam pads so that the whole lung is included on the radiograph.

Supplementary views

Supine antero-posterior. This view should be taken of all patients who are to undergo thoracic surgery, for use as a control for future post-operative radiographs. It should be taken also of patients with chest injuries who may develop mediastinal haematomata.

Penetrated postero-anterior and lateral (to demonstrate (a) the carina and main bronchi (b) the paraspinal region (c) cardiac calcification (d) the lungs in patients with pathological conditions which increase the opacity of the chest contents and (e) the lung bases in patients with dense breast shadows). Positioning is as for the basic views. High kilovoltage (100 to 150 kV) is needed and so either a secondary radiation grid or an air gap (p. 183) is used.

Antero-posterior (to demonstrate the lung apices, lesions in the posterior part of the chest or to distinguish between opacities within and outside the lungs). The patient is positioned with his back to the cassette. In all other respects the positioning is as for the postero-anterior view.

Postero-anterior view on expiration (to demonstrate pneumothorax, emphysema, collapse due to an inhaled foreign body, diaphragmatic movement, or to distinguish between opacities in a rib or in a lung). Positioning is as for the basic view. The kilovoltage is increased by 5.

A small pneumothorax is best demonstrated on *expiration* because the intrapleural pressure is then increased and tends to compress the collapsed lung and thus make the pneumothorax bigger.

Apical (Plate XXV) (to demonstrate the lung apices). The patient is positioned with his back to the cassette and about 25 cm (10 in) away from it, leaning back so that only the shoulders are in contact with the cassette which should be displaced cephalad (Fig. 32). The arms are positioned as for the postero-anterior view.

Centre in the mid-line at the level of the sternal angle, with the tube angled 30° cephalad.

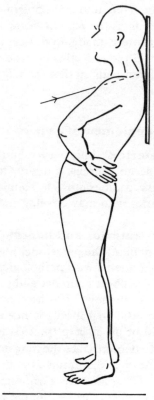

Fig. 32

Posterior oblique (to demonstrate lower lobe collapse). The patient is positioned with his back to the cassette and is then rotated 45° so that the side being examined is against the cassette. The arms are held away from the sides so that they do not obscure the lung fields.

Centre to the cassette, which is placed so as to include the whole chest, or a specific part as indicated on the basic views.

Left posterior oblique. To demonstrate a foreign body in the oesophagus.

Lateral decubitus (to demonstrate pneumothorax or effusion in an ill patient). The patient lies (*a*) on the affected side—to demonstrate fluid in the pleural cavity or (*b*) on the non-affected side—to demonstrate air in the pleural cavity. He should be raised from the table-top on foam pads so that the whole of the chest is included on the radiograph. The cassette is placed vertically behind or in front of him. The arms should be placed on the pillow or round the cassette.

Centre to the cassette, using a horizontal beam.

TO DEMONSTRATE INTERLOBAR EFFUSION

A lordotic view is rarely taken but a 'reverse' lordotic view may be useful. The patient is positioned with his back against the cassette, leaning back slightly so that only the shoulders are in contact with it. The cassette is displaced cephalad and should be large enough to include the whole chest.

Centre to the xiphisternum, with the tube angled 30° cephalad (Fig. 32).

TO ASSESS CARDIAC SIZE AND SHAPE

Anterior obliques with barium. For the left anterior oblique view, the patient faces the cassette and is then rotated approximately 75°, so that the left shoulder is against the cassette. The right hand is placed on the head or on the cassette stand. For the right anterior oblique view, the positions are reversed and the right shoulder is placed against the cassette, the degree of rotation being about 65°.

Centre to the cassette which is placed so as to include the whole chest.

Left lateral with barium. The positioning is the same as for the basic lateral view.

For each of these three views, the patient is given a spoonful of barium paste to chew and swallow immediately before the exposure is made. The radiographs should show a column of barium in the oesophagus, between the heart and the vertebral column. (If the degree of obliquity is insufficient, the barium will appear superimposed on the vertebral column. The exact degree of obliquity required for an individual patient can only be determined by fluoroscopy.)

ADDITIONAL EXAMINATIONS
Fluoroscopy. Tomography (p. 47). *Computed tomography* (p. 52).

Macroradiography (p. 38). *Angiocardiography* (p. 228). *Selective arteriography* (pulmonary and bronchial). *Scintigraphy* (p. 63) to demonstrate pulmonary emboli. *Ultrasonography* (p. 70) to demonstrate pericardial effusion.

DIAPHRAGM

Anatomy. The diaphragm is the musculo-fibrous division between the chest and abdomen. It forms part of the respiratory mechanism, being lowered on inspiration to increase the capacity of the chest. In an erect view of the chest, the upper border of the diaphragm is seen at the level of the tenth and eleventh ribs on inspiration, and the ninth and tenth ribs on expiration. The diaphragm is rarely the site of primary disease but it may be affected by pleural or peritoneal disease or by phrenic nerve damage and it may be the site of trauma or of congenital deficiency. The main purpose for radiographic examination of the diaphragm is the investigation of the structures above and below it.

Basic views

Postero-anterior. The patient is positioned as for the basic postero-anterior view. A 30 × 40 cm (15 × 12 in) or 35 × 43 cm (17 × 14 in) cassette is used transversely, with its lower border at the level of the lower costal margin. If investigation of the respiratory movement of the diaphragm is required, fluoroscopy is the examination of choice but if fluoroscopy equipment is not available, two exposures are made on one film, one taken on full inspiration using two-thirds of the total required exposure and the other taken on full expiration using one-third. A grid is used unless the patient is very slim.

Centre to the xiphisternum.

Lateral. The patient is positioned as for the basic lateral view (p. 184 and Fig. 31).

Centre to the axilla, at the level of the xiphisternum.

Special circumstances

To show gas under the diaphragm in an ill patient, a lateral decubitus view is taken, with the patient lying on the left side in order to distinguish between gas under the diaphragm and gas in the stomach. A horizontal beam is used. The grid cassette is supported vertically in front of the patient who must be raised from the table-top on foam pads so that the whole diaphragm is included. The lower border of the cassette is placed at the level of the lower costal margin.

Centre to the cassette, using a horizontal beam.

ADDITIONAL EXAMINATIONS

Fluoroscopy to assess diaphragmatic movement and to distinguish between paralysis of the diaphragm (caused e.g. by carcinoma of the bronchus with invasion of the mediastinum) and non-paralytic abnormality (caused e.g. by intra-abdominal pressure) (Carmichael, 1976). *Other examinations* appropriate for the site of primary diseases in the chest or abdomen.

RIBS

Anatomy. There are 12 pairs of ribs. The first seven pairs, termed 'true ribs', are attached by their costal cartilages directly to the sternum, the next three pairs are each attached by their costal cartilages to the cartilages of the ribs directly above them and the last two pairs, termed 'floating ribs', are free at their anterior ends.

The ribs slope downwards so that the anterior ends are considerably lower than the posterior and it is important to remember this when examining the ribs radiographically.

Although the ribs are flexible and resilient, fractures are common, particularly of the middle ribs in the axillary line, which is the point of greatest weakness. Trauma to the thoracic or abdominal viscera may be associated with injury to the ribs.

Radiographs must show the whole length of the ribs under examination and preferably several above and below. Radiography is made more difficult by the curved shape of the ribs, their position in relation to the lungs and diaphragm, their obliquity and the attachment of the costal cartilages (which may become calcified). To show as many ribs as possible above the diaphragm, views for the upper ribs are taken on inspiration. To show as many ribs as possible below the diaphragm, views for the lower ribs are taken on expiration.

Upper ribs

Basic views

Postero-anterior. As for basic view of the chest (p. 184). The kilovoltage is increased by 5.

Oblique. For the left ribs, a left posterior oblique or a right anterior oblique view (depending on the site of interest) is taken. For the right ribs, a right posterior oblique or a left anterior oblique view is taken. The patient is rotated 45° from the antero-posterior or postero-anterior positions, as the case may be. A grid cassette is used which should be large enough to include the whole chest. The upper border of the cassette is placed 2·5 cm (1 in) above the level of the top of the shoulders.

Centre in the mid-clavicular line of the side under examination, at the level of the middle of the cassette.

Lower ribs

Basic views

Antero-posterior. The patient lies supine on the X-ray table. A 30 × 40 cm (15 × 12 in) cassette is placed transversely, with its lower border 5 cm (2 in) below the lower costal margin.

Centre in the mid-line at the level of the middle of the cassette.

Oblique. From the antero-posterior position, the patient is rotated 45° so that the side being examined is nearer the table.

Centre in the mid-clavicular line of the side being examined, at the level of the lower costal margin.

Special circumstances

If the patient's condition precludes turning on to the injured side, an oblique view of the ribs can be taken by angulation of the tube across the patient, making sure that the cassette is sufficiently displaced so that the lateral border of the thorax is included on the radiograph. If a grid is used, the grid lines must run transversely.

Supplementary views

Oblique. Additional information may be obtained by taking the opposite oblique view, e.g. left anterior oblique in addition to right anterior oblique.

Lateral. To demonstrate the anterior ends and distal thirds of the lower six ribs, the patient stands or lies in the lateral position, with the arms over the head. The lower border of the cassette is placed 5 cm (2 in) below the level of the lower costal margin.

Centre in the mid-axillary line, at the level of the lower costal margin.

STERNUM

Anatomy. The sternum is composed of three parts, the manubrium sterni, the body and the xiphisternum. The lateral borders of the sternum have a serrated appearance, the curved parts being for the articulation of the first seven pairs of costal cartilages. The sternum is a thin, flat bone and in the antero-posterior position it is overshadowed by the denser vetebral column and mediastinum. It is easily palpable for radiographic positioning.

Basic views

Either **anterior oblique with patient rotated.** The patient stands or sits facing the grid cassette or vertical Bucky stand and is rotated about 40° until the sternum is no longer superimposed by the thoracic vertebrae. A long exposure time of at least 2 seconds is used, during which the patient breathes gently, to blur out lung markings. Therefore it is important that there should be no other movement by the patient and to ensure this he should hold on to the cassette stand for support and be made to feel relaxed and secure.

Centre 5 cm (2 in) caudad to the level of the sternal notch, about 10 cm (4 in) away from the mid-line, on the side further from the cassette, and thus directly through the sternum.

Or **anterior oblique with tube angled.** A grid cassette is used with the grid lines running transversely. The patient stands or lies facing the cassette, with the sternum in the middle of the cassette. A long exposure time of at least 2 seconds is used, during which the patient breathes gently, to blur out lung markings. He must be comfortable and immobilised if necessary, to avoid unsharpness due to movement blur.

Centre 5 cm (2 in) caudad to the level of the sternal notch, about 10 cm (4 in) away from the mid-line, with the tube angled 20° towards the mid-line—hence the need for the grid lines to run transversely.

Lateral. The patient stands in the lateral position with one shoulder against the cassette. The shoulders are drawn well back and the chin is raised. A long, 150 cm (60 in), focus-film distance is used, so as to avoid magnification due to the large object-film distance.

Centre to the sternal angle.

ADDITIONAL EXAMINATION

Tomography (p. 47), particularly inclined frontal plane tomography (Plate XXVI).

STERNO-CLAVICULAR JOINTS

Anatomy. These are gliding synovial joints formed by the medial ends of the clavicles articulating with the manubrium sterni and with the upper surfaces of the first costal cartilages. The clavicles project further anteriorly than the sternum does. The medial ends of the clavicles are separated by the suprasternal notch and are easily palpable.

Basic view

Postero-anterior obliques. Both left and right anterior oblique views are taken. The patient sits or stands facing the grid cassette or vertical Bucky stand and is rotated about 45° to each side in turn. A long exposure time of at least 2 seconds is used, during which the patient breathes gently, to blur out lung markings. Therefore it is important that there should be no other movement by the patient and to ensure this he should hold on to the cassette stand for support. A narrow transverse aperture is used so as to include both joints. The centre of the cassette is placed at the level of the sternal notch.

Centre about 10 cm (4 in) lateral to the spinous processes, on the side further from the cassette, and thus directly through the joint on that side.

Supplementary view

Lateral. The patient stands in the lateral position with one shoulder against the cassette. The shoulders are drawn well back and the chin is raised. A long, 150 cm (60 in), focus-film distance is used, so as to reduce magnification. A small aperture is used.

Centre to the sternal notch.

ADDITIONAL EXAMINATION
Tomography (p. 47).

26

Abdomen

Radiological examination of the abdomen is usually undertaken in an acute surgical emergency. Plain films of the abdomen are also taken before many radiological procedures and are frequently required as follow-up examinations.

Abdominal examinations may be divided into two categories each requiring different basic views:

Those for the gastro-intestinal tract which require supine and erect antero-posterior views of the whole abdomen. Such views are also needed for gynaecological problems.

Those for the urinary tract and retro-peritoneal structures which require views of the kidneys, ureters and bladder (K.U.B.). Included in this category are organs such as the liver, spleen and supra-renal glands, which require very similar views.

Radiographs of the abdomen must include both the diaphragm and the symphysis pubis. The kidney outlines, psoas muscle shadows, soft tissues and the pro-peritoneal fat line in the lateral abdominal wall should all be demonstrated. Exposure factors must be chosen to give optimum soft tissue differentiation. Low kilovoltage (60 to 65 kV) is usually employed. For most examinations of the abdomen, exposures are made on arrested expiration but occasionally radiographs may have to be taken on arrested inspiration, e.g. to determine the relationship of a kidney to an opacity. The liver and spleen are better demonstrated if the radiograph is taken on arrested full inspiration (Chesney, 1967).

To show small renal calculi, or other calcification, there must be no movement or respiratory blur. The highest output unit available must always be used in the radiographic investigation of acute conditions of the abdomen so that short exposure times can be used. Rare earth or very fast tungstate screens which permit the use of low kilovoltage and short exposure times should be used, particularly for a very ill patient.

The examination of a patient with acute abdominal symptoms is performed preferably when he is en route to a ward or operating theatre so as to cause as little disturbance to the patient as possible. Views taken with a mobile unit are seldom of the required quality and attempts to interpret them are more likely to be misleading than helpful.

Care of the patient. The patient presenting with acute abdominal symptoms is often very ill and gentle treatment is imperative. He should be moved on to the X-ray table and disturbed as little as possible afterwards. If a drip infusion or drainage tube is present, particular attention must be paid to it so as to ensure that its function is not impaired when the patient is moved on to the X-ray table, or when he is moved from the supine to the erect position or when turned into the lateral position.

The patient should be undressed and wear a suitable gown. Thick folds of sheet or blanket must be avoided so as to prevent artefacts obscuring soft tissue detail on the radiograph.

In cases of suspected intestinal obstruction or perforation of viscera, the examination must include a view taken with a horizontal beam and the whole of the abdomen must be clearly seen in order to show the presence of any fluid levels or free peritoneal gas.

When the patient is to be examined in the erect position, it must be ascertained before moving him that he is able to stand or sit. When a tilting table is used, the foot-rest and hand-grips should be suitably positioned and the table gently brought into the vertical position.

If the patient is able to stand easily for the erect view, a postero-anterior view is taken in preference to an antero-posterior view. The patient faces the cassette and puts both arms round the cassette and is asked to press his abdomen tightly against it. In this way, movement blur is minimised because the patient feels more secure, and better definition is obtained because of the compression (applied by the patient himself).

If the patient is unable to stand and a tilting table is not available, some method of supporting the patient in the sitting position must be provided. A means of supporting the cassette in the vertical position behind the patient and at a suitable height must also be provided. The methods chosen will depend on the accessories available and on the condition of the patient. Each department will have a routine method of providing the necessary support.

In the examination of the acute abdomen, a view of the chest is taken as an integral part of the examination because primary intra-thoracic disease may present with symptoms indistinguishable from an abdominal emergency.

Infants. A baby's abdomen is almost as wide as it is long and the width of the abdomen is greater than the width of the pelvis. That part of a baby's abdomen which is wider than the pelvis contains organs—not just fat as with an adult. Therefore the light beam diaphragm must be collimated to the full width of the abdomen, not to the width of the pelvis (Gyll, 1977). A baby's diaphragm is higher and the kidneys are lower than in an adult. The abdomen is as deep as it is wide, so the exposure factors are more than might be expected. A grid is normally used.

GASTRO-INTESTINAL TRACT

Basic views

Supine antero-posterior. The patient lies supine on the X-ray table, with the knees flexed over a small pillow for comfort. A 35 × 43 cm (17 × 14 in) cassette is used, positioned so that its lower border includes the symphysis pubis. In the case of small patients, at 100 cm (40 in) focus-film distance, the diaphragm may be included. In the case of tall or large patients, an additional radiograph using a 35 × 43 cm (17 × 14 in) cassette placed transversely will be necessary. The lower border of this cassette is placed at the level of the iliac crests.

Centre in the mid-line at the level of the middle of the cassette for each view.

Erect antero-posterior. If his condition allows it, the patient should be raised to the sitting or standing position and comfortably supported. The cassette is placed so that its upper border is 5 cm (2 in) above the xiphisternum so that the diaphragm is included.

Centre in the mid-line at the level of the middle of the cassette.

Antero-posterior view of the chest. The patient should remain in the same position as for the erect view, with the hands placed so as not to obscure the lung fields. A long focus-film distance, preferably 150 cm (60 in), is used. The upper border of the cassette should be 5 cm (2 in) above the level of the shoulders so that the lung apices are included. The exposure is made on arrested full inspiration.

Centre in the mid-line at the level of the middle of the cassette.

Special circumstances

1. If the patient is too ill to sit upright a lateral decubitus view should be taken. The patient should lie on one side, preferably raised from

the table-top on foam pads. The left lateral decubitus position is usually preferred when the presence of free gas is suspected, as the film will not then include the confusing gastric gas bubble. The hands are placed by the head so that they do not obscure any part of the abdomen. The cassette is supported vertically behind or in front of the patient, with its upper border 5 cm (2 in) above the level of the xiphisternum so that the diaphragm is included. A horizontal beam is used.

Centre in the mid-line at the level of the middle of the cassette.

2. If the patient is too ill to sit up, a supine view of the chest is taken.

Supplementary view

Prone. With children, the use of the prone position is recommended to detect the site and presence of an obstruction and to separate bowel loops and free gas (Berdon *et al.*, 1968). The child lies prone, with the pelvis positioned symmetrically. A cassette large enough to include the whole abdomen is used, with its lower border at the level of the symphysis pubis.

Centre in the mid-line at the level of the middle of the cassette.

URINARY TRACT

Basic views

Antero-posterior (K.U.B.). The patient lies supine with the pelvis positioned symmetrically and the knees flexed over a small pillow for comfort. Two radiographs are taken:

1. A 35 × 43 cm (17 × 14 in) cassette is used, with its lower border including the symphysis pubis.

Centre in the mid-line at the level of the middle of the cassette.

2. A 24 × 30 cm (12 × 10 in) cassette is used for the kidney region. It is placed transversely with its lower border 2·5 cm (1 in) below the iliac crests. For a very large patient a 30 × 40 cm (15 × 12 in) cassette may be needed.

Centre in the mid-line at the level of the middle of the cassette.

Supplementary views

LIVER
This is seen as an area of increased density on the right side of the upper abdomen. It extends from the right dome of the diaphragm,

across the mid-line and down to the lower costal margin. Its lower border is usually visible because of adjacent pericolic fat.

Antero-posterior. The patient lies supine. A 35 × 43 cm (17 × 14 in) cassette is used transversely with its lower border at the level of the iliac crests. Low kilovoltage (50 to 60 kV) is used for maximum soft tissue differentiation.

Centre in the mid-line at the level of the middle of the cassette.

SPLEEN

This is situated on the left side of the upper abdomen, under the diaphragm, and may be visible in obese patients because of adjacent pericolic fat.

Antero-posterior. The patient lies supine. A 24 × 30 cm (12 × 10 in) cassette is used, with its lower border at the level of the lower costal margin. Low kilovoltage is used.

Centre in the mid-clavicular line, at the level of the middle of the cassette.

SUPRA-RENAL GLANDS

These are small endocrine glands situated one above each kidney.

Antero-posterior. The patient lies supine. A 24 × 30 cm (12 × 10 in) cassette, placed transversely, is used, with its lower border at the level of the lower costal margin.

Centre in the mid-line at the level of the middle of the cassette.

ADDITIONAL EXAMINATIONS

Scintigraphy (p. 63). *Ultrasonography* (p. 70). *C.T. scanning* (p. 52). *Other examinations* appropriate for the site of primary disease in the abdomen.

27

Skeletal survey

A skeletal survey is the radiographic demonstration of the whole skeleton. It is performed:

1. To exclude the possibility of a specific disease, e.g. Paget's disease in a patient with suspected osteomalacia.

2. To demonstrate further evidence of a specific disease, in which case the examination is limited to those areas most likely to show it, e.g. the joints in a patient with generalised arthropathy.

3. To exclude the possibility of metastases in a patient with a known primary neoplasm or to demonstrate the axial skeleton in a patient with known metastases—but in both these cases bone scintigraphy (if available) followed by radiography of suspicious areas, is often preferred instead.

The type and extent of the examination must be determined by the radiologist for each particular case. It may be (*a*) a bone survey or (*b*) a joint survey, either of which may be a full or a limited examination, depending on the patient's presenting clinical problem.

The examination is bound to be a lengthy one. It should therefore be planned carefully in advance so as not to take longer than necessary and to involve the minimum number of moves for the patient, thus causing him as little pain or distress as possible.

If available, an X-ray table with a sliding top should be used as this makes the examination easier for both patient and radiographer. All necessary accessories, e.g. foam pads, sandbags, gonad protection, should be at hand.

The radiographic technique depends on the extent of the survey and the condition of the patient. Before commencing the examination, the radiographer must know the precise scope of the examination and the specific views that are required and the order in which they are going to be taken.

If a full skeletal survey is required, each bone and each joint must be demonstrated on at least one radiograph but, by taking unorthodox views, it may be possible to include more than one joint or bone on the same radiograph. If the patient's condition permits, the following scheme will serve as a basis, but with experience the radiographer will vary this scheme to suit the apparatus and other facilities available.

The patient standing:

1. Chest, postero-anterior (p. 184).
2. Cervical spine, lateral (p. 110).
3. Skull, lateral (p. 92).

These radiographs are processed and checked.

4. Hands and wrists, dorsi-palmar (p. 143).

The patient is then placed on the X-ray table.

The patient lying supine, with the knees flexed and the soles of the feet on the table:

5. Thoracic spine, antero-posterior (p. 118).
6. Lumbar spine, antero-posterior (p. 120).

These two radiographs are processed and checked for (*a*) tube/grid alignment (*b*) artefacts and (*c*) exposure factors, which depend on the patient's bone condition, e.g. Paget's disease (for which increased kilovoltage is needed) or osteomalacia (for which decreased kilovoltage is needed).

7. Feet, dorsi-plantar (p. 160).

The patient lying supine, with the legs extended:

8. Pelvis and upper femora, antero-posterior (p. 147).
9. Femora, antero-posterior from the knees upwards (for which a 35×43 cm cassette is needed).
10. Tibiae, fibulae and ankles, antero-posterior (for which a 35×43 cm cassette is needed).
11. Right humerus and scapula, antero-posterior (for which a 35×43 cm cassette is needed).
12. Right radius and ulna, antero-posterior (p. 139).
13. Left radius and ulna, antero-posterior (p. 139).
14. Left humerus and scapula, antero-posterior (for which a 35×43 cm cassette is needed).

These radiographs are processed and if an abnormality is demonstrated on any of the radiographs, a full radiographic examination of that area is carried out.

If the patient is unable to stand, it will probably be found convenient to take the radiographs in the following order:

(*a*) Supine views 5 to 14.
(*b*) Lateral views 2 and 3, using a horizontal beam.
(*c*) Antero-posterior view of the chest taken with the patient sitting if possible, otherwise lying supine.
(*d*) Dorsi-palmar view 4.

Part III

RADIOLOGICAL PROCEDURES

28

Contrast media

The absorption of X-rays by the tissues of the body, and thus their radiographic density, depends on the atomic weight of the principal substances of which the tissues are composed. With the exception of bone and certain calcified structures that contain calcium and other radiopaque salts, most of the tissues (including the skin, muscle and abdominal viscera) are composed of carbon, hydrogen and oxygen which have low atomic weights and display very small differences in density. Bone is intrinsically denser than other tissues; fat and gas are less dense.

The differences in density (i.e. radiographic contrast) between bone, muscle, fat and gas form the basis of plain film radiography. Bone, which besides having a high inherent density is surrounded by soft tissues and is filled with bone marrow, provides a wide range of densities. Certain structures that contain air, such as the lungs and the paranasal sinuses, provide high contrast with adjacent bony structures. The outline of the kidney is visible on a plain film because it is surrounded by peri-nephric fat, but the pelvi-calyceal pattern is not visible. Similarly, the fine structures of many organs are not delineated by adjoining fat and bone, and detail is not visible because of lack of contrast. Artificial methods of delineating such organs are required and so a suitable contrast medium is employed.

The contrast medium may have either a high atomic weight and provide positive contrast or a low atomic weight and provide negative contrast. Examples of positive contrast media are barium sulphate and organic iodine compounds. Examples of negative contrast media are gases such as air, oxygen and carbon dioxide.

The contrast medium may be introduced by one of several methods. It may be (a) injected intra-vascularly (b) administered and then concentrated or excreted by the organ under examination, as in excretion urography and cholecystography (c) ingested, as in a barium meal examination (d) injected directly into the site of interest, as in retrograde pyelography or (e) injected and then caused to move (usually by postural means) to the site of interest, as in pneumography.

All these methods demonstrate the anatomy of the required part; some also test function.

The selection of the appropriate contrast medium is governed by five important factors:

1. It must be non-toxic and must be safe both locally where administered, and elsewhere if there is a possibility of leakage.

2. It must produce adequate contrast. A very dense contrast medium must be used in cases where the contrast medium will be diluted immediately after injection (as in percutaneous transplenic portal venography) or where the vessel being examined has a very small calibre (as in sialography). In some examinations (e.g. choledochography) the contrast medium must not be too dense or small calculi may be obscured.

3. It must have a suitable viscosity. For some examinations (e.g. angiocardiography) a highly fluid contrast medium must be used so that there is no resistance to the contrast medium in the catheter. For examinations where the contrast medium is injected and stays in the organ or dissipates slowly from it (e.g. urethrography or hystero-salpingography) a more viscous contrast medium can be used.

4. It must have a suitable persistence. Some contrast media remain in the body for several years (e.g. after being injected into an abscess in the brain or into the lymphatic system) and are thus of use in assessing progress by continuing to show any change in the size of the contrast-filled lesion, without further injection. If a rapidly dispersing contrast medium is used, a repeat injection is possible within a reasonable length of time if the first attempt proves unsuccessful; thus, for example, an arthrogram can be repeated about 30 minutes after an unsuccessful one.

5. It must have miscibility or immiscibility, as appropriate. For some examinations (e.g. renal cyst puncture) the contrast medium must mix with the contents of the structure into which it is injected. For other examinations it must remain in a bolus; thus in myelography it must not mix with the cerebro-spinal fluid into which it is injected.

Constant research is being undertaken in the improvement of the drugs used as contrast media. Great advances have been made in recent years, particularly in decreased toxicity and increased density. Various pharmaceutical firms manufacture very similar contrast media. With the exception of barium sulphate in suspension, which is used for examination of the alimentary tract, most of the positive contrast media are organic iodine compounds. Detailed description of the chemical composition of these is not within the scope of this book and reference should be made to the literature supplied with their products by the pharmaceutical firms. Reference should also be made to detailed works on the subject (e.g. Miller and Skucas, 1977) or to specialised chapters in certain books (Grainger, 1970; Sutton, 1975). The general groups of contrast media, the concentration of iodine, the proprietary names of commonly used contrast media and the purposes for which they are employed are as follows:

Contrast media in common use

		Iodine content
Alimentary tract		
Barium sulphate suspension		
Numerous proprietary preparations, including amongst those most commonly used:		
Micropaque (colloidal)		
Baritop (with carbon dioxide)		
E-Z-Paque (with sorbitol, smethicone and a dispersing agent)		
E-Z-EM (with flavouring)		
Gastrografin (sodium and meglumine diatrizoate)	76% w/v	370 mg/ml
Gastro-conray (sodium iothalamate)	60% w/v	360 mg/ml
Biliary tract		
(*a*) Oral		
Biloptin (sodium ipodate)		61·4% w/w
Telepaque (iopanoic acid)		66.7% w/w
(*b*) I/V or Infusion		
Biligrafin Forte (meglumine iodipamide)	50% w/v	250 mg/ml
Biligram (meglumine ioglycamide)	35% w/v	176 mg/ml
Biligram (100 ml infusion)	17% w/v	85 mg/ml
Bronchography		
Dionosil aqueous (propyliodone and carboxymethyl cellulose)	50% w/v	280 mg/ml

		Iodine content
Dionosil oily (propyliodone suspension in arachis oil)	60% w/v	340 mg/ml
Lipiodol viscous		540 mg/ml

Hystero-salpingography

Diaginol viscous (sodium acetrizoate plus dextran)	40% w/v	260 mg/ml
Lipiodol viscous		540 mg/ml
Urografin 60 (sodium and meglumine diatrizoate)	60%	292 mg/ml

Laryngography and nasopharyngography

Dionosil aqueous (propyliodone and carboxymethyl cellulose)	50% w/v	280 mg/ml

Lymphography

Lipiodol ultra-fluid (iodised ethyl esters of fatty acids of poppy seed oil)	40% w/v	480 mg/ml

Sialography and dacryocystography

Lipiodol 'F'		520 mg/ml

Myelography

Myodil (mixture of isomers of ethyl iodo-phenyl undecyclate)		300 mg/ml
Pantopaque (iophendylate)	30·5% w/v	300 mg/ml

Radiculography

Dimer X (meglumine iocarmate)	60% w/v	280 mg/ml

Vascular and urographic agents

Angiografin (meglumine diatrizoate)	64%	305 mg/ml
Conray 280 (meglumine iothalamate)	60%	280 mg/ml
Conray 420 (sodium iothalamate)	70%	420 mg/ml
Conray 480 (sodium iothalamate)	80%	480 mg/ml
Cardio-Conray (sodium and meglumine iothalamate)	78%	400 mg/ml
Hypaque 25 (sodium diatrizoate)	25%	150 mg/ml
Hypaque 45 (sodium diatrizoate)	45%	270 mg/ml
Hypaque 65 (sodium and meglumine diatrizoate)	65%	390 mg/ml

		Iodine content
Hypaque 85 (sodium and meglumine diatrizoate)	85%	440 mg/ml
Urografin 30 (sodium and meglumine diatrizoate)	30%	150 mg/ml
Urografin 45 (sodium and meglumine diatrizoate)	45%	220 mg/ml
Urografin 60 (sodium and meglumine diatrizoate)	60%	290 mg/ml
Urografin 76 (sodium and meglumine diatrizoate)	76%	370 mg/ml
Urovison (sodium and meglumine diatrizoate)	58%	320 mg/ml

Miscellaneous

(*a*) Cystography
Steripaque (sterile barium sulphate) 100% w/v

(*b*) Urethrography
Umbradil viscous (diodone in carboxymethyl cellulose jelly) 35% w/v 180 mg/ml

29

Emergencies in the X-ray department

Radiological contrast media containing iodine occasionally cause sensitivity reactions, usually following intravenous injection of the medium. Local anaesthesia may also occasionally cause sensitivity reactions. Reactions to contrast media now occur rarely, as great improvements have been made in recent years to decrease the toxicity of the drugs. Sometimes emergencies occur in the X-ray department which are not directly due to the administration of contrast medium but are due to the patient's presenting illness. Although emergencies are fortunately rare, they do nevertheless occur and every member of the staff of the X-ray department must be familiar with the location of necessary equipment and the routine procedure for dealing with any emergency.

Reactions to contrast media

Minor reactions include urticaria, sneezing, flushing, nausea and vomiting. Usually no treatment is needed other than reassurance and the provision of a vomit bowl.

Major reactions include (a) bronchospasm causing wheezing (b) laryngeal angioneurotic oedema causing choking (c) vascular collapse, when the patient is pale and sweating, has a thready pulse and may lose consciousness. This can lead to cardiac arrest (d) respiratory failure, when the patient becomes cyanosed and may stop breathing and (e) convulsions and coma. All these major reactions require prompt and efficient treatment if the patient is to survive.

The nature of the reactions to contrast media is not fully understood. They are usually of an allergic nature, often Type I—anaphylactoid.

Formerly, prophylactic anti-histamine treatment was often recommended for patients with a history of hay-fever, asthma, eczema or previous reaction to contrast media. Many radiologists now consider this treatment unhelpful (Davies et al., 1975). Special care is needed for infants, the elderly and patients with renal or hepatic failure, mye-loma, heart disease or a history of previous major reaction.

Treatment of reaction. Any emergency is a medical problem and a doctor must be sent for *immediately*. Efficient treatment for a patient who has collapsed depends on the immediate availability of the necessary drugs and equipment. Whenever a contrast medium is being administered, emergency drugs and a supply of oxygen must

---

TREATMENT OF SEVERE REACTIONS FOLLOWING INJECTION OF CONTRAST MEDIA

Severe reactions are predominantly of four types

In any severe reaction:

(a) Release compression
(b) Administer 100% oxygen by face mask and bag
(c) Fetch crash box from . . . .
(d) Emergency Number .

Type	Treatment
GROUP A Anaphylactic type. Mild cases have urticaria, etc. Bronchospasm, oedema of glottis or pulmonary oedema may occur in severe cases.	(a) Piriton 10 mg intravenously. (b) Adrenaline 0·5 ml of 1:1000 subcutaneously. (c) Methyl Prednisolone sodium succinate (Solu-Medrone) 40 mg I/V *or* Hydrocortisone succinate 100 mg I/V. (d) Large French's needle into trachea, via crico-thyroid membrane and give 100% oxygen through it.
GROUP B Generalised convulsions.	(a) 10 mg Diazepam intravenously. Repeat as necessary.
GROUP C Hypotensive with peripheral circulatory failure.	(a) Elevate feet 18 in. (b) Vasoxine 5 mg intravenously and repeat every 3 minutes depending on response. (c) Hydrocortisone succinate 100 mg intravenously. Repeat up to 3 times.
GROUP D Cardiac arrest.	(a) Thump praecordium. External cardiac massage. Elevate feet 18 in. (b) Mouth to mouth respiration. —Air Viva resuscitator (in crash box) —intubate (c) Fetch crash box. Send for ECG and defibrillator.

Fig. 33

CARDIAC ARREST

SIGNS

ALWAYS :   No Pulse - Carotid ... Femoral ... Aorta

Colour   - Pale ... Cyanosed

PERHAPS :   Pupils   - Dilated ... Fixed

In doubt ? ACT NOW think later

① Put patient on hard surface e.g. bed board or floor

② Cardiac massage :

Press hard on lower ⅓ of sternum with heels of both hands 60 times a minute. Allow period for lung inflation.

③ Clear the airway :

Extend head
Push lower jaw forward

④ Inflate the lungs : Use mouth to... { nose / mouth mask Brook airway

or (best) Air Viva with oxygen 12 times a minute

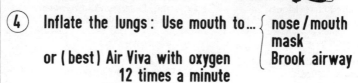

Gary H James

DON'T GIVE UP

Now dial
or   say "Cardiac arrest.................... Ward".

then send for your crash box from ....

and your E.C.G. from ....

Fig. 34

be readily accessible. Oxygen cylinders must be regularly checked and suitable masks and tubing must be available. Emergency drugs are not often required in an X-ray department but the drug cupboard and emergency tray must be regularly checked and drugs must be replaced well before their expiry date.

The radiographer must (*a*) know where the nearest oxygen supply is and how to administer it (*b*) know where the emergency drugs and the key of the D.D.A. drug cupboard are kept (*c*) be able to communicate with the radiologist and be able to get help without leaving the patient, or the room and (*d*) know where to get immediate further help, such as an anaesthetist and a 'crash set'.

Clearly worded instructions are prominently displayed in many hospitals. They usually give information on treatment and how to obtain immediate help. A typical example is shown in Figure 33. Sometimes details of how to carry out external cardiac massage are also given (e.g. Fig. 34).

Basic emergency equipment

Oxygen

If a piped supply is not available, a cylinder of oxygen with about 2 to 3 m (6 to 9 ft) flexible tubing and with suction catheter attached, is needed.

Face masks for adults and children
Airways for adults and children
Anaesthetic rebreathing bag
Endotracheal tubes
Lubricating jelly

Drugs

Piriton
Phenergan
Adrenaline 1:1000
Diazepam
Methyl prednisolone sodium succinate
Hydrocortisone
Aminophyline
Atropine
Aramine
Calcium chloride
Vasoxine

Rogitine
Water for injection
Normal saline
Dextrose injection, 50% w/v, 50 ml

Equipment

Syringes: 2 ml and 10 ml
Intravenous giving set
Endotracheal tubes: various sizes
Disposable needles: various sizes
Disposable drawing-up cannulae
Files for opening ampoules
Scissors
Sphygmomanometer
Stethoscope
Drip stand
Sterile pack containing scalpel and French's needle

30

Angiography

Angiography is the radiographic demonstration of the circulatory system by means of the injection of contrast medium into an artery.

The injection may be made by direct puncture of the required artery or by catheterisation from a distant artery. To demonstrate the circulation adequately, contrast medium must be injected rapidly. Hand injection is adequate for selective injections but an automatic pressure injector is necessary when a large quantity of contrast medium must be injected quickly. This may be either a simple pump (e.g. the Talley Anaesthetic Co. pump) or a more complicated one (e.g. the Gidlund pump or the Cordis pump).

General anaesthesia is often used for angiographic procedures because the injection of contrast medium may cause pain and thus result in movement by the patient. However, the examination can be carried out on adults under local anaesthesia and adequate premedication. Children usually require a general anaesthetic.

A rapid series of films is needed to record full arterial, capillary and venous phases in one region, or the arterial phase only along the whole path of the limb arteries. A hand-changer or single films are adequate for many purposes. In some examinations, particularly angiocardiography, it is preferable to take films in two planes simultaneously, so a bi-plane rapid serial changer is used. Additionally, cinéfluorography and video-tape recording are employed in some cases.

Short exposure times are required to enable several films per second to be taken when a rapid serial changer is used and to avoid recording both arterial and capillary phases on the same film. The generators used must be capable of providing adequate output to allow the required number of films to be taken at very short intervals, particularly when a high milliamperage is being used to keep the exposure time as short as possible.

Preliminary films are taken before all angiographic examinations. They are essential in order to (*a*) check exposure factors, positioning of the patient, coning and preparation of the patient (*b*) select the level for the puncture in aortography and (c) detect any abnormality that may subsequently be seen to be overlying the vessels.

During insertion of the needle, the patient or tube may accidentally be moved and the centering altered. All these points must be checked by the radiographer before the injection is given. If, as sometimes happens, the generator and control panel for one of the tubes in a bi-plane changer are situated in an adjoining room, precautions must be taken to ensure that the control panel is not altered inadvertently once it has been set for the angiogram.

Surgical equipment required. The specific equipment required for each type of angiographic examination depends on the preference of the radiologist but the basic necessities for the sterile trolley are listed where appropriate. When angiography is carried out frequently, the instruments and accessories for the sterile shelf are packed in boxes or bags and autoclaved together so that preparation of the trolley is a relatively simple matter of opening the appropriate boxes and laying out the contents (Chesney and Chesney, 1978).

Aseptic precautions. The X-ray table, X-ray tubes, cables and all accessories should be dusted and wiped with an antiseptic-impregnated cloth some time before the start of the examination. Angiography is performed under strict aseptic precautions. The area of the puncture site is cleansed with a suitable antiseptic (e.g. Hibitane) and the patient is covered with sterile towels.

Contrast medium. The meglumine and/or sodium salts of diatrizoate or iothalamate (e.g. Angiografin, Conray 280 or 420) are normally used, the quantity and strength depending on the part of the vascular system being investigated.

Reactions to contrast medium. These occur less frequently when it is injected into an artery than when it is injected intravenously (Lang, 1965). Hypersensitivity to the contrast medium may result in a minor or major reaction. Oxygen, resuscitation drugs and equipment must always be readily available in any room where angiography is carried out (pp. 211 and 212).

Radiation protection. All X-ray staff and others assisting at the examination, and remaining in the vicinity of the patient when the exposures are made, must wear protective lead aprons, under sterile gowns if these are worn. Lead panels, often suspended from the ceiling on pulleys, are placed round the patient. It is usually possible to cover the patient's pelvis with lead rubber except during examination of the pelvic vessels. This protection must be secured in position before the examination is commenced. Patients undergoing examination of the lower limb vessels are often elderly but with other regions (particularly the heart) patients may be young and unnecessary irradiation of the gonads must be avoided.

Management of a hand-changer. When a hand-changer is used, all those assisting must know the routine of the particular examination. The precise technique will vary with different examinations but there must be a trained team having particular functions and all understanding the simple words of command used (e.g. 'take', 'pull') so that there is no confusion. A trial run, without radiation, will ensure that any new member of the team understands the exact sequence of events.

When several exposures are to be made in quick succession, using a hand-operated exposure switch, the machine must be kept in the 'prepare' position between each exposure.

After-care of the patient. A patient who has just undergone angiography must remain in bed after the investigation so that he can be observed closely for several hours. He usually remains in hospital for 24 hours. When the patient returns to the ward, instructions to the nursing staff must always include frequent observation of the puncture site. Pulse and blood pressure are recorded every 15 minutes for 4 hours, after which they are usually recorded every 4 hours. Temperature and respiration are also usually recorded every 4 hours for 24 hours after the angiogram. Inspection of the puncture site is especially important after catheterisation, when the hole made is larger than that made by direct puncture by a needle.

Further details of patient care following angiography will be found in the works of Saxton and Strickland (1972) and Chesney and Chesney (1978).

Detailed description of all the varieties of angiography will be found in specialised works on the subject (e.g. Sutton, 1962) and the precise procedure is decided by the radiologist carrying out the examination.

Examples will be given of typical examinations using each of the various methods of angiography, namely:

Carotid angiography. Direct puncture of a palpable artery, all films being taken at the same site.

Femoral arteriography. Direct puncture of a palpable artery, a series of films being taken down the length of the limb.

Translumbar aortography. Direct puncture of a non-palpable artery, a test dose being an integral part of the examination.

Arch aortography. Catheterisation from the femoral artery.

Renal arteriography. Selective arteriography from femoral catheterisation, localised views of the renal area being taken. This may be carried out on a screening apparatus.

Angiocardiography. Selective angiography from catheterisation of an arm vein, or sometimes the femoral artery, views in two planes being taken simultaneously.

CAROTID ANGIOGRAPHY

Carotid angiography is used to demonstrate abnormalities of the blood supply to the anterior and middle parts of the brain. The area particularly evaluated by this method is the supratentorial region. The abnormalities which can be detected include vessel occlusion, aneurysms, angiomas and clots. Space-occupying lesions such as cysts, abscesses and tumours can be accurately located by vessel displacement and tumours may also be located by tumour circulation. Haematoma due to bleeding into the extradural or subdural spaces, can also be accurately diagnosed and located for surgical treatment.

If available, C.T. scanning (p. 52) is the investigation of choice for many of the conditions for which carotid angiography would otherwise be performed.

Carotid angiography is carried out either by direct injection of contrast medium into the carotid artery following needle puncture or cannulation, or by a catheter technique from the femoral artery with the tip of the catheter in the common carotid artery. It is usually carried out on a sedated patient under local anaesthesia but children under about 17 years of age and adults who are unable or unwilling to co-operate require general anaesthesia.

A manual film-changer which takes either three or five films can be used but a rapid serial changer may be preferred by the radiologist. The injection is given by hand or by means of a pump. Subtraction (p. 41) is valuable in visualising the vascular pattern, particularly where the image of a vessel (e.g. the ophthalmic artery) is overshadowed by the images of other structures.

Macroangiography (macroradiography, p. 38) improves radiographic definition and can reduce the radiation dose to the eyes by as much as 40 per cent of that received during conventional radiography using a grid. The skull table can be modified quite simply for macroangiography (Lloyd and Ardagh, 1972) and the technique allows vessels as small as 100 μ diameter to be visualised (Hungerford, 1975).

Preparation of the patient

1. Basic skull and chest films must be taken in advance.
2. The patient must have nothing to eat or drink for five hours.
3. All radiopaque objects (e.g. dentures, hairpins) must be removed.

Premedication such as Omnopon and Nembutal is given.

Contrast medium. Angiografin or its equivalent, 10 ml per injection.

Preliminary film (using a basic skull unit). The patient lies supine with the top of the head near the top of the skull table so that later, when positioning for the antero-posterior view, the need for further movement of the patient is minimised. The chin is raised and foam pads are placed under the shoulders and neck so that the neck can be extended. A foam block is placed under the head to raise it from the table so that the whole head is included on the lateral view. The lateral cassette box is pushed down firmly against the patient's shoulder so that the needle point can be seen on the films taken after injection of the contrast medium. The head must be positioned symmetrically, with the median sagittal plane vertical. The X-ray tube is directed horizontally and centred 1 cm ($\frac{1}{2}$ in) above the external auditory meatus. The cone, or light beam diaphragm aperture, should be just large enough to cover the head, the latter being immobilised with a head-band of the type which encircles the head.

Technique. The carotid artery is punctured and saline is infused. The position of the patient's head and the centering of the tube are checked before the protective panels are lowered into position. The injection is made by hand and radiographs are taken to show arterial (Plate XXVII), capillary and venous phases. The intervals between the exposures therefore depend on the patient's circulation rate. Usually the first exposure is made when there are about 2 ml of contrast medium left in the syringe, the next exposure 1 to 2 seconds later and the third (to show the venous phase) 2 seconds later again. If a changer with five cassettes is used, the films are exposed more rapidly. A lateral view of the neck may be required at this stage to show the bifurcation of the common carotid artery, in which case a further injection of contrast medium is given. The needle point must be shown and therefore the cassette must be pushed down into the patient's shoulder and supported. The X-ray tube is centred to the middle of the neck.

For the antero-posterior views, the patient's head is supported by an assistant, the table is lowered and the foam pads are removed, with the exception of a thin wedge-shaped one which is retained under the patient's head. The table is then raised gently and angled slightly (5° to 10°) so that it is easier for the patient to be positioned with the chin tucked in. The tube is then rotated 90° and angled 25° caudad and centred 5 cm (2 in) above the glabella. The head must be positioned symmetrically. The cone or aperture is adjusted to the smaller dimension of the head in this projection. A further injection of contrast medium is given and the antero-posterior series of radiographs is taken. Oblique views may be required at this stage, particularly to obtain further information about an aneurysm. For this, the head is rotated 30° away from the side under examination. The tube is centred 5 cm (2 in) above the mid-point of the superior orbital margin of the side being examined. Further oblique views or per-orbital views may also be required. Saline is infused throughout the examination to keep the needle clear. When all the radiographs have been taken and seen, the needle is removed and pressure applied to the puncture site for at least 5 minutes.

After-care of the patient. See page 215.

Basic trolley setting

Upper (*sterile*) *shelf*

> Angiography needles (e.g. Lindgren)
> Flexible connections, Luer-lok, male to female adaptors
> One 10 ml syringe
> Three 20 ml syringes
> One 2 ml syringe
> Drawing-up cannula
> Two lotion bowls
> Gallipot
> Towels
> Gauze swabs
> Small plastic or mackintosh sheet

Lower (*unsterile*) *shelf*

> Skin cleanser (e.g. Hibitane 0·5% in industrial spirit, blue stain)
> Local anaesthetic (e.g. Procaine 2%)
> Ampoules of contrast medium in bowl of warm water
> Saline
> File (for opening ampoules)
> Disposable needles
> EMERGENCY DRUGS

VERTEBRAL ANGIOGRAPHY

Vertebral angiography is used to demonstrate abnormalities of the blood supply to the posterior part of the brain. It requires almost identical radiography with the exception of increased caudad tilt for the antero-posterior view. Subtraction (p. 41 and Plate II) is frequently used. The examination is usually carried out under general anaesthesia and may be performed by direct puncture of the artery in the neck or by selective catheterisation from the femoral artery.

FEMORAL ARTERIOGRAPHY

Femoral arteriography is performed to investigate the arteries of the lower limb. The whole length of the limb, from the hip joint to the foot, is usually examined.

The examination is usually carried out under local anaesthesia and sedation, but general anaesthesia is necessary for children under about 17 years of age and for apprehensive adults.

Preparation of the patient

1. The patient must have nothing to eat or drink for five hours.
2. Local preparation of the injection site, including shaving of the groins, is carried out.
3. The patient should micturate immediately before the examination.

Premedication. If the examination is being carried out under general anaesthesia, the anaesthetist will prescribe the premedication. If under local anaesthesia, premedication such as Omnopon and Scopolamine is given.

Contrast medium. 20 to 30 ml Conray 280 or its equivalent.

Apparatus. A series of overlapping films is required. A hand-changer which is linked to the tube column can be employed and a series of about five films is taken, the position of the X-ray tube and film being changed for each exposure. An alternative method is to use a film changer which is programmed by a punch card. The punch card controls the exposure sequence, commencement of injection, reduction of exposure factors (if needed) during the series of exposures and the movement of the table-top over the fixed serial changer. The start of transit of the punch card initiates the first exposure.

Preliminary film. The patient lies in the supine position on the

X-ray table, with the limb under examination in the centre of the table. The foot is rotated inwards to separate the leg arteries. It is immobilised in this position with foam pads and sandbags. A preliminary film of the upper thigh is taken. When a non-automatic changer is used, exposure factors for the rest of the limb can usually be easily adjusted from the thigh exposure but if there is any doubt about them further preliminary films must be taken. With a hand-changer, the size of the film is usually 35×43 cm (17×14 in). The upper border of the film is placed at the level of the anterior superior iliac spine.

If a hand-changer is used, the position of the tube for each of the overlapping films is decided and the positions are marked while the preliminary film is being processed. If the tube is floor-mounted, this is most easily carried out by placing markers on the floor. A typical series of films is (a) hip and upper thigh (b) thigh (Plate XXVIII) (c) lower thigh and knee (d) knee and calf and (e) calf and ankle.

A well-trained team is required, a system of verbal commands being used for making the exposures, changing the cassettes and moving the tube. Usually at least four people (radiologist, nurse and two radiographers) are needed unless the movement of the tube or of the table-top is motorised. Exposure factors for each film are in descending order and preferably only one factor (usually the kilovoltage) is changed each time. The anode must be kept rotating throughout the series and the machine is sometimes modified so that it can be kept in the 'prepare' position without pressure on a button having to be maintained, or it may be electronically controlled.

If a punch card programmed changer is used, the movements and exposures are controlled automatically but care is necessary to ensure that everything is correctly set.

Technique. After the anaesthetic (general or local) has been given, the femoral artery is punctured and saline is infused to keep the needle clear. The position of the patient is checked, the lead protection screens are lowered into position and the contrast medium is injected. The series of films is taken according to the pre-arranged plan. After viewing the films, the radiologist may decide to take a further series, according to a different plan, e.g. when the femoral artery is occluded, the circulation is slow and delayed films may be necessary to show the arteries below the occlusion.

At the end of the examination, the needle is withdrawn and pressure is exerted on the injection site for at least five minutes, and longer in certain cases.

After-care of the patient. See page 215.

Basic trolley setting

Upper (sterile) shelf

Two arteriogram needles, with stilettes
Flexible connection, Luer-lok, male to female adaptors
Two 50 ml syringes, all glass
One 10 ml syringe
One 2 ml syringe
One-way tap, male to female, Luer-lok
Drawing-up cannula
Sponge forceps
Two lotion bowls
Gallipot
Gauze swabs
Towels
Gowns

Lower (unsterile) shelf

Skin cleanser (e.g. Hibitane 0·5% in 70% industrial spirit, blue
    stain)
Local anaesthetic (e.g. Lignocaine 2%)
Ampoules of contrast medium in bowl of warm water
Saline
Disposable needles
File (for opening ampoules)
EMERGENCY DRUGS

TRANSLUMBAR AORTOGRAPHY

Translumbar aortography is performed to investigate the aorta and
its major branches, chiefly in the investigation of ischaemic lesions
of the lower aorta and of the iliac arteries. It is particularly useful
when femoral catheterisation is contra-indicated by iliac or femoral
atheroma. It is usually carried out under general anaesthesia.

Preparation of the patient

1. If possible the patient should take a suitable aperient on each
    of the preceding two nights. Sometimes an enema is given
    instead.
2. The patient must have nothing to eat or drink for five hours.

3. Local preparation of the injection site, including shaving if necessary, is carried out.
4. The patient should micturate immediately before the examination.
5. If there is a possibility of barium in the alimentary tract, a plain film of the abdomen must be taken the day before the examination.

Premedication. If the examination is being carried out under general anaesthesia, the anaesthetist will prescribe the premedication. If under local anaesthesia, premedication, such as Omnopon and Scopolamine, is given.

Contrast medium. 20 to 30 ml Conray 420 or its equivalent.

Preliminary film. The patient lies prone with the head turned to one side. The hands are placed above the head or by the sides. Depending on the apparatus being employed, a 35×43 cm (17×14 in) or 35×35 cm (14×14 in) film is used. The lower border of the film is placed at the level of the symphysis pubis. A strip of three metal markers, each 4 cm ($1\frac{1}{2}$ in) apart, is placed on the patient's back with the lowest marker at the level of the fifth lumbar vertebra. The position of each marker is marked on the patient's skin. The X-ray tube is centred to the middle marker. Low kilovoltage, usually about 65 to 70 kV, is used to obtain an image with maximum contrast.

Technique. If the examination is being carried out under general anaesthesia, the preliminary film is taken after induction. When the whole limb is being examined, a series of overlapping films is taken as in femoral arteriography. A hand-changer linked to the tube column can be used, the position of the film and tube being changed before each exposure. Alternatively, a programmed serial changer (p. 219) can be used. A series of five films is taken.

While the preliminary film is being processed, the position of the tube for each film in the series is decided as in femoral arteriography but the positions are slightly different. Usually the lower border of the first film is at the level of the posterior iliac spines, the second includes the whole pelvis and upper femora, the third covers the femora, the fourth the knees and upper part of the legs and the fifth, if used, includes as much as possible of the calves. The exposure factors for the series are in descending order but it must be noted that the second film in the series is of the pelvis and requires adequate exposure.

The abdominal aorta is punctured using a special long (20 or 22 cm) aortogram needle. A test injection of 4 ml of contrast medium is given and one (or sometimes two) radiographs taken and processed without delay. Some radiologists routinely take two films, one during the injection and the other at the end of it, so that it can be seen not only that the needle is correctly sited but also that the contrast medium disperses quickly.

When the needle has been correctly sited, the injection of contrast medium is given by hand as quickly as possible or by a pump.

An intermittent injection of saline, approximately 1 ml per minute, is given throughout the examination. The radiologist may decide to take a further series of films at different intervals. When all the necessary films have been taken, the needle is withdrawn.

After-care of the patient. See page 215.

Basic trolley setting

Upper (sterile) shelf

> Two aortogram needles (Luer-lok, short bevel and flush-fitting stilettes)
> Flexible connection, Luer-lok, male to female adaptors
> Two 50 ml syringes
> Two 20 ml syringes
> One-way tap, male to female, Luer-lok
> Drawing-up cannula
> Sponge-holding forceps
> Gallipot
> Two lotion bowls
> Gauze swabs
> Towels
> Gowns

Lower (unsterile) shelf

> Skin cleanser (e.g. Hibitane 0·5% in 70% industrial spirit, blue stain)
> Ampoules of contrast medium in bowl of warm water
> Saline
> Disposable needles
> File (for opening ampoules)
> Adhesive strapping
> EMERGENCY DRUGS

ARCH AORTOGRAPHY

Arch aortography is performed to investigate abnormalities of the aorta and major branches of the arch, namely the innominate, left subclavian and left carotid arteries. It is carried out by catheterisation from the femoral, or axillary, artery. It is usually performed under local anaesthesia and sedation.

A rapid serial changer is used whenever possible but the examination can be carried out with a manual changer. The progress of the catheter is always under fluoroscopic control, preferably with image intensification and television. Subtraction (p. 41) is frequently employed.

Preparation of the patient

1. The patient must have nothing to eat or drink for five hours.
2. Local preparation of the injection site, including shaving of the groins, is carried out.
3. The patient micturates immediately before the examination.

Premedication. Premedication such as Omnopon and Scopolamine is given.

Contrast medium. 40 ml Conray 420 or its equivalent.

Preliminary film. The patient lies supine, with the thorax over the serial changer, and is then rotated about 45° on to the right side into the right posterior oblique position and is supported in this position by foam pads. The upper border of the film is placed at the level of the lower border of the pinna so that the root of the neck is included on the film. The centering point and limit of the light beam aperture are marked on the patient's skin for speedy centering later.

Technique. The femoral, or axillary, artery is punctured and a guide wire inserted through the needle which is then removed. The guide wire is wiped with a saline-impregnated swab and the catheter is threaded over the guide wire and advanced under fluoroscopic control until the tip of the catheter is in the ascending aorta. A test injection of 5 ml of contrast medium is given and watched on the television monitor. Infusion of heparinised saline is maintained throughout the examination. Although the test dose is usually screened, if there is any doubt whether the catheter has been correctly sited a further test dose is given and a radiograph taken using the undercouch tube. When the catheter is positioned correctly, the patient and the tube are re-positioned and centred and the serial changer is prepared.

The contrast medium is injected using a pressure injector to produce a bolus of contrast medium in the aortic arch. The series of films is taken, usually at 4 per second for 4 seconds. The films are then processed rapidly and when they have been seen, the catheter is removed and pressure applied to the puncture site for at least fifteen minutes, or until there is no further bleeding.

After-care of the patient. See page 215.

Basic trolley setting

Upper (sterile) shelf

Seldinger arterial cannula and trochar *or* Seldinger/Sutton needles (P.E. 160)
Catheter of appropriate size and length (usually Kifa radiopaque catheter)
Guide wire of appropriate size and length
Polythene leader of appropriate length
Connector to fit catheter
Two 50 ml syringes
Two 20 ml syringes
One 2 ml syringe
Drawing-up cannulae
Bard Parker scalpel handle
Surgical ruler
One large receiver
Two lotion bowls
Two gallipots
Sponge-holding forceps
Four towel clips
Operating sheet
Towels
Gauze swabs
Gowns

Lower (unsterile) shelf

Skin cleanser (e.g. Hibitane 0·5% in 70% industrial spirit, blue stain)
Local anaesthetic (e.g. Lignocaine 2%)
Ampoules of contrast medium in bowl of warm water
Heparin
Saline

Disposable needles (for local anaesthetic)
Disposable scalpel blade
File (for opening ampoules)
Adhesive strapping
EMERGENCY DRUGS

INTRAVENOUS AORTOGRAPHY

When direct puncture of the aorta and arterial puncture with insertion of a catheter into the aorta are both unsuccessful (or contraindicated) intravenous aortography is sometimes performed (Ahlberg *et al.*, 1968). In this method, a large quantity of contrast medium (e.g. 100 ml Urografin 76 per cent) is injected via two catheters. These are inserted into the femoral veins so that the tips of the catheters are immediately caudal to the right atrium.

The contrast medium is injected by a pressure pump and delayed films are taken.

SELECTIVE RENAL ARTERIOGRAPHY

Renal arteriography is used in the investigation of space-occupying lesions of the kidney and suspected renal arterial lesions. It is usually carried out under local anaesthesia and sedation, and the radiographs are taken using the under-couch tube and fluoroscopy unit. It is not often necessary to use a rapid serial changer.

Preparation of the patient

1. The patient must have nothing to eat or drink for five hours.
2. Local preparation of the injection site, including shaving of the groins, is carried out.
3. The patient micturates immediately before the examination.

Premedication. Premedication such as Omnopon and Scopolamine is given.

Contrast medium. Conray 280 or its equivalent, 6 to 8 ml per injection.

Preliminary film. The patient lies supine on the screening table. The over-couch tube is used for the preliminary film and a 24×30 cm $(12 \times 10$ in) cassette is placed transversely with its lower border at the level of the iliac crests. Low kilovoltage, about 65 to 70 kV, is used.

Technique. The catheter used has a curved tip. Disposable, pre-formed curved catheters are now available in a range of sizes and shapes of curve. Alternatively, the catheter may be shaped by the radiologist immediately before the examination. This is done by inserting the end of the catheter into boiling water, bending it to the required shape and then immersing it in cold sterile water to stabilise the curve.

The catheter is inserted into the femoral artery by the Seldinger technique and the catheter is adjusted under fluoroscopic control into the orifice of each renal artery in turn. The position of the tip of the catheter is checked by a test injection which is observed on the screen. The tube is then centred to the kidney and the cassette placed in the serial device which is locked into position. The anode is then rotated, the injection is given and the film exposed during the injection to show the arterial branches. The cassette is then changed quickly and a second exposure is made to show the nephrogram phase, the renal vein sometimes being demonstrated as well. These radiographs are examined and further injections are given if needed. Approximately 6 to 8 ml of contrast medium are injected each time.

After-care of the patient. See page 215.

Basic trolley setting

The basic trolley setting is the same as for arch aortography (p. 225).

RENAL MACROANGIOGRAPHY

This is used in the investigation of the small vessel pattern of the kidney, which may help to distinguish between hypertensive and chronic pyelonephritic changes.

The examination is always preceded by standard aortography and selective renal arteriography.

For renal macroangiography, a high speed X-ray tube with a fine focus of 0.28 mm^2 is used, which rotates at 8,500 revs. per minute. It is used in conjunction with a three-phase generator. The focus-film distance is 112·5 cm (45 in) and the focus-patient distance is 37·5 cm (15 in) giving a magnification of 3 : 1 (Sidaway, 1972).

A preliminary film is taken and the field is marked on the patient's skin. Selective arteriography is performed, from which is ascertained the interval elapsing between the injection and the filling of the small vessels in the late arterial phase.

The apparatus is then set up for macroangiography, as for the preliminary film. A further injection of contrast medium is given and, after the appropriate interval previously ascertained, the exposure is made. Usually only one exposure is necessary.

ANGIOCARDIOGRAPHY

Angiocardiography is the radiographic demonstration of the anatomy and functioning of the heart and great vessels, following injection of contrast medium.

Angiocardiography is usually preceded by cardiac catheterisation. This is a combined haemodynamic-radiological study and the role of radiology is (a) to help in directing the catheter through the heart and great vessels (b) to locate the optimum anatomical sites from which blood sampling should be taken and to determine whether this objective has been achieved and (c) to recognise and record when the catheter takes an abnormal course (e.g. from the pulmonary artery through a patent ductus arteriosus to the ascending aorta) (Gordon and Ross, 1977).

During cardiac catheterisation, pressures within the chambers of the heart and great vessels are recorded, samples of blood are taken to measure oxygen saturation and test doses of contrast medium are injected at various sites within the heart and great vessels.

The series of films during angiocardiography is taken using a bi-plane rapid serial changer. Ciné-fluorography is used also (to record dynamic and physiological functions of the heart) with simultaneous video-tape recording so that the ciné 'run' can be viewed on video-tape immediately, without waiting for the ciné film to be processed. Test doses of contrast medium are recorded on video-tape also and played back before each new manœuvre is carried out.

A pressure pump is used for making the injection. This is needed in order to inject a large enough bolus of contrast medium rapidly into a heart chamber so as to avoid too much dilution of the contrast medium and therefore loss of radiopacity.

The examination is usually carried out under local anaesthesia and sedation, except with children, for whom general anaesthesia is required.

Preparation of the patient

1. The patient should have nothing to eat or drink for five hours.

2. When a femoral artery is to be catheterised, the groins must be shaved, if applicable.
3. The patient should micturate immediately before the examination.

Premedication. Premedication such as Omnopon and Scopolamine is given. The examination is usually performed under antibiotic cover.

Contrast medium. Conray 420, Cardio-Conray or their equivalent is used; 1 to 1·5 ml per kg body weight is given, depending on the age of the patient. The quantity may need to be reduced for pulmonary artery and for aortic injections. The maximum volume of contrast medium per injection is usually restricted to 50 ml.

Preliminary films. The patient lies supine on a foam mattress on the angiography table. The arms are placed above the head and the patient is positioned so that the heart is centred to the serial changer. In most departments two or sometimes three control films are taken with differing exposure factors. The selection of exposure factors is based on experience with patients of similar age and weight. The centering points and limits of the light beam diaphragm are marked on the patient's skin for speedy centering later.

Technique. The examination is a relatively long one and the patient must be made as comfortable as possible. The site of insertion of the catheter depends on the particular examination and the diagnostic problem. The catheter is inserted via a vein in the arm or groin for right heart studies and via a brachial or femoral artery for left heart studies. A catheter with a sealed end and six side holes is used. A side-hole catheter is less likely to cause damage to the endocardium than an end-hole catheter because the force of the injection is spread over a wider area. As large a catheter as possible is used in order to obtain the fastest rate of injection of the contrast medium.

The catheter is adjusted under fluoroscopic control using image intensification and television and the position of the tip of the catheter is checked by a test injection of contrast medium which is watched on the screen. When the catheter has been correctly sited, the patient is moved back over the serial changer and the centering is checked. The pressure injector and serial changer are prepared. If local anaesthesia has been used, the patient is warned of the noise that will follow and of a sensation of warmth in the chest that will be felt when the contrast medium is injected. All staff then retire behind lead screens, the injection is given and the series of films is taken. The sequence of films depends on the problem involved but a typical sequence would be 6 films per second for 3 seconds, followed by 1 per second for 6 seconds. After these films have been taken and while they are being processed, the patient is screened again to ensure that no mechanical damage has been done to the heart. In infants, the urinary tract is later screened in order to visualise renal pathology (e.g. congenital abnormality), if present.

After-care of the patient. See page 215.

Basic trolley setting

Upper (sterile) shelf

Cardiac catheter
Catheter extension
Dissecting forceps
Artery forceps (large curved)
Artery forceps (small curved)
Stitch scissors
Retractors
Hooks (sharp and blunt)
Bard Parker scalpel handle and blade
One 10 ml syringe
One 5 ml syringe
Drawing-up cannula
Towel clips
Two-way tap
Three lotion bowls
Three gallipots
Three 20 ml syringes
Gauze swabs
Towels
Gowns
Gloves
Suturing equipment

Lower (unsterile) shelf

Skin cleanser (e.g. Hibitane 0·5% in 70% industrial spirit)
Local anaesthetic
Ampoules of contrast medium in bowl of warm water
Normal saline
Heparinised saline
Disposable needles
EMERGENCY DRUGS

Sterile tray for injection

Syringe for Gidlund or Cordis pump
Two-way tap
Two 50 ml syringes
Drawing-up cannula
Gallipot
Gauze swabs

Additional equipment

Anaesthetic trolley
Defibrillator
Sucker
Electrocardiograph apparatus (for connecting with catheter)
Video-tape recording apparatus

CORONARY ARTERIOGRAPHY

Coronary arteriography is the radiographic demonstration of the coronary arteries by selective catheterisation and injection of contrast medium into each artery. The examination is performed (*a*) where diagnosis of ischaemic heart disease is uncertain on clinical or electro-cardiographic evidence (*b*) where differentiation between ischaemic heart disease and congestive cardiomyopathy is difficult (*c*) before re-vascularisation procedures (e.g. aorto-coronary bypass) are considered (*d*) after re-vascularisation procedures to show patency of the graft(s) and to demonstrate whether there is stenosis or occlusion at the insertion(s) or (*e*) before aortic valve surgery.

The examination is performed under fluoroscopic control, using image intensification and television. If possible, a 'C' arm intensifier is used so that oblique and lateral views can be taken without moving the patient. If this is not available, an X-ray table with a curved top ('cradle') is used, which allows the patient to be rotated into different positions easily and without discomfort. He is made secure in the cradle by means of webbing straps which are fastened by radiolucent 'Velcro'. Before the examination begins, the movement of the cradle should be explained and demonstrated to the patient so that he will not be alarmed when he is rotated during the examination.

A circular collimator for the under-couch tube provides more effective collimation to the shape of the heart and avoids including lung in the area for ciné-fluorography as this will influence the 'E' metre.

Full resuscitation facilities must be immediately available. E.C.G. and catheter pressures are monitored throughout the procedure. The series of injections is recorded by ciné-fluorography and on video-tape. In some departments, a rapid serial changer and 35×35 cm films are used.

Preparation of the patient

1. The patient must have nothing to eat or drink for 4–6 hours.
2. The groins must be shaved.
3. If the patient is on β-blocker drugs (e.g. propanalol) they should not be given for at least 24 hours before the examination, unless such drugs are essential.
4. Postero-anterior and left lateral views of the chest must be taken within the previous 24 hours.
5. The patient should micturate immediately before the examination.

Premedication. Premedication such as Diazepam is given.

Preliminary films. No preliminary films are needed.

Contrast medium. Urografin 370 or its equivalent. A 200 ml bottle for infusion is used and 8–10 ml are injected each time. Fifty ml of Cardio-Conray, or its equivalent, are used for the left ventricular angiogram.

Catheters. There are several types of catheter currently available for coronary arteriography, e.g. Judkins (for the femoral approach and differently shaped for the left and right coronary arteries) and Sones (for the brachial approach and the same shape for each artery). For the left ventricular angiogram which usually completes the examination, a 'pig-tail' catheter is used. This has a curved tip and 12 side holes.

Contrast medium, saline and a manometer line are connected to the catheter by a multi-way connector.

Technique. A method using the femoral approach for catheterisation and employing a curved table-top and ciné-fluorography will be described.

The patient lies supine, covered with a light-weight blanket or sheet so that the straps do not injure his skin, and is made as comfortable and secure as possible. The femoral artery is catheterised by the Seldinger method and the appropriate catheter for the first artery to be demonstrated is manipulated into the ascending aorta and the guide wire is removed. For catheterisation of the right coronary artery, the patient is rotated on to his left side and his hands are placed on his head. The 'E' metre reading is taken at this stage for ciné-fluorography later. The under-couch tube is centred to the heart and the whole of the likely territory of the coronary arteries must be included. The reading is taken on deep arrested inspiration.

When the artery has been catheterised, contrast medium is injected by hand and recorded on ciné film (Plate XXIX) and video-tape. The basic views are usually lateral and right anterior oblique views for the right coronary artery, lateral and both anterior oblique views for the left coronary artery.

More views may be required depending on what has been demonstrated on fluoroscopy. These may include magnified views which are useful to demonstrate graft insertions and to show the left main stem and its branches.

The patient is then rotated back into the supine position, the guide wire is re-inserted into the catheter and the catheter changed. With the patient still in the supine position, the catheter is manipulated into the ascending aorta and the guide wire is removed. When the catheter has been positioned in the left coronary artery, the patient is rotated into the oblique position with his left side raised. Contrast medium is injected and recorded by ciné-fluorography and on video-tape.

On the routine views, the left main stem coronary artery appears foreshortened. For a complete demonstration, a further view—usually a hemi-axial view—is sometimes required. This is most easily performed by using a 'C' arm intensifier. If this is not available, the catheter is removed from the coronary artery and the patient is raised 30–40° into a semi-recumbent position and supported, preferably on an air-filled wedge. The catheter is re-positioned in the left coronary artery and a further injection of contrast medium is made and recorded.

When the coronary arteries have been satisfactorily demonstrated, a pig-tail catheter is positioned in the left ventricle and left ventricular angiography is performed to demonstrate ventricular function. Fifty ml of contrast medium are injected via a pressure injector, at a rate of 10–15 ml per second.

At the end of the examination, the catheter is removed and pressure is applied to the puncture site for about 15 minutes or until there is no further bleeding.

After-care of the patient

1. The patient must lie flat in bed for 24 hours.
2. Temperature, pulse, respiration and blood pressure are

recorded every 15 minutes for 4 hours and then every 4 hours for 24 hours.
3.   The puncture site must be observed regularly.

Basic trolley setting

The basic trolley setting is the same as for arch aortography (p. 225) plus a multi-way connector and appropriate catheters.

OCCLUSION ARTERIOGRAPHY

Trans-catheter occlusion of abdominal arteries may be performed (*a*) to control bleeding—either from the gastro-intestinal tract or from tumour or (*b*) to control the size of a tumour and the symptoms arising from it.

Appropriate selective arteriography is performed and occlusion is achieved by injecting either pharmacological vasoconstrictors (Chuang *et al.*, 1976) or solid particles (e.g. metallic coils, metal or silastic spheres or Gelfoam) to occlude the artery (Goldstein *et al.*, 1976).

31

Venography

PERCUTANEOUS TRANSPLENIC PORTAL VENOGRAPHY

In the portal system, venous blood from the capillaries of the stomach and of the large and small intestine is collected by the portal vein and passes into the liver before returning to the heart. In the liver, the portal vein branches into capillaries and sinusoids within the hepatic tissue. These finally join to form the hepatic veins and pass into the inferior vena cava.

Percutaneous transplenic portal venography is the radiological examination of the portal system following direct injection of contrast medium into the spleen (Plate XXX). The examination is performed mainly to ascertain whether the portal vein is patent and to distinguish intra-hepatic portal obstruction (which is suitable for a portocaval shunt) from pre-hepatic portal obstruction (which is not suitable). It is also performed after a portocaval shunt operation, to show the patency of the vessel. The examination will also demonstrate intra-hepatic portal veins.

Percutaneous transplenic portal venography is usually carried out under local anaesthesia and sedation, except for patients under about 17 years of age who require general anaesthesia. The examination is carried out only on an 'in-patient' so that he can be closely observed afterwards.

Preparation of the patient

1. If there is a possibility of barium in the alimentary tract, a plain film of the abdomen must be taken the day before the examination.
2. If possible, the patient should take a suitable aperient on each of the preceding two nights.
3. The prothrombin time should be checked and corrected if necessary.

4. The patient should have nothing to eat or drink for five hours.
5. The patient should micturate immediately before the examination.

Premedication. If the examination is being carried out under general anaesthesia, the anaesthetist will prescribe the premedication. If under local anaesthesia, premedication such as Omnopon and Scopolamine is given.

Contrast medium. Usually 30 ml of Hypaque 85 per cent or its equivalent.

Radiation protection. Lead rubber is placed over the patient's pelvis, just below the level of the anterior superior iliac spines. Protective lead panels, usually suspended on pulleys from the ceiling, are placed round the patient before the injection is given. All staff remaining in the vicinity must wear lead aprons.

Preliminary film. The patient lies supine. Either a 35 × 43 cm (17 × 14 in) or a 35 × 35 cm (14 × 14 in) film is used, depending on whether a manual or an automatic serial changer is being employed. The lower border of the film is placed at the level of the anterior superior iliac spines. The diaphragm must be included on the film. Some radiologists require a radiopaque marker to be placed on the left tenth rib in the mid-axillary line and its position marked on the patient's skin. The patient is asked to breathe in and out gently and the exposure is made on arrest of this shallow breathing. Low kilovoltage (about 65 kV) must be used to provide optimum contrast which is very important but which may be difficult to obtain in a patient who has ascites.

Management of a hand-changer. As in all examinations where several films are taken using a hand-changer, there must be a routine that is understood by all concerned and the words of command used must be known by all members of the team (p. 215).

Technique. After the anaesthetic (general or local) has been given, an exploring needle with a short bevel (or a needle-catheter) is inserted well into the spleen and as soon as it is correctly sited, the positions of the patient and of the tube are checked. The protective panels are lowered into position and the contrast medium is injected by hand. There should be as little delay as possible between inserting the needle and taking the radiographs. The needle is withdrawn immediately after the injection. (If a catheter is used instead of a needle, the catheter can be left *in situ* and gently perfused with saline while the films are being processed.)

The number of radiographs and the rate at which they are taken is determined by the radiologist for each patient. When a rapid serial changer is used, a typical sequence is one film per second for 10 seconds, followed by six films at two-second intervals. When a hand-changer is used, the films are individually timed by the radiologist, five films usually being taken within 10 seconds. Usually the first three are taken at short intervals, followed by two at longer intervals.

The radiographs are checked and if necessary a second puncture and injection are given.

After-care of the patient

1. The patient must keep still in bed for about 5 hours and must remain in bed for 24 hours.
2. Pulse and blood pressure are recorded every 15 minutes for 4 hours, then pulse, respiration, temperature and blood pressure every 4 hours for 24 hours.
3. If contrast medium has leaked, the patient may have severe pain on return to the ward and appropriate analgesics will be required.

Basic trolley setting

Upper (sterile) shelf

Exploring-type needle with short bevel (Luer-lok, 15 B.W.G. $\times 3\frac{1}{2}$ in) and with flush-fitting stilette
Flexible connection, Luer-lok, male to female adaptors
Two 50 ml syringes
Two 2 ml syringes
Drawing-up cannula
Gallipot
Lotion bowl
Sponge-holding forceps
Gauze swabs
Towels
Gown

Lower (unsterile) shelf

Skin cleanser (e.g. Hibitane 0·5% in 70% industrial spirit, blue stain)
Local anaesthetic (e.g. Lignocaine 2%)

Saline

Ampoules of contrast medium in bowl of hot water (Hypaque 85% or Conray 70% crystallises and must be heated to 43°C, 110°F)

Disposable needles

File (for opening ampoules)

Adhesive strapping

EMERGENCY DRUGS

PERIPHERAL VENOGRAPHY

Peripheral venography is the radiographic examination of the venous system of a limb following injection of contrast medium. The examination is usually carried out on the lower limb, to determine the patency of the deep veins, the competence of valves and the site of incompetent perforating veins. It is also indicated in cases of acute deep vein thrombosis, with or without pulmonary embolism, and of unexplained oedema which may be due to deep vein thrombosis.

The examination is usually carried out under local anaesthesia. The progress of the contrast medium is under fluoroscopic control by the radiologist, preferably using an image intensifier and television.

If possible, the patient is examined in the semi-erect position because this lessens the difficulties of obtaining an adequate demonstration of the deep venous system and is of great value in functional studies of incompetence (Pim, 1972). However, this position is not always possible, especially when the patient has acute venous thrombosis and may be too incapacitated to stand, but in such cases the patient can usually be tilted 20° to 30° feet-down.

Preparation of the patient

1. The patient must have nothing to eat or drink for five hours.
2. The patient should micturate immediately before the examination.

Premedication. Usually, premedication such as Omnopon is given.

Contrast medium. 30 to 50 ml meglumine iothalamate 60 per cent (e.g. Conray 280).

Preliminary film. A postero-anterior view of the knee is taken, using the under-couch tube. The exposure factors required for the thigh and leg can be determined from this and further preliminary films are not usually taken.

Technique. To occlude the superficial veins, compression is applied just above the ankle and, in some cases, just below the knee also. This compression is most satisfactorily carried out by inflatable cuffs about 5 cm (2 in) wide. The patient is then instructed in the Valsalva technique which is required for each film. This is most easily explained by asking the patient to take a deep breath and then to breathe out hard while keeping the mouth closed and pinching the nose between the fingers. This manœuvre has the effect of distending the veins and demonstrating the efficiency of the valves.

The leg being examined is internally rotated to separate the images of the tibia and fibula. The ankle is compressed in order to engorge the veins of the foot. A small needle attached to a flexible polythene connection (or a 'Butterfly' needle) is inserted into a vein on the dorsum of the foot and is firmly strapped in position by adhesive tape. Saline is infused throughout the examination. The cuffs are fully inflated and the injection of contrast medium is given. The progress of the contrast medium along the limb vessels is watched on the television monitor and 35 × 43 cm (17 × 14 in) films are taken as required, using the under-couch tube, one of the first being of the ankle to see if occlusion of the superficial veins has been satisfactory. Before each radiograph is taken the patient is asked to perform the Valsalva manœuvre. When all the required radiographs have been taken and seen, the needle is removed.

Usually, by controlling the cuffs and the tilt of the table, it is possible to demonstrate the iliac veins satisfactorily as far as the origin of the inferior vena cava.

After-care of the patient. As soon as the effects of the premedication have worn off, the patient is encouraged to walk about, in order to prevent phlebitis.

Basic trolley setting

Upper (sterile) shelf

Scalp vein set *or* 'Butterfly' needles, sizes 19 and 23
Two 20 ml syringes
Two 50 ml syringes
Flexible connections
'Y'-shaped connector
Drawing-up cannula
Gallipot

Towels
Gauze swabs
Gown

Lower (unsterile) shelf

Skin cleanser (e.g. Hibitane 0·5% in 70% industrial spirit)
Local anaesthetic (e.g. Lignocaine 1%)
Ampoules of contrast medium in bowl of warm water
Disposable needles
File (for opening ampoules)
Saline
Adhesive strapping
EMERGENCY DRUGS

INTRA-OSSEOUS VENOGRAPHY

Intra-osseous venography is used mainly to demonstrate venous networks, such as the vertebral plexus and the lumbo-azygos system, that cannot be demonstrated by other means. It is also used to replace or supplement conventional venography (Isherwood, 1964) and is particularly useful in demonstrating the inferior vena cava, often combined with synchronous femoral venography of the opposite limb, when other techniques have not succeeded.

When contrast medium is injected into the bone marrow it is taken up by the local venous drainage. There are several sites possible for injection (Schobinger, 1960) and the site selected will depend on the clinical problem and the region to be demonstrated. The most usual sites are the vertebral spinous processes (to show the vertebral and lumbo-azygos systems), the ribs (to show the superior vena cava), the greater trochanters (to show the pelvic veins and the inferior vena cava) and the malleoli (to show the veins of the lower limbs).

The examination is performed under general anaesthesia. If the patient is not already an 'in-patient' he should be admitted for the nights before and after the examination and remain in hospital for about 24 hours after it.

The technique employed in cases where the injection is made into a spinous process will be described here. The whole spine must have been examined radiographically before the examination is performed.

Preparation of the patient

1.   The patient must have nothing to eat or drink for five hours.
2.   The patient should micturate before the examination.

   Premedication. Premedication will be prescribed by the anaesthetist.
   Contrast medium. 20 ml Hypaque 45 per cent or its equivlaent.
   Apparatus. If available, a bi-plane serial changer is used; if not,
a manual changer.
   Preliminary films. The patient lies prone. A postero-anterior
view, and a lateral view using a horizontal beam, are taken. The level
of the injection and thus the area covered by the films will depend
on the clinical problem and the technique being employed. The purpose of the lateral view is to assess the angle of inclination of the
spinous processes.
   Technique. For injection into the thoracic or lumbar regions, the
patient lies prone. For injection into the cervical region, the sitting
position is usually preferred.
   A bone marrow needle is inserted into the selected vertebral
spinous process and heparinised saline is gently infused throughout
the examination.
   A test injection, of 5 ml contrast medium, is given and a lateral
view is taken using a horizontal beam. If this shows the needle to be
correctly sited, the full dose of contrast medium is given and a series
of films is taken. If a bi-plane rapid serial changer is being used, about
10 films are taken at one-second intervals. If a manual changer is
being used, about five films are taken at two-second intervals and
a second injection is then given and a series of lateral films taken.
   When the radiographs have been viewed a further series of films
with the patient in the oblique position may be necessary. When all
the required radiographs have been taken, a further injection of
heparinised saline is given and the needle is then removed.

After-care of the patient

1.   Pulse and respiration are recorded every 15 minutes for 4
      hours.
2.   After the patient has recovered from the anaesthetic, he need
      not necessarily remain in bed.

Basic trolley setting

Upper (sterile) shelf
   One bone marrow needle (e.g. Lea Thomas needle)

Polythene connection 60 cm (24 in) long, male to female
    connection, Luer-lok
Two-way tap
Two 30 ml syringes
Two 20 ml syringes
Drawing-up cannula
Lotion bowl
Gallipot
Gauze swabs
Towels
Gown

Lower (unsterile) shelf

Skin cleanser (e.g. Hibitane 0·5% in 70% industrial spirit)
Ampoules of contrast medium
Disposable needles
Saline
File
Masks
EMERGENCY DRUGS

FRONTAL VENOGRAPHY
(Orbital phlebography)

This examination is performed in the radiological investigation of
proptosis. By demonstrating the position of the orbital veins, it helps
to identify the exact location of an abnormal mass in the orbit. In
addition to the venous system of both orbits, the cavernous sinus,
inferior petrosal sinus and jugular bulb are demonstrated (Lloyd,
1972).

Subtraction (p. 41) plays an important part in the examination.
Macroradiography (p. 38) is also recommended (Lloyd, 1972) to
demonstrate the very small-calibre vessels.

Either a manual film-changer which takes three or five films, or
a rapid serial changer, may be used.

Preparation of the patient

1.   Recent radiographs of the skull, including occipito-mental
     and over-tilted occipito-mental views (p. 95) must be
     available.

2. All radiopaque objects (e.g. dentures, hair pins) must be removed.

Premedication. Usually no premedication is required, but children may require sedation.

Contrast medium. 10 to 15 ml mcglumine diatrizoate (e.g. Angiografin).

Preliminary film. An under-tilted submento-vertical (over-tilted occipito-mental) view is taken. The patient lies supine, with the chin raised and the neck hyper-extended. The X-ray tube is angled cephalad so that it makes an angle of 75° to the base line.

Centre to the lower border of the orbits.

Technique. A thick rubber band is placed round the forehead at the hair margin, to prevent reflux of contrast medium over the scalp. The injection of contrast medium is given by hand, into the frontal or supra-orbital vein, using a scalp vein needle. During the injection, the flow of blood in the facial veins is occluded by finger pressure, by the patient himself (Lloyd, 1970). The series of radiographs is taken and these are subtracted.

A series of lateral radiographs may then be required, for which a further injection of contrast medium is given. A horizontal beam is used.

After-care of the patient. Usually no special after-care is necessary.

Basic trolley setting

Upper (sterile) shelf
  One scalp vein needle
  One 30 ml syringe
  One 20 ml syringe
  One 10 ml syringe
  Drawing-up cannula
  Gallipot
  Gauze swabs
  Gown
  Towels

Lower (unsterile) shelf
  Skin cleanser
  Local anaesthetic
  Contrast medium
  Disposable needles
  EMERGENCY DRUGS

JUGULAR VENOGRAPHY

This examination is performed to demonstrate glomus jugulare tumours, which grow into the jugular bulb at the point where it passes through the jugular foramen. Jugular venography is carried out by direct puncture of the jugular vein in the neck. The vein must be occluded between the puncture site and the clavicle and the contrast medium is injected retrogradely. A series of radiographs of the skull is taken.

Retrograde catheterisation of the jugular vein can also be performed, usually for the purpose of taking blood samples at different levels in order to locate the site of a parathyroid tumour.

PARATHYROID VENOGRAPHY

The purpose of this examination is to locate suspected parathyroid tumours pre-operatively. Veins draining the parathyroid glands can be catheterised selectively via the femoral vein, using the Seldinger technique. Samples of blood are withdrawn and the level of parathormone is assayed. It is also possible to demonstrate tumours by hand injection of contrast medium into the thyroid and parathyroid glands. Conray 280, or its equivalent, is used and serial films are taken.

SUPERIOR VENA CAVOGRAPHY

The purpose of this examination is to assess superior vena cava thrombosis or compression of the superior vena cava by carcinoma of the bronchus. It is occasionally performed before and after radiotherapy on patients with carcinoma of the bronchus.

A catheter is inserted into each subclavian vein by the Seldinger technique and advanced under fluoroscopic control to the level of the axillary veins. The two catheters are attached to a 'Y'-shaped connector and contrast medium (50 ml Hypaque 45 per cent or its equivalent) is injected into both arms simultaneously. A series of radiographs of the chest, usually at 6 per second for 4 to 6 seconds, is taken using a rapid serial changer.

INFERIOR VENA CAVOGRAPHY

This examination is performed to demonstrate (*a*) displacement or compression of the inferior vena cava by tumour and (*b*) thrombus formation in the iliac veins or vena cava.

Both common femoral veins are punctured directly and the needles are connected via flexible polythene tubing to a 'Y'-shaped connector attached to a syringe. The contrast medium (50 ml Conray 420 or its equivalent) is injected simultaneously and a series of radiographs of the abdomen, usually at 1 to 2 per second for 10 seconds, is taken using a rapid serial changer.

RENAL AND ADRENAL PHLEBOGRAPHY

This examination is performed (*a*) to investigate cases of renal vein thrombosis (*b*) to demonstrate adrenal tumours by adrenal vein blood sampling (*c*) to assess prospective renal transplant donors and (*d*) occasionally, but now less frequently, to demonstrate renal or other retro-peritoneal tumours.

A pre-curved renal catheter is inserted into the renal artery by the Seldinger technique and the catheter is adjusted under fluoroscopic control until it is in the orifice of the renal artery. The femoral vein is then catheterised by the Seldinger technique and a catheter with a long curve is introduced into the main renal vein. 20 mg adrenaline in saline are injected through the arterial catheter and, 20 to 30 seconds later, the contrast medium (15 to 20 ml Conray 420 or its equivalent) is injected into the renal vein at a pressure of 4 kg per cm².

A series of radiographs, usually 1 per second for 6 seconds, is taken using a rapid serial changer.

32

Lymphography

Lymphography is the radiographic examination of the lymphatic system following the injection of contrast medium. The injection is given after cannulation of a lymph vessel, usually on the dorsum of the foot, although the hand, mastoid area, or spermatic cord is sometimes used.

Lymphography is undertaken in the investigation of disease of lymph vessels or lymph nodes, including metastatic carcinoma, sarcoma or multiple myeloma. In cases of lymphoma, it is particularly helpful in demonstrating whether the abdominal lymph nodes are involved—even if there is no clinical evidence—thus staging the disease.

Lymphography is most frequently performed on adults, usually under local anaesthesia. A child can usually be examined under heavy sedation but general anaesthesia may be necessary. A nurse must remain with the child throughout the examination.

Contra-indications

The examination is contra-indicated in patients (*a*) with impaired respiratory function (*b*) in heart failure (*c*) who have recently received radiotherapy to the chest or to the lymph nodes being investigated (*d*) who have recently been treated with anti-metabolic drugs or (*e*) who have a known sensitivity to any of the agents used in the examination.

The method of pedal lymphography (i.e. the injection being into a lymphatic vessel in the foot) in an adult is as follows:

Preparation of the patient

1. It must be ensured that there are no contra-indications to the examination.
2. If there is oedema of the legs, they should be elevated for at least 24 hours before the examination and in severe cases

bound with crêpe bandages from thighs to toes. For this, the patient may have to be admitted to hospital.

3. The patient must have had a recent radiograph of the chest. Usually this is taken immediately before the lymphogram.
4. The feet must be shaved if necessary.
5. The procedure must be carefully explained to the patient, including the necessity for keeping the feet perfectly still during the cannulation and injection. He should be warned that he may look ill for 24 hours owing to the absorption of the blue dye and that his urine will be blue. Both he and his relatives should be reassured about this.
6. The patient should be told that the examination will take a long time and be invited to bring something to read.
7. The patient should micturate immediately before the examination.
8. If the patient is not already an in-patient, he is usually admitted to hospital for the night following the first part of the examination.

Premedication. Premedication is not usually necessary because lymphography should be a painless procedure but if the patient is unduly apprehensive sedation is given. If he has pain, particularly spinal pain, analgesics are needed to enable him to lie perfectly still on his back for the necessary time.

Contrast medium. An oil-based contrast medium (e.g. Lipiodol Ultra Fluid) is nearly always used. Most of the contrast medium outlines the lymphatic vessels. Within 15 minutes or so of completing the injection, the cisterna chyli and thoracic duct can be shown, particularly if the patient is active during this interval. From the thoracic duct, minute globules of contrast medium are discharged slowly into the subclavian vein. These globules are too large to traverse the pulmonary capillaries and 24 hours after the injection pin-point high-density opacities can usually be seen in a chest radiograph. Their presence in the lungs causes temporary depression of respiratory function which is greatest within the first day or so and is not noticed by the patient unless he already has poor respiratory function. The remainder of the contrast medium outlines the abdominal lymph nodes and is released more slowly over several months or even a year.

Water-soluble contrast medium (Kinmonth and Taylor, 1954) has been used to demonstrate the distal lymphatic vessels but, because it diffuses so rapidly into the circulation, it cannot demonstrate the lymphatic nodes.

Method of injection. The viscosity of the oily contrast medium and the time taken for it to pass through the catheter and the lymphatic vessels make an automatic injector essential (Kinmonth, 1972). Because the injection must be given over a period of one to two hours, it is impossible to maintain a steady injection by hand, especially when contrast medium is being injected into both legs simultaneously. The injector used is usually either electrically driven or of the simple gravity-feed type. In the former, the syringes are horizontal and the rate of injection can be controlled by means of a variable ratio gear box. In the latter, the syringes are vertical and a number of 5 kg weights placed on the plungers control the rate of injection.

Preliminary film. An antero-posterior view of the abdomen is taken. The patient lies supine. A 35 × 43 cm (17 × 14 in) cassette is used, with its lower border at the level of the symphysis pubis.

Centre in the mid-line, at the level of the iliac crests.

Technique. Usually, an attempt is made to cannulate a vessel in each foot. Occasionally—e.g. if the patient has diminished respiratory reserve—one side only may be examined at a time, in which case it is usually preferable to do the right side first because the incidence of cross-over of lymph vessels from the right to the left side of the abdomen is greater than from the left to the right (Jackson and Kinmonth, 1974).

Two ml of patent blue violet dye (2·5 per cent) are mixed with an equal volume of local anaesthetic (e.g. Lignocaine 1 per cent). Under aseptic conditions, 0·5 ml of this mixture is injected into the two medial web spaces of each foot. These injections can be given in the ward, about one hour before the patient comes to the X-ray department. The patient is encouraged to move both his feet freely so that the dye is absorbed by the lymphatics thus making them visible.

The patient is made as comfortable as possible on the X-ray table. The feet are supported and immobilised. A convenient method of achieving this is by means of a large foam polythene pad, which has depressions cut in it to accommodate the feet. This pad rests on a rigid plastic 'tunnel' under which a cassette can be placed without disturbing the patient's feet (Fig. 35). Foam pads are placed under the calves, knees and thighs so that he is supported as comfortably as possible and can keep the feet and legs still for the required length of time. The patient's position is not moved again until the injection of contrast medium is completed.

The examination is carried out under strict aseptic conditions.

The feet are cleansed with a suitable antiseptic and are placed in sterile towels on the foam support. Local anaesthetic is injected and an incision is made over one of the lymphatic vessels (visible as thin

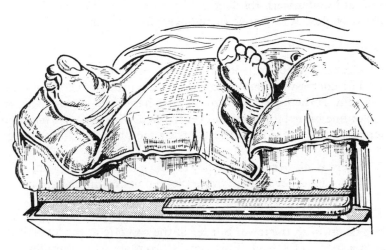

Fig. 35

blue lines stained by the blue dye), usually over the navicular bone. The vessel is cleared from surrounding tissue.

Various methods of cannulation are practised. In some departments, a needle attached to a long polythene connection is used (Kinmonth, 1972) while in others a fine polythene catheter, which may be inserted for some distance, is used. Before inserting either the needle and connection or the catheter, the whole system must be tested for leaks by filling with saline. A lymphatic vessel in each foot is cannulated in almost all cases. A bright light is essential for this part of the examination and some radiologists wear magnifying spectacles.

When the vessel has been cannulated, and the needle or catheter tied in place with silk, the syringe containing contrast medium is attached to the end of the polythene connection or catheter and the injection is started. The time when the injection is started and the amount of contrast medium in each syringe are noted. If the patient experiences pain due to the injection, this may be caused (*a*) by contrast medium having extravasated (when the rate of injection should be decreased) or (*b*) by dermal back-flow (when it may be necessary to stop the injection).

On completion of the injection, the needles or catheters are removed and, if necessary, a further injection of local anaesthetic is given, and the incisions are sutured and covered with dry dressings which can be held in place by transparent adhesive tape strapped round and underneath the feet.

Film series. A sequence of radiographs is taken:

To control injection

Control of the injection is important to ensure that:

1. The contrast medium is going into a lymphatic vessel and not into a vein. If the injection is into a lymphatic, the appearances are those of fine branching vessels, evenly filled with contrast medium, whereas if it is into a vein, the contrast medium will form 'beads' and pool.
2. There is no dermal back-flow.
3. There is no abnormal lymphatic-venous communication.
4. The correct volume of contrast medium is injected.

Foot and ankle. An antero-posterior view of the foot, ankle and calf is taken, with the lower border of the cassette at the level of the plantar aspect of the heel. This view is taken about 10 minutes after the start of the injection because that is the time required for the contrast medium to displace the saline in the polythene connection or catheter and reach the foot.

Knees. A few minutes later, an antero-posterior view of the knees is taken, using the Bucky grid and a 35×43 cm (17×14 in) cassette placed transversely.

Centre between the knees at the level of the lower border of the patellae.

Thighs. About five minutes later, an antero-posterior view of the thighs is taken, using a 35×43 cm (17×14 in) cassette with its upper border at the level of the anterior superior iliac spines.

Centre between the thighs, at the level of the middle of the cassette.

Pelvis and upper thighs. About 10 minutes later, an antero-posterior view of the pelvis and upper thighs is taken, using a 35×43 cm (17×14 in) cassette placed transversely. Its upper border is placed at the level of the iliac crests.

Centre in the mid-line, at the level of the middle of the cassette.

Abdomen. About 10 minutes later, an antero-posterior view of the abdomen is taken, using a 35×43 cm (17×14 in) cassette. The light-beam diaphragm is restricted laterally so that the area covered on the radiograph is a little wider than the sacro-iliac joints. The exposure is made on arrested expiration.

Centre in the mid-line, at the level of the iliac crests.

Views of the abdomen are taken every 15 minutes or so until the contrast medium has reached the level of LV3 or the maximum dose (5–7 ml per side if both sides have been injected or 10 ml if only one side has been injected) has been given.

Macroradiography (p. 38) can be used to demonstrate small filling defects in the nodes.

Two hours after completion of the injection

Pelvis and upper thighs (Plate XXXI). As for control of injection.

Abdomen. As for control of injection but centred to the level of the lower costal margin.

Chest. The patient remains in the supine position. The upper border of a 35×43 cm (17×14 in) cassette is placed at the level of the angle of the jaw. The exposure is made on arrested inspiration. The exposure factors required are the same as those for an antero-posterior view of the thoracic spine. The thoracic duct is usually demonstrated, superimposed on the thoracic spine and curving to the left where it enters the subclavian vein.

Centre to the cassette.

24 hours after the injection

Chest. An erect postero-anterior view of the chest is taken. There must be no movement blur. Low kV, 60–65 kV, will show the small oil emboli more readily.

Pelvis and upper thighs. The patient lies supine. A 35×43 cm (17×14 in) cassette is used, with its upper border at the level of the iliac crests.

Centre in the mid-line, at the level of the middle of the cassette.

Abdomen. The patient lies supine. A 35×43 cm (17×14 in) cassette is used. This radiograph serves also as the preliminary film for the excretion urogram, so the kidney area must be demonstrated.

Centre in the mid-line, 2·5 cm (1 in) cephalad to the iliac crests.

Excretion urography. This is not performed routinely but is of value if (*a*) the lymphogram shows an abnormality or suspected abnormality—to demonstrate whether there is any displacement of the urinary tract by abnormal nodes (*b*) the position of the kidneys has not been shown on earlier radiographs but is necessary clinically, e.g. for radiotherapy planning or (*c*) there are clinical indications, e.g. in a patient with carcinoma of the bladder or cervix (Walker *et al.*, 1977). Excretion urography is not performed on patients whose abnormalities are only congenital.

Full-length views are taken, using 35 × 43 cm (17 × 14 in) cassettes. No compression is used. Usually 60 ml of Conray 420, or its equivalent, are injected intravenously. A radiograph of the abdomen is taken immediately after the injection is completed, to show the nephrogram phase. Further antero-posterior radiographs are taken at five and 15 minutes. As soon as the ureters are well filled with contrast medium—usually between 10 and 15 minutes—the following views are taken:

1. *Posterior obliques*. The patient is rotated 45° towards each side in turn and is supported on foam pads.

Centre in the mid-clavicular line of the raised side, at the level of the iliac crest.

2. *Lateral*. The patient lies on his side, with the knees flexed slightly to aid balance, and with the hands on the pillow. A narrow light-beam diaphragm aperture is used to reduce secondary radiation and improve definition.

Centre 10 cm (4 in) anterior to the spinous processes, at the level of the iliac crest.

3. *Antero-posterior*. The patient lies supine.

Centre in the mid-line, at the level of the iliac crests.

When these radiographs have been checked, the patient is asked to empty the bladder and a full-length post-micturition view is taken.

Follow-up films

These are taken to elucidate equivocal changes in the nodes and to show the response of the disease to treatment.

An antero-posterior view of the pelvis and upper thighs and an antero-posterior and both posterior oblique views of the abdomen are taken at two, four and eight weeks after the lymphogram. Lateral views are sometimes required.

If any abnormality is demonstrated in the leg, thigh or cisterna chyli, 'coned' views of the area must be taken and these should be repeated at each follow-up examination.

After-care of the patient

1. The patient is told to avoid getting his feet wet (which usually precludes taking a bath) until after the stitches have been removed. This is because healing should be by primary intention, but the site is under tension and subject to trauma and the patient's response to inflammation or infection may be reduced by subsequent radiotherapy.

2. Water-proof adhesive dressing must not be used over the

incisions. When the dry dressings come off, usually in a day or two, the area should be left uncovered, or another dry dressing applied.

3. The sutures are removed after seven to ten days.

Basic trolley setting

Upper (sterile) shelf

Two McCarthy's disposable lymphangiogram sets
One pair plain McIndoe's dissecting forceps
One pair toothed McIndoe's dissecting forceps
Two Kilner's skin hooks (one sharp, one blunt)
One small aneurysm needle (fine)
Mosquito artery forceps
Two pairs iris forceps
One Blalock's needle holder
Two pairs iris scissors (one sharp, one blunt)
One lacrimal sac dilator
One 10 ml syringe
One 20 ml syringe
Two 10 ml glass syringes
Bard Parker scalpel handle
Stitch scissors
Gallipot
Sterile adhesive tape
Gauze swabs
Towels
Gown
Suturing equipment (4/0 and 2/0 silk)

Lower (unsterile) shelf

Skin cleanser (e.g. Hibitane 0·5% in 70% industrial spirit)
Local anaesthetic (e.g. Lignocaine 1%)
Patent blue violet dye (2·5%)
Ampoules of contrast medium
Drawing-up cannula
Disposable needles
Disposable scalpel blades
20 ml ampoules of saline
Plastic dressing spray
Transparent adhesive strapping
EMERGENCY DRUGS

33

Gastro-intestinal tract

Anatomy. The gastro-intestinal tract may be conveniently divided into three regions, each of which is examined by a different radiological technique.

Upper alimentary tract. This comprises the oesophagus, the stomach and the duodenum as far as the duodeno-jejunal flexure.

The oesophagus extends from the neck to the fundus of the stomach and passes through the chest in the posterior mediastinum slightly to the left of the mid-line.

The fundus of the stomach lies in the left hypochondrium and the body of the stomach usually in the left half of the abdomen but its shape and position vary considerably between individual subjects. The duodenal cap lies just to the right of the spine and the duodenal loop extends across the upper abdomen to the duodeno-jejunal flexure which lies in the left hypochondrium, behind the stomach. Radiological examination of the upper alimentary tract is by barium swallow and meal and is under direct fluoroscopic control by the radiologist.

Small bowel. This comprises the duodenum, jejunum and ileum. It extends from the duodenal cap to the ileo-caecal valve. From the duodeno-jejunal flexure in the left hypochondrium, the jejunum extends downwards and towards the right. The small bowel has a long mesentery and the mid-jejunum and ileum are often in the pelvic cavity. The terminal ileum is relatively fixed at its junction with the caecum in the right iliac fossa. The duodenum is C-shaped and within the curve lies the head of the pancreas.

The small bowel is investigated either (a) by barium follow-through examination, either separately or combined with a barium meal. This method usually takes several hours, unless some form of accelerator is used which shortens the examination slightly. Although fluoroscopy is used from time to time during the examination, most of the radiographs are taken at specific intervals by the radiographer, or (b) by intubation whereby barium is injected or infused directly into the duodenum. This method takes only a short time because it is independent of pyloric control over the passage of barium to the area being examined. It is performed under fluoroscopic control and most of the radiographs are taken using the under-couch tube.

Large bowel. This comprises the caecum, colon and rectum. The caecum lies in the right iliac fossa. From the caecum, the colon ascends to the hepatic flexure and passes across the mid-abdomen, as the transverse colon, to the splenic flexure which is usually higher than the hepatic flexure. From the splenic flexure, the descending colon passes to the left iliac fossa where it becomes the sigmoid colon. This loops upwards and towards the mid-line before descending to join the rectum in the region of the pelvic inlet and thence to the anal canal.

The large bowel is investigated by a barium enema examination which is performed under fluoroscopic control, radiographs being taken using the under-couch tube during the injection of contrast media and using the over-couch tube after the completion of the injection of contrast media.

Care of the patient. During examinations of the alimentary tract, particularly barium meal and enema examinations, much of the investigation is performed by the radiologist using fluoroscopy and some of the usual radiographic problems of centering, coning and positioning of the patient are performed by the radiologist. But the radiographer has increased duties in looking after the patient.

In most departments, barium examinations are carried out in 'lists', several examinations being performed consecutively by one radiologist. It is therefore essential that great care be taken to identify each patient to ensure that the correct examination is being carried out.

Each radiologist has a standard routine procedure, varied for particular problems, and for the smooth running of the session the radiographer must know the routine of the radiologist. This includes having an adequate supply of cassettes, preferably sufficient for more than one examination so that there need be no delay. Because of the similarity of all barium meals and the probable impossibility of distinguishing between them if they are incorrectly named, it is of extreme importance that the radiographer should have an infallible method of knowing which cassettes in the screening room are exposed and which are unexposed and that the set of films for each patient should be correctly named.

When image intensification and television are not available and fluoroscopy is carried out in a darkened room, certain problems arise. These are mainly associated with the very old or very young patients and with those who are deaf, who do not understand the language or who are particularly apprehensive.

The alteration in the position of the fluoroscopy table from horizontal to vertical may cause distress to the patient, so reassurance and a supporting hand are necessary. Before beginning to move the table into the vertical position, the patient's feet should be placed firmly on the platform and the hand-grips adjusted to a position convenient for the patient to hold them. Before the vertical position is reached, the pillow should be removed and it should be confirmed that the patient's feet are firmly on the platform and the knees straight in order to support the weight of the body. When the table is lowered to the horizontal position, the patient should again be reassured and a pillow placed under the head.

The very ill patient is most likely to be examined in the horizontal or semi-recumbent position. Care must be taken to ensure that a drip infusion is not impeded and that the drip-stand is placed out of the way of the X-ray apparatus, particularly when the position of the table is altered.

Care of the diabetic patient. Diabetic patients present special problems for barium meal examinations, owing to the necessity to abstain from food for several hours and the diabetic's reliance on a properly controlled diet. Patients who receive daily insulin are told to omit the morning dose on the day of the examination and to bring this and their normal breakfast with them. Alternatively, a meal may be provided for them by the hospital diet kitchen. Diabetic patients should be placed first on the 'list' and the examination completed as quickly as possible, so that they may receive insulin and food.

After-care of the patient. Although a barium examination is not usually an ordeal for the patient, it must be confirmed that the patient is fit to leave the department at the end of the examination. The patient should be advised to take a meal as soon as possible, and perhaps a hot drink before leaving the hospital.

BARIUM MEAL

The barium meal examination is the basic method of investigation of the upper alimentary tract. In every case the oesophagus, stomach and duodenum are all examined.

Single contrast technique can be used but the double contrast technique is now more often preferred (Saxton, 1977). Double contrast technique involves the use of (*a*) barium sulphate suspension that has good coating qualities (*b*) a gas-producing agent and (*c*) a drug that causes transient gastric atony. It produces excellent demonstration of the gastric mucosal surface (Plate XXXII) and allows detection of very small abnormalities (de Lacey, 1977a). It is particularly valuable in detecting early gastric carcinoma.

For a female patient, the 10-day rule should be observed if the degree of clinical urgency permits.

Preparation of the patient

1. The patient must have nothing to eat or drink for at least five hours before the examination.
2. Patients are often advised to stop taking 'doctors' medicines' but this applies *only* to radiopaque substances, such as bismuth, and the patient must not stop taking essential drugs such as digitalis or steroids, or the contraceptive pill.
3. The patient should be warned that he or she may be in the department for some time.

Premedication. None is required.

Contrast medium

1. *Single contrast examination.* Initially 60 ml barium sulphate suspension (100 per cent w/v) to show the gastric mucosal pattern, followed by 180–240 ml diluted barium sulphate suspension (more if necessary) to distend the stomach.

2. *Double contrast examination.* About 200 ml barium sulphate suspension which should have low viscosity, high density and good coating qualities. A gas-producing agent—often in the form of tablets—to give 200–300 ml of gas in the stomach.

Great care must be taken where there is a possibility of (*a*) aspiration of contrast medium into the trachea (*b*) perforation or (*c*) subacute large bowel obstruction. If perforation or obstruction is suspected, water-soluble medium (e.g. Gastrografin) is used. If there is danger of aspiration, oily medium (e.g. Dionosil) is used. As each of these has an unpleasant taste, the addition of a small quantity of concentrated orange or blackcurrant juice makes the examination easier for the patient.

Equipment. Barium meal examinations are performed by the radiologist, using fluoroscopy, preferably with image intensification and television, and combined with either conventional under-couch radiography, 70 or 100 mm radiography or ciné-fluorography. If available, a video-tape recorder may be used also.

The ancillary equipment required includes a sufficient quantity of barium, cups, feeding cups and flexible straws. The patient is examined in the erect and horizontal positions, and a pillow, foot-rest and hand-grips must be provided. Compression devices must be available and, as some radiologists consider palpation an essential part of the examination, lead rubber gloves must therefore be available for their use. In the investigation for hiatus hernia, the radiologist may require the patient to sip water while in the prone position (Linsman, 1965) or he may place a pillow or firm pad under the patient's abdomen (Saxton, 1977). The radiographer should know the radiologist's requirements for this examination so that the necessary equipment is readily available. An adequate supply of lead coats must be available for any staff or other persons who have to remain in the fluoroscopy room.

Exposure factors

1. *Single contrast method.* High kilovoltage (120 kV or more) is used to penetrate the barium.

2. *Double contrast method.* Lower kilovoltage (85–100 kV) is used because there is only a thin layer of barium adhering to the mucosal surface and the stomach is distended with gas, not barium. Smaller exposures are needed than for the single contrast method because of the extra radiolucency provided by the gas.

Short exposure times are needed. When possible, rare earth or very fast tungstate screens are used, thus allowing the use of the fine focus also. The differences between the exposures needed for the single and double contrast methods are greater than the inexperienced radiographer might expect.

A photo-timer is a great advantage but if this is not available the radiographer must observe the patient's size and physique before the examination. During the examination, the size of the aperture, the amount of barium present, the degree of obliquity and whether or not the screen is in close contact with the patient must all be taken into consideration when choosing exposure factors.

Examination of the oesophagus is carried out routinely during a barium meal examination. However, when the oesophagus requires special investigation, either ciné-fluorography or several 'split' 24 × 30 cm (12 × 10 in) films are used. The use of a 70 mm camera allows six films per second to be taken for optimum visualisation of the oesophagus. When ciné-fluorography is not available, short exposure times are essential to show a bolus of barium in the oesophagus.

Technique. For the double contrast examination, the patient is first of all given an intravenous injection of a drug—either Glucogon (Goldsmith *et al.*, 1976) or Buscopan (Kreel *et al.*, 1973)—which causes transient gastric atony so that the stomach can be examined free from muscle spasm. Buscopan (Hyoscine-N-Butylbromide) is an anticholinergic drug and is contra-indicated for patients with acute glaucoma, prostatism or uncompensated cardiac failure. It may cause blurring of vision. The atonic effect of each of these drugs lasts about 15 minutes.

The patient is positioned for fluoroscopy. If gas-producing tablets are to be used, he is asked to swallow about 20 of them with a sip of barium or water. They must all be swallowed at the same time and the patient is told that they will fill his stomach with gas and is asked not to expel it. The fundus of the stomach is soon distended with gas and the examination can then proceed. The patient is given a small quantity of barium, the table is tilted into the horizontal position and he is turned prone. He is then rotated round once or twice so that barium is 'washed' across the surface of the stomach, leaving a thin layer on the gastric mucosa. This thin layer is outlined by gas. More barium is given by means of a straw and the oesophagus is examined.

For the examination of the stomach, the patient is given more barium—about 200 ml in total—and is examined in the prone, supine, oblique and erect positions.

Under-couch views are taken when required, some with compression. Compression pushes the anterior and posterior walls of the stomach together and makes it possible to detect small abnormalities which may not have been adequately demonstrated earlier, particularly if they are on the anterior wall and poorly coated with barium.

Trolley. A sterile trolley is not required for barium meal examinations but everything needed for the session should be placed in readiness and in such a position that the radiographer can find it in the dark when conventional screening is used.

After-care of the patient. No special after-care is usually needed but a patient who has received Buscopan and in whom blurring of vision occurred, must wait in the department until his vision has returned to normal.

Special circumstances

1. A modified double contrast examination is usually performed on an ill patient, e.g. following haematemesis or malaena. The patient is propped up to drink the barium and swallow the gas-producing tablets and is given an injection of Glucogon. The fluoroscopic examination is performed with the patient lying in the supine position and he is rotated gently as necessary.

2. If investigation to exclude a gross lesion in the upper gastro-intestinal tract is needed in a very ill patient, a modified single contrast method is usually the examination of choice.

ADDITIONAL EXAMINATION

Parietography. This is a method of demonstrating the stomach wall by filling with gas simultaneously the peritoneal cavity and the lumen of the stomach. When the pneumoperitoneum has been achieved (normally using about 1,500 ml oxygen) the stomach is inflated by means of tartaric acid followed by sodium bicarbonate in a little water. The patient is then tomographed in the supine or oblique position (Köhler, 1965).

BARIUM GRANULE MEAL

This examination (Horton *et al.*, 1965) measures the gastric emptying time by the radiographic observation of enteric-coated granules of barium sulphate.

Preparation of the patient. As for barium meal examination (p. 257).

Contrast medium. The barium granules are made up of barium sulphate with sucrose and acacia, giving a final content of 50 per cent barium sulphate w/v. The granules are coated with cellular acetate phthalate. This enteric coating protects the granules from breakdown in the stomach.

Technique. The patient has a breakfast of porridge, bacon, egg, toast and tea. The granules are mixed with the porridge and the patient is asked to swallow it at intervals during the meal in an attempt to distribute the granules evenly throughout the food in the stomach. To preserve the enteric coating, the patient is asked not to chew the porridge. If he has had a gastrectomy, he is admitted to hospital because the first radiograph must be taken half an hour after the meal.

A series of radiographs is taken at intervals, as directed by the radiologist. The intervals depend on the rate at which the stomach evacuates its contents. If the stomach is intact, the first radiograph is usually taken three hours after the meal. Further radiographs are taken at hourly or two-hourly intervals until the stomach is empty. The patient lies prone on the X-ray table. For the first radiograph, a 35×43 cm (17×14 in) cassette is used, with its lower border at the level of the symphysis pubis.

Centre in the mid-line, at the level of the middle of the cassette.

After inspection of the first radiograph, the position and shape of the stomach can be seen, e.g. whether it is high up under the diaphragm or low in the pelvis. Thus centering can be adjusted if necessary for subsequent radiographs. The satisfactory centering point is marked on the patient's skin.

The gastric emptying time is usually found to be within four to eight hours, usually five to six hours. It is considerably slower after vagotomy and faster after gastrectomy.

ACID-BARIUM TEST

This examination (McCall *et al.*, 1973) is used to test the sensitivity of the oesophagus to acid. The commonest cause of such sensitivity is reflux of gastric contents. Usually such reflux gives rise to typical symptoms and the acid-barium test has little to add. Less often, reflux gives rise to symptoms that are atypical and mimic those of other conditions, e.g. chronic laryngitis, globus pharyngis, or pulmonary fibrosis. The acid-barium test is a simple way of showing if reflux is likely to play a part in these symptoms.

A conventional barium meal examination of the upper alimentary tract (p. 256) is performed first and the acid-barium test is carried out immediately afterwards. The latter cannot form part of the basic examination, because acid-barium does not coat the gastric mucosa.

If available, a video-tape recorder is used.

Contrast medium

1. Neutral barium sulphate suspension, e.g. dilute Micropaque.

2. Acid-barium sulphate suspension, e.g. 1 ml of concentrated HCl (37 per cent) in 100 ml barium sulphate or 25 ml of 1·4 per cent HCl in 100 ml barium sulphate. The mixture must be made up before each examination because it becomes too thick if it is allowed to stand.

Technique. After the basic examination of the upper alimentary tract has been completed, the patient is placed in the prone position on the fluoroscopy table and the examination proceeds as follows:

1. The patient is given a mouthful of the neutral barium sulphate suspension from which he is required to swallow once only, during which he is screened. This serves as the control. The rest of the mouthful, if any, can then be swallowed.

2. He is then given a mouthful of the acid-barium sulphate suspension to swallow, during which he is screened again.

The test is positive if the oesophagus responds to the swallowing of the acid-barium by having periods of aperistalsis and non-peristaltic contractions lasting 20 to 30 seconds, associated with regurgitation and delayed emptying, and terminating with a peristaltic wave (Donner *et al.*, 1966).

3. The patient is given 30 ml antacid, e.g. aluminium hydroxide, to drink.

4. Finally, the patient is given another mouthful of the neutral barium sulphate suspension and the procedure in paragraph 1 is repeated. This is to see whether any abnormality revealed by the acid-barium has been reversed or improved by the antacid.

HYPOTONIC DUODENOGRAPHY

Hypotonic duodenography is the radiographic examination of the duodenal loop by outlining it in a flaccid state, free from peristaltic movement. This atonicity is produced by the injection of an anticholinergic drug such as Hyoscine-N-Butylbromide (Buscopan) (Ayre-Smith, 1976), or Glucogon.

Usually a double contrast technique is employed, whereby the duodenal mucosa is coated with barium and the duodenal loop is distended with gas. By forcing the inner wall of the duodenal loop against the pancreas, the duodenal mucosa is clearly visualised and early lesions of the pancreas and papilla of Vater may be shown.

The examination may be carried out by intubation of the duodenum and the injection of barium down the tube. An anticholinergic drug is injected intravenously and as soon as duodenal atony occurs air or oxygen is injected down the tube. But recently duodenography has been carried out without intubation, by using gas-producing tablets, as for the double contrast barium meal (p. 259) and this is the method that is now described.

Hypotonic duodenography is not used instead of conventional barium meal studies but gives additional information where there is suggestive, but inconclusive, evidence of a duodenal lesion or where a lesion of the head of the pancreas is suspected clinically (Grech, 1973).

For a female patient, the 10-day rule should be observed if the degree of clinical urgency permits.

Preparation of the patient. The patient must have nothing to eat or drink for five hours.

Premedication. No premedication is usually required.

Contrast medium. 100 ml barium sulphate suspension. 40 gas-producing tablets.

Technique. The patient is given the barium and the gas-producing tablets to swallow and he then lies on his right side on the fluoroscopy table. He is screened intermittently until the barium outlines the duodenal loop. The anticholinergic drug is then injected. The patient is rotated once or twice so that gas escapes from the distended stomach into the duodenal loop. Radiographs are taken in the supine, prone and oblique positions, usually with the under-couch tube (Plate XXXIII). Occasionally over-couch radiographs—using 30×40 cm (15×12 in) cassettes placed transversely—may be needed, in which case a marker can be placed on the patient's abdomen to correspond with the duodenal loop as seen on the screen, to assist with centering.

BARIUM FOLLOW-THROUGH

This examination is used to demonstrate the whole of the small bowel from the duodeno-jejunal flexure to the ileo-caecal valve. A combination of fluoroscopy and over-couch radiography is usually employed.

For a female patient, the 10-day rule should be observed if the degree of clinical urgency permits.

Preparation of the patient

1. A suitable aperient should be taken on each of the preceding two nights.
2. The patient must have nothing to eat or drink for at least five hours.

Premedication. None is required.

Care of the patient. As this is a lengthy examination, with long periods of inactivity for the patient, comfortable waiting accommodation must be provided. When the appointment is made, the patient should be warned that the examination may take all day and should be advised to bring something to help pass the time, e.g. books, knitting, etc.

Contrast medium. The type and quantity of barium sulphate suspension is decided by the radiologist. Usually a barium sulphate suspension that does not flocculate is used, in quantities from 60 to about 500 ml. An accelerator may be used to reduce the time taken for the examination by increasing the speed of gastric emptying and the rate of transit through the small bowel. The accelerator can be (*a*) taken orally, either before or with the barium sulphate or (*b*) given intravenously. The use of an accelerator is decided by the radiologist.

Technique. After ingestion of the barium, the patient lies prone or on the right side until the barium has left the stomach. The aim is to produce a continuous column of barium in the small bowel. Over-couch radiographs are taken with the patient in the prone position, until the contrast medium reaches the terminal ileum.

Either the series of radiographs can be taken at set times or each radiograph can be assessed to decide the timing of subsequent radiographs. Usually radiographs are taken at 15-minute intervals for the first hour because transit of barium through the proximal part of the small bowel is very rapid. Thereafter radiographs are taken at half-hourly intervals because transit through the distal small bowel is less rapid.

When the stomach is empty, the patient may, with advantage, take lunch. This not only makes the examination more tolerable for the patient but also accelerates the transit of barium through the small bowel. Fluoroscopy may be required at any point during the examination and is usually performed routinely when the barium has reached the terminal ileum.

High kilovoltage (120 kV or more) is employed so that short exposure times can be used to avoid blur due to respiration or peristalsis and also to reduce the radiation dose to the patient.

Prone view. The patient lies prone in the mid-line of the X-ray table. A 35 × 43 cm (17 × 14 in) cassette is used. For early radiographs when the stomach is still full, the lower border of the cassette is placed at the level of the posterior iliac spines. When the stomach is empty, the lower border of the cassette is placed at the lower margin of the symphysis pubis.

Centre in the mid-line, at the level of the middle of the cassette.

Erect view. This view is occasionally required to show fluid levels particularly in the presence of jejunal diverticulosis. The patient stands with his back against the erect Bucky or grid cassette. The lower border of a 35×43 cm (17×14 in) cassette is placed at the level of the symphysis pubis. The kilovoltage required is about 8 more than for the prone view. An obese patient will require further increase to compensate for the loss of the compression afforded by the prone view.

Centre in the mid-line, at the level of the iliac crests.

Prone view for the terminal ileum. The patient lies on the left side and a pad is placed in the right iliac fossa. The patient is then rolled into the prone position with the pad held firmly in place to prevent the small bowel falling back against the caecum and thus obscuring the terminal ileum. A 30×40 cm (15×12 in) cassette placed transversely is used, with its lower border at the level of the symphysis pubis.

Centre in the mid-line, at the level of the middle of the cassette.

BARIUM FOLLOW-THROUGH (CHILDREN)

For examining the small bowel in children, the following simple method avoids injection or intubation and affords an excellent demonstration of the small bowel.

Preparation of the patient

1. A suitable aperient should be taken on each of the preceding two nights.
2. The child should have nothing to eat or drink for eight hours.

Premedication. None is required.

Contrast medium. The type of barium sulphate suspension is decided by the radiologist. It is usually one that does not flocculate. It may be flavoured with orange or chocolate if the child is reluctant to drink it. The quantity varies with the age of the child—about 60 ml are required for a child aged two, and proportionately more for older children, depending on the size of the patient and the nature of the small bowel abnormality. An accelerator is not usually required.

Technique. After drinking the barium mixture, the child lies on the right side for 15 minutes before the first radiograph is taken. Initially, radiographs are taken at 15-minute to 20-minute intervals. After the first two radiographs have been seen, it can be decided whether more contrast medium is necessary. After about 30 minutes, the child is asked to micturate, as a distended bladder can result in many segments of small bowel being superimposed.

The barium usually takes between 45 and 90 minutes to reach the caecum. The child is then placed on the right side for about one minute. A firm pad is placed in the right iliac fossa, just medial to the right anterior iliac spine. The child is then rolled into the prone position, with the pad held firmly in place, and a further radiograph is taken.

Views. Prone views of the abdomen are taken, the whole abdomen being included on each radiograph. The lower border of a suitably-sized cassette is placed at the level of the symphysis pubis. As for all barium examinations, high kilovoltage technique is used, together with fast screens and films, to reduce the radiation dose to the child.

SMALL BOWEL ENEMA

The examination of the small bowel by intubation is replacing the conventional barium follow-through as it avoids the disadvantages of (*a*) pyloric control over the rate of transit and (*b*) the obscuring of individual coils of small bowel by the complete filling of the tract with barium. The examination is sometimes used also as a follow-up to a conventional barium follow-through examination to localise a lesion or to examine particularly a section of the small bowel where a lesion is suspected from another investigation.

There are a number of duodenal tubes that can be used and most radiologists will have a preference, e.g. one with a guide wire such as a modified Bilbao-Dotter tube (Sellink, 1976) or the Scott-Harden double-lumen tube (Scott-Harden, 1960). Careful positioning of the tube under fluoroscopic control enables barium sulphate suspension to be injected or infused at the required site, usually the duodeno-jejunal flexure.

For a female patient, the 10-day rule should be observed if the degree of clinical urgency permits.

Preparation of the patient. The patient must have nothing to eat or drink for at least five hours before the examination.

Premedication. None is required.

Contrast medium. 600 to 1,200 ml of barium sulphate suspension, diluted to a specific gravity of about 1·3. Up to 1,000 ml of water is sometimes used as an accelerator. It also washes away the barium from the small bowel proximal to the column of barium.

This allows clear visualisation of a required segment of the small bowel without superimposition of other coils. It causes distension of the intestinal loops and provides double contrast.

If peristaltic movement is inadequate, an accelerator such as metaclopromide (Maxalon) may sometimes be needed, in which case 20 ml are mixed with the barium sulphate suspension being infused (Nolan, 1978).

Exposure factors. High kilovoltage (120 kV or more) is used for single contrast studies, to penetrate the barium. Rare earth or very fast tungstate screens permit short exposure times to avoid blurring caused by peristaltic movement and also allow the more frequent use of the fine focus.

Technique. The patient either sucks an anaesthetic lozenge to reduce the sensitivity of the pharyngo-oesophagus, or the radiologist sprays the pharynx and larynx with a topical anaesthetic. The tube is manipulated into the stomach, the guide wire acting as a stiffener to prevent coiling. The guide wire is removed before the tube enters the duodenum. The tube is advanced as far as the ligament of Treitz. The patient lies supine. Six hundred to 1,200 ml of barium suspension are infused at a rate of about 80–100 ml per minute, the infusion continuing until the column of barium reaches the terminal ileum (Plate XXXIV). If, when 1,200 ml have been infused, the terminal ileum has not been reached, about 600 ml of water are infused (Sanders and Ho, 1976).

When the infusion has been completed the patient is turned into the prone position.

During the infusion, localised views are taken as necessary, using the under-couch tube. Localised views are taken also when the terminal ileum has been filled. Compression is needed to separate the superimposed coils of small bowel.

Over-couch radiographs with the X-ray tube angled cephalad and/or caudad may assist by separating superimposed coils (Sanders and Ho, 1976). Tilting the patient 40–80° head downwards (with him supported by a myelography harness) may also assist by separating barium-filled loops within the pelvis (Dodds et al., 1975).

ADDITIONAL EXAMINATIONS

1. For the diagnosis of disaccharidase deficiency, an additional examination is performed using a disaccharide barium sulphate mixture as the contrast medium (Laws et al., 1967). The results are compared with those of the routine follow-through examination previously performed.

The patient must have nothing to eat or drink for at least five hours before this additional examination. The contrast medium used is 120 ml Micropaque to which 25 g of a test sugar have been added. In some cases, the examination is repeated with a different sugar.

The patient lies on the right side for 45 minutes after ingestion of the contrast medium. A supine view of the abdomen is taken 15 minutes later. For this, a 35 × 43 cm (17 × 14 in) cassette is used with its lower border at the level of the symphysis pubis.

2. Reflux small bowel examination is recommended by some authorities (Miller, 1965) to localise total or partial bowel obstruction and to find extremely small lesions. A maximum of 4,500 ml of 20 per cent w/v barium sulphate is used in retrograde manner.

BARIUM ENEMA

The barium enema examination is the method of investigation of the colon by retrograde injection of contrast medium. The procedure usually involves the use of both radiopaque and radiolucent contrast media, thus producing double contrast.

For a female patient, the 10-day rule should be observed if the degree of clinical urgency permits.

Preparation of the patient

1. The patient should keep to a low residue diet for four days before the examination.
2. The colon must be empty when the examination is carried out. Different methods are used in different departments, no method being entirely satisfactory with every patient. The most usual methods are (a) an aperient taken on each of the preceding two nights or (b) an aperient taken about 48 hours before the examination and a high colonic washout given two or three hours before the examination.
3. The patient should have nothing to eat or drink for four to six hours before the examination.
4. The patient must undress completely and wear an open-backed gown. Shoes, stockings or socks should be removed in case of accidental soiling by barium.

Premedication. None is required, but intravenous injection of Glucogon is sometimes recommended (Harned et al., 1976; Meeroff et al., 1975) to reduce smooth muscle spasm and thus give better colonic filling and make the examination more comfortable for the patient. One mg is injected about 10 minutes before the examination.

Contrast medium. Barium sulphate suspension is used. It should have high density, low viscosity and should coat the mucosa well and evenly, without flocculation or flaking (de Lacey, 1977b). Three pints of barium sulphate suspension are usually required, but in certain cases (e.g. megacolon) a larger quantity may be necessary.

Usually a double contrast technique is used whereby after the colon has been evacuated of barium it is distended with air. Small defects that may have been obscured by the large amount of barium previously injected, may become visible by double contrast. The air is injected under the control of the radiologist, the quantity being determined by him for each patient.

Ancillary equipment. The enema container must be large enough to hold about three pints (2 litres) and it should be adjustable in height. Attached to it is a long tube to which the catheter is connected. If a Higginson syringe is to be used for air insufflation, a Y-shaped connector is needed for attachment of the catheter and the syringe to the tube. Clips or Spencer Wells forceps are used to clip off the part not required. By using such a connector, barium and air can each be injected without change of equipment and, if required, barium can be run out of the patient without his getting off the table. More sophisticated methods of evacuation are available, e.g. an extractor using water suction. Alternatively, a special valve (Templeton and Addington, 1951) may be used which permits immediate selection of barium injection, air insufflation or suction drainage. This valve may be used in conjunction with a water suction extractor which can be built into the wall.

Several kinds of disposable enema administration sets are now available, comprising the container, tubing and often the catheter as well. Some also contain barium sulphate powder to which must be added sufficient water to provide a suspension of suitable specific gravity. Some containers are designed so that, after the barium has been run back into them, they can be inverted and used for air insufflation.

Care of the patient. In most general departments, barium enema examinations are carried out frequently and it is sometimes overlooked that the examination can be an uncomfortable and embarrassing one for the patient and may be quite an ordeal for an old or frail person. As the co-operation of the patient is essential for the success of the examination it is important that he should understand what is going to happen and what he is required to do. Lavatories must be sited as near as possible to the screening room so that the patient has only a very short distance to walk, though this is less important if most of the barium has been run out during the examination. If the colon has been filled with barium and the patient is required to go to the lavatory to get rid of the barium, he should not be left long without surveillance as on occasions a patient may become weak or even collapse.

At the end of the examination, it must be ascertained that the patient is fit to leave the department. The provision of a hot drink is usually welcomed.

Exposure factors. High kilovoltage (about 120 kV) is used for single contrast examinations. Lower kV (85–100) is used when there is a large quantity of air present as for barium meal examinations (p. 258).

Technique. A little barium is run through the tube and catheter to make sure there are no blockages. The X-ray table is covered with a sheet on top of which is placed a disposable polythene sheet covered by an incontinence sheet. The patient is told exactly what is going to happen and is then positioned on his side with the knees flexed. The catheter (well lubricated) is inserted approximately 10 cm (4 in) into the rectum. The patient is then turned into the prone position. The tubing is adjusted so that the barium will be able to flow easily, i.e. there must be no kinks in the tubing and the patient must not be lying on it. The height of the enema container is then adjusted to about 100 cm (40 in) above the table-top.

Some radiologists still prefer the conventional method of using the under-couch tube for most of the radiographs, but now many prefer to use the over-couch tube for the double contrast views (de Lacey, 1977b). By this method the entire colon from the sigmoid region to the splenic and hepatic flexures is demonstrated on each 35 × 43 cm (17 × 14 in) radiograph.

In each method, the table is tilted so that the patient is lying 10° head downwards. Under fluoroscopic control, barium is run in under gravity, slowly at first—or it will not be retained—until it reaches the level of the iliac crests. The tube is then clipped off but the barium already in the colon will continue to flow a little further. More barium is run in slowly, a little at a time, until it reaches the splenic flexure. The tube is clipped off again, the table is returned to the horizontal position and the patient is turned on to his right side. Barium in the colon will fill the hepatic flexure and ascending colon. If the hepatic flexure does not fill, a little more barium is run in. Thereafter the alternative methods are:

1. *Using mainly under-couch views*. While the colon is being filled with barium, under-couch views are taken by the radiologist, as required. Usually postero-anterior, oblique and lateral views are taken.

Over-couch films may sometimes be required before the patient is allowed to get off the table and go to the lavatory or the colon is otherwise evacuated.

a. *Antero-posterior view*. The patient lies supine in the mid-line of the table. A 35×43 cm (17×14 in) cassette is used, with its lower border at the level of the symphysis pubis.

Centre in the mid-line, at the level of the middle of the cassette.

b. *Outlet view*. A pedestal Bucky is ideal for this view. If this is not available, the patient may sit on a grid cassette at the end of the X-ray table. The patient sits on the pedestal Bucky, or cassette, with the knees parted and bends forward as far as possible so that the spine is parallel with the table. A 35×35 cm (14×14 in) cassette is used, with its posterior border level with the edge of the soft tissues of the buttocks.

Centre mid-way between the posterior iliac spines.

Sufficient time should then be allowed for all or as much as possible of the barium to be got rid of. When this has been achieved the patient is again placed on the X-ray table and a 'post-evacuation' radiograph is taken. This may be taken by the radiologist using the under-couch tube, or an over-couch radiograph may be required. For the over-couch radiograph the position and centering are the same as for the antero-posterior view taken before evacuation. The kilovoltage should be decreased by 5.

If air insufflation is to be performed, a catheter is inserted as before. Air is gently pumped into the rectum by means of the Higginson's syringe. By rotating the patient, the air is manoeuvred round the colon which has previously been coated with barium. Small defects that may have been obscured by the large amount of barium previously injected, may now become visible. Under-couch radiographs are taken by the radiologist, the kilovoltage necessary being 8 to 10 less than for the filled colon. At the end of the examination, the catheter is removed and the patient is directed to the lavatory again to get rid of the air. He is then allowed to leave the department, if fit.

2. *Using mainly over-couch views*. While the colon is being filled with barium, under-couch views are taken by the radiologist, as required. When sufficient barium has been introduced, the table is tilted so that the patient is lying $10°$ feet downwards and barium is

allowed to run back into the enema container or into a receiver. When sufficient barium has been removed, the patient is turned into the prone position and air insufflation is carried out either by using a Higginson's syringe or by inverting the enema bag (if of the appropriate type) and squeezing it intermittently. While air is being insufflated, the patient is turned first on to his right side—to fill the splenic flexure—and then on his left side—to fill the hepatic flexure. Insufflation is continued until air has filled the caecum, at which stage the patient is rotated several times so that the colon is thoroughly coated with barium and air.

The catheter is then removed and the following views are taken, using the over-couch tube and $35 \times 43\,cm$ ($17 \times 14\,in$) cassettes:

a. *Antero-posterior*. The patient lies supine. The lower border of the cassette is placed at the level of the symphysis pubis.

Centre in the mid-line, at the level of the iliac crests.

b. *Left posterior oblique*. From the supine position, the patient is rotated 30°, with his right side raised and supported on a foam wedge.

Centre in the mid-clavicular line of the raised side, at the level of the iliac crest.

c. *Right posterior oblique*. The patient is rotated so that the left side is raised 30° and is supported on a foam wedge.

Centre in the mid-clavicular line of the raised side, at the level of the iliac crest.

d. *Postero-anterior* ('angled prone view'). This view demonstrates the recto-sigmoid region (Plate XXXV). The patient lies prone. The pelvis must be positioned symmetrically. The upper border of the cassette is placed at the level of the anterior superior iliac spines. The mA.s should be four times that needed for the non-angled views.

Centre in the mid-line, at the level of the iliac crests, with the tube angled 45° caudad.

e. *Left lateral decubitus*. The patient lies on his left side with his arms on the pillow above his head, so that their image does not appear on the radiograph. The grid cassette is supported vertically (preferably in a cassette holder) either anterior or posterior to the patient. A horizontal beam is used.

Centre in the mid-line, at the level of the iliac crests.

f. *Right lateral decubitus* (Plate XXXVI). The patient lies on his right side. The procedure is as for the left lateral decubitus view (above).

g. *Antero-posterior erect*. Either the fluoroscopy table is tilted into the vertical position or the patient stands in front of an erect Bucky stand or a vertically placed grid cassette.

Centre in the mid-line, at the level of the iliac crests.

This series of radiographs is viewed by the radiologist and if no further views are required, the patient is allowed to go to the lavatory and then if fit, to leave the department.

Modifications

Infants. The barium sulphate suspension should be mixed with saline and not with tap water as for adults. Barium suspended in water and given as an enema, is hypotonic and can cause excessive absorption of water from the colon especially if the colon is dilated and a large quantity of barium has been needed to fill it (Gordon and Ross, 1977). 10 g of salt should be added to every litre of enema fluid to ensure that the enema is isotonic.

Ileostomy and colostomy patients. Examination of the colon distal to the site of an ileostomy or colostomy is usually performed by infusing barium via the rectum. It is usually infused until it reaches the site of the ileostomy or colostomy. When the examination is performed on a patient who has undergone a sigmoid colectomy and temporary colostomy, water-soluble contrast medium (e.g. Urografin 30 or Hypaque 25%) is used instead of barium. This precaution is taken to avoid the risk of barium leaking from the anastomosis site and pooling outside the lumen of the bowel.

Occasionally, the proximal colon needs to be investigated. If so, the barium sulphate suspension is infused via the colostomy opening (stoma). A soft Foley catheter is used, with the balloon already inflated. The tip of the catheter is inserted into the colostomy opening and the balloon is held, or taped, into position *outside* the colostomy. Alternatively, the Foley catheter can be threaded carefully a little way into the colon. The balloon is never inflated inside the colon.

Basic trolley setting

Although a sterile trolley is not required for barium enema examinations, everything used must be hygienically clean and carefully washed after use. Unless the disposable type is used, the catheters must be sterilised after use.

Enema container with suitable length of tubing
Means of support for container so that it can be adjusted in
    height—usually 100 cm (40 in)
Y-shaped connector *or* special valve
Polythene connection between tubing and catheter
Catheters (if a disposable enema set is used, the container and
    tubing are supplied and are ready for use)

Barium sulphate (made up to correct temperature, 38°C or
    100°F, immediately before inserting catheter)
Plastic sheeting
Incontinence sheet
Cellulose wadding
Gauze swabs
Lubricating jelly
Clips or Spencer Wells forceps
Dressing towels
Receivers

A bed-pan and cover must be readily available.

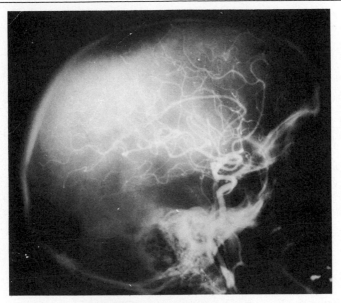

PLATE XXVII. Carotid angiogram, arterial phase (p. 217).

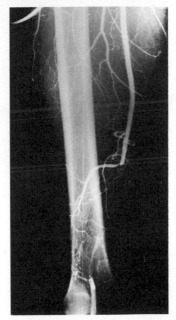

PLATE XXVIII. Femoral arteriogram (p. 220), showing obstruction at adductor canal.

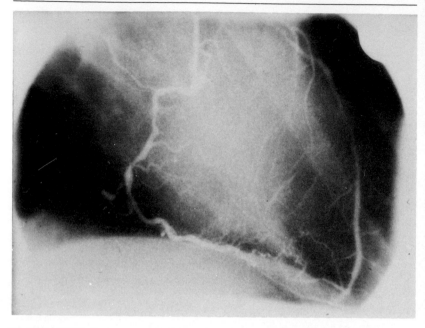

PLATE XXIX. Coronary arteriogram (p. 233), right anterior oblique view. Right coronary artery injected. Marked atheromatous disease of the right coronary artery is shown with several critical stenoses.

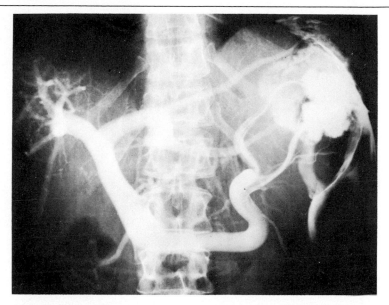

PLATE XXX. Percutaneous transplenic portal venogram (p. 235).

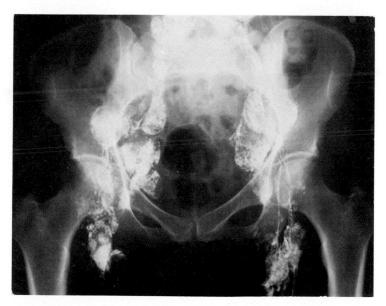

PLATE XXXI. Lymphogram, taken two hours after injection (p. 251), showing a form of Hodgkin's disease.

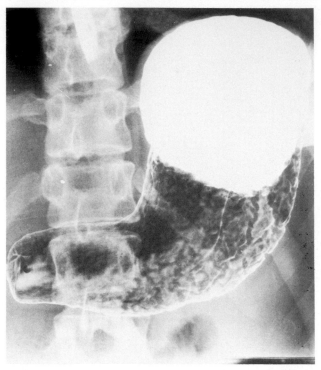

PLATE XXXII. Double contrast barium meal (p. 257), showing normal gastric mucosal pattern.

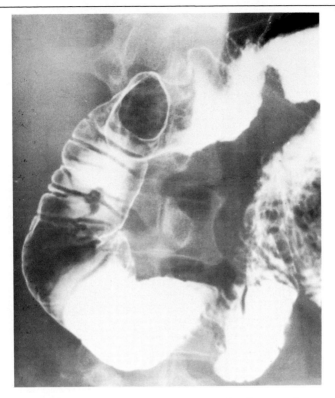

PLATE XXXIII. Hypotonic duodenogram (p. 263), showing normal appearances.

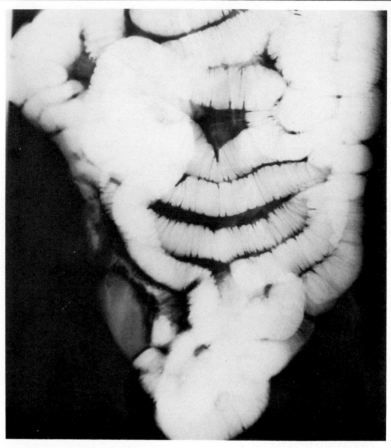

PLATE XXXIV. Small bowel enema (p. 267), showing normal appearances.

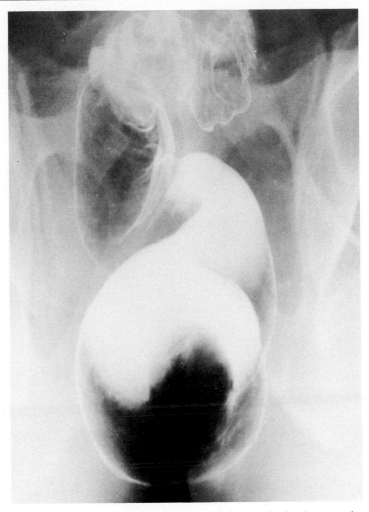

PLATE XXXV. Barium enema, angled prone view (p. 272), showing a carcinoma which was not shown on other views.

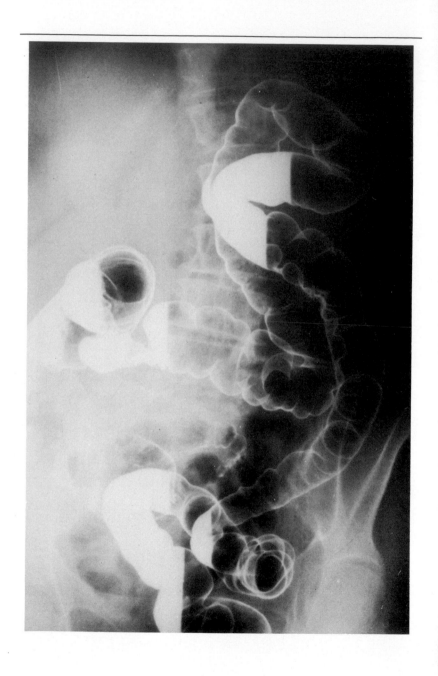

PLATE XXXVI. Barium enema, right lateral decubitus view (p. 272).

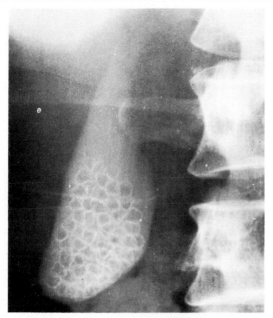

PLATE XXXVII. Oral cholecystogram (p. 277), showing gall-stones.

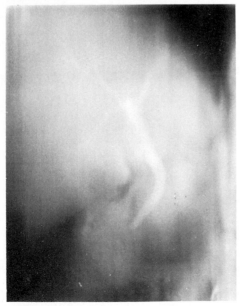

PLATE XXXVIII. Infusion choledochogram (p. 280). Tomogram showing normal appearances after cholecystectomy.

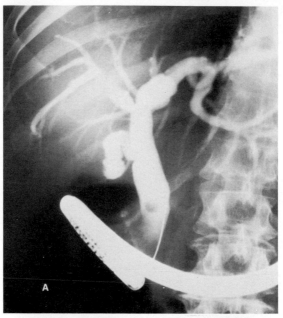

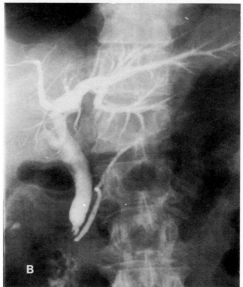

PLATE XXXIX. Endoscopic retrograde choledocho-pancreatograms (pp. 283, 284).

A. Dilated common bile duct with a translucent filling defect due to a calculus (endoscope in position).

B. Simultaneous filling of the pancreatic duct and the biliary tree (endoscope removed).

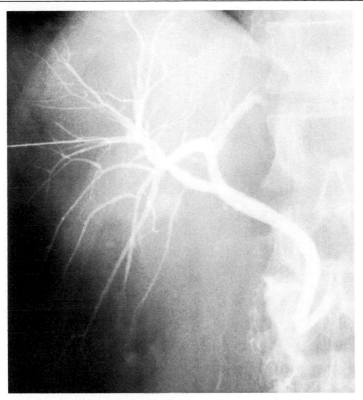

PLATE XL. Percutaneous transhepatic choledochogram (p. 286), showing normal duct system.

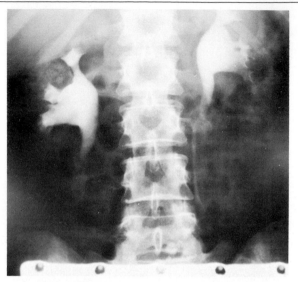

PLATE XLI. Excretion urogram, 15 minutes after injection, compression device *in spu* (p. 293).

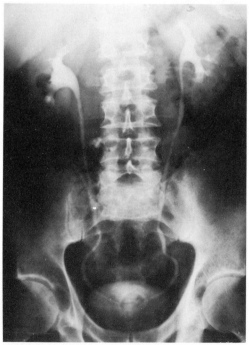

PLATE XLII. Excretion urogram, after release of compression (pp. 294, 295).

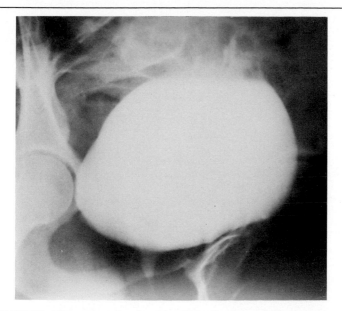

PLATE XLIII. Micturating cystogram (p. 305), showing normal appearances in a female.

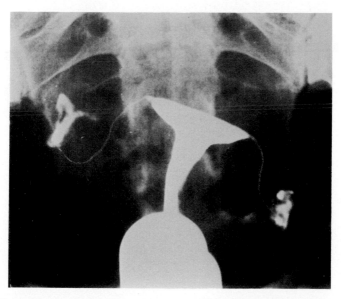

PLATE XLIV. Hystero-salpingogram (p. 314), showing normal appearances.

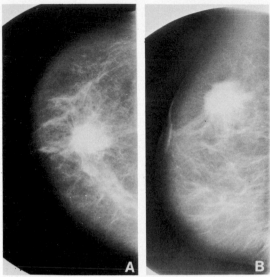

PLATE XLV. Mammograms (pp. 325, 326), showing a neoplasm in a post-menopausal breast. A. Supero-inferior view. B. Lateral view.

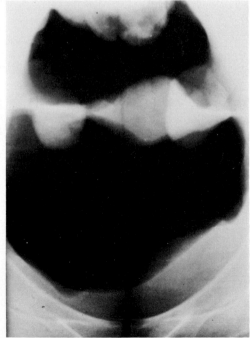

PLATE XLVI. Gynaecogram (p. 331), showing enlargement of the left ovary.

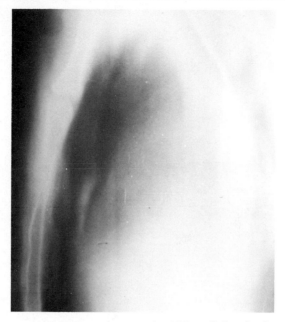

PLATE XLVII. Mediastinal pneumogram (p. 336), outlining the thymus gland.

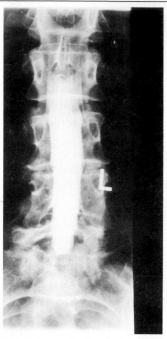

PLATE XLVIII. Radiculogram (p. 347), showing normal appearances.

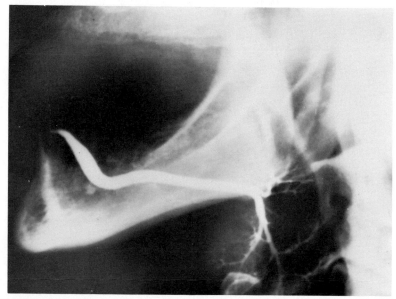

PLATE XLIX. Submandibular sialogram (p. 354), showing sialectasis.

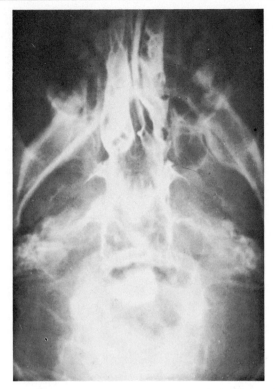

PLATE L. Nasopharyngogram (p. 357). Submento-vertical view showing normal appearances.

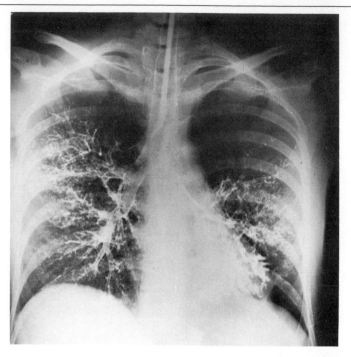

PLATE LI. Bronchogram (p. 360), showing left lower lobe bronchiectasis.

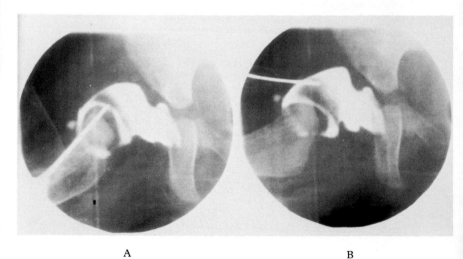

A   B

PLATE LII. A and B. Arthrograms (p. 369), showing congenital dislocation of the
right hip. A. Internal rotation. B. External rotation.

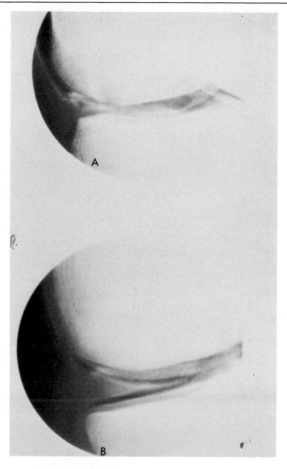

PLATE LIII. Double contrast arthrogram of the knee (p. 372). Medial meniscus.
A. Anterior horn tear. B. Normal posterior horn.

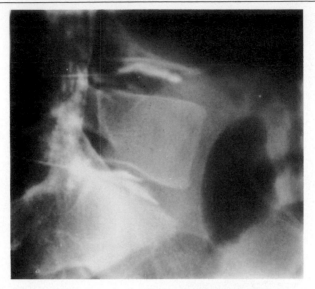

PLATE LIV. Discogram (p. 375), showing prolapsed disc at L4/5 and degenerate disc at L5/S1.

34

Biliary tract

Anatomy (Fig. 36). The intrahepatic bile ducts drain into the left and right hepatic ducts which leave the liver at the porta hepatis and join to form the common hepatic duct. The gall-bladder is a hollow pear-shaped viscus consisting of a body, fundus and neck. The cystic duct leads from the neck and joins the common hepatic duct to form the common bile duct. Just before its termination, the common bile duct is usually joined by the pancreatic duct to form the ampulla of Vater and it enters the second part of the duodenum at the duodenal papilla.

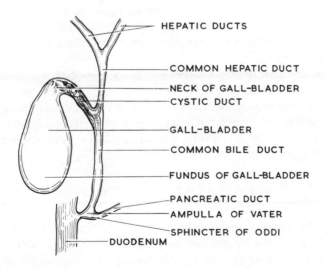

HEPATIC DUCTS
COMMON HEPATIC DUCT
NECK OF GALL-BLADDER
CYSTIC DUCT
GALL-BLADDER
COMMON BILE DUCT
FUNDUS OF GALL-BLADDER
PANCREATIC DUCT
AMPULLA OF VATER
SPHINCTER OF ODDI
DUODENUM

Fig. 36

The position of the gall-bladder varies in different subject types. Usually the gall-bladder is approximately parallel with the spine and near it, to the right of the second and third lumbar vertebrae. But, it may be as high as the tenth rib and lie almost transversely or it may be as low as the right sacro-iliac region.

The normal biliary tract is of soft tissue density and is thus not demonstrable by plain film radiography. Radiographic examination of the biliary tract is usually required to show function and to demonstrate anatomical abnormalities, particularly calculi. Biliary calculi (cholelithiasis) can be found in the gall-bladder or in the ducts and they are more often radiolucent than radiopaque. Contrast medium is therefore needed to demonstrate them and it may be given (a) orally (b) intravenously (c) by retrograde cannulation of the papilla of Vater (d) percutaneously into the hepatic ducts (e) by direct injection at operation or (f) through a drainage tube after operation.

The biliary tract may also be examined by scintigraphy (p. 63) and by ultrasonography (p. 70).

Oral contrast medium is excreted by the liver and enters the gall-bladder where it is concentrated. A healthy gall-bladder is necessary to concentrate it and the process takes several hours. Prior to concentration in the gall-bladder, the concentration of contrast medium in the bile is too low for it to be demonstrable radiographically.

Intravenous contrast medium is excreted by the liver sufficiently concentrated to be demonstrable radiographically and will outline an inert gall-bladder. The process takes about three hours but the ducts are usually visible about 20 minutes after the contrast medium has been injected.

As the contrast medium never reaches a very high concentration, low kilovoltage must be used for all examinations of the biliary tract.

The term choledochography is used in this chapter, rather than cholangiography, which although perhaps better known is less accurate because it is the biliary ducts and not biliary vessels that are opacified.

ORAL CHOLECYSTOGRAPHY

This is the initial examination for the investigation of the biliary tract in a patient who has not undergone cholecystectomy.

For a female patient, the 10-day rule (p. 19) should be observed if the degree of clinical urgency permits.

Preparation of the patient

1. The patient should take a suitable aperient on each of the two nights preceding the examination.

2. For the day before the examination, a fat-free diet should be taken.
3. The patient should take the contrast medium 14 hours before the examination. The capsules should be taken with a light fat-free evening meal.
4. The patient should have nothing further to eat until after the examination but should be encouraged to drink freely as this lessens the remote chance of renal complications (Kreel, 1973).

Premedication. No premedication is required.
Contrast medium. Biloptin or Telepaque, 6 capsules (3 g).
Preliminary film. A prone oblique view is usually taken when the appointment is made. The patient lies prone, with the right side raised about 20°. The necessary degree of obliquity depends on the physique of the patient, a slim patient needing a greater degree of obliquity than an obese one to avoid superimposition of the gall-bladder on the vertebral column. The area covered by the preliminary film must include the eleventh and twelfth ribs, the right side of the spine, the right iliac crest and the lateral abdominal wall.
Centre 7·5 cm (3 in) to the right of the spinous processes, 2·5 cm (1 in) cephalad to the level of the lower costal margin.
Technique. A prone oblique view is taken as for the preliminary film 14 hours after ingestion of the contrast medium (Plate XXXVII). The centering point and limits of the light-beam diaphragm are marked on the patient's skin.

If the gall-bladder has concentrated the contrast medium, and is thus shown on the radiograph, a coned view is then taken also. The position of the gall-bladder should be noted from the first radiograph and the centering adjusted accordingly.

The patient is usually then screened in the erect position and a series of radiographs is taken. Compression may be necessary to displace bowel gas. If fluoroscopy is not available, an erect view is taken, the centering point being 5 cm (2 in) lower than for the prone view.

A fatty meal (such as bacon and eggs or a proprietary fat emulsion) is then given to the patient. Usually two coned views of the gall-bladder are taken after the fatty meal. The first (to demonstrate the cystic and common bile ducts) is taken 15 minutes after the fatty meal and the second (to see if the gall-bladder has contracted) is taken 15 minutes later. Filling of the ducts is often helped by the patient's lying supine for about 10 minutes before the prone view is taken. If the gall-bladder has failed to contract, the patient is given further fat and another radiograph is taken 30 minutes later.

If the gall-bladder has not concentrated the contrast medium and so is not shown on the radiograph, a view of the whole abdomen is taken, using a 35×43 cm (17×14 in) cassette. This is done to see if the gall-bladder is located in an abnormal position, e.g. on the left side.

If the gall-bladder is still not visible, a 'double dose' examination is sometimes carried out, for which the patient takes, in all, twelve capsules of contrast medium, six capsules being taken on each of the two nights preceding the examination. (Thus if the examination is performed on the day following the unsuccessful one, only six further capsules are taken.) Alternatively, a 'four-day' examination may be carried out, for which the patient keeps to a fat-free diet and takes two capsules after each meal (i.e. six capsules a day) for each of the four days preceding the examination. The contrast medium thus taken is adsorbed on to the surface of any gall-stone present, thereby rendering it radiopaque.

However, it has been suggested (Grainger, 1972) that these repeated or multiple doses of cholecystographic agents should not be used because (a) they are rarely effective if a single dose has been ineffective and (b) they increase the hazard of renal failure, this being rare with the contrast medium used for cholecystography but more likely if the hepato-biliary disease is of increasing severity, if the patient has had a recent intravenous choledochogram or if he is dehydrated.

INTRAVENOUS CHOLEDOCHOGRAPHY

This examination is performed: (a) when oral cholecystography has failed (b) when demonstration of the ducts is required in a patient who has undergone cholecystectomy and has symptoms of biliary tract disease (c) when choledocholithiasis is suspected or (d) in acute cholecystitis.

The traditional method of injecting the contrast medium intravenously is by a syringe but this procedure produces an unacceptable degree of nausea and vomiting. Recently it has been shown that diluting the contrast medium, and injecting it slowly by drip infusion, usually overcomes this problem.

The examination is performed on an X-ray table equipped for tomography.

The examination must not be performed within 48 hours of the patient's having had an oral cholecystogram (Kreel, 1973).

For a female patient, the 10-day rule should be observed if the degree of clinical urgency permits.

Preparation of the patient

1. The patient should take a suitable aperient on each of the two nights preceding the examination.
2. The patient's diet should not be restricted. The examination should be performed only on a non-fasting and well-hydrated patient (Kreel, 1973).

Premedication. No premedication is required.

Contrast medium. Meglumine iodipamide (Biligrafin) or meglumine ioglycamide (Biligram). One hundred ml bottles for infusion are obtainable. Alternatively, ampoules of contrast medium are used, mixed with a suitable diluent, the quantities being from 10 ml (Ansell and Faux, 1973) to 1 ml/kg body weight (Nolan and Gibson, 1970), mixed with 250 ml normal saline.

When given intravenously, these contrast media combine readily with albumin. The process of protein binding is slow but ultimately about 92 per cent combines. Protein-bound contrast medium is secreted by the liver and non-bound contrast medium is excreted by the kidneys in the same way as urographic contrast media. If the contrast medium is injected at a rate faster than that of protein binding, the non-bound contrast medium is lost through the kidneys. At all dose levels of contrast medium, the injection rate should not exceed that of protein binding. The infusion of contrast medium is therefore given over a period of from 30 minutes to one hour.

Contra-indications. The examination is usually contra-indicated in patients (*a*) with known sensitivity to contrast media or other drugs (*b*) who have asthma, combined severe renal and liver disease, or serum bilirubin above 3 to 4 mg per cent or (*c*) in whom hypotension would be dangerous (e.g. who have ischaemic heart disease).

Preliminary film. Usually a prone oblique view is taken, as for oral cholecystography (p. 277) but for an obese patient the prone position is preferable because the natural compression afforded by the prone position improves definition by reducing tissue thickness and scattered radiation (Bryan, 1971). The centering point and limits of the light-beam diaphragm are marked on the patient's skin. Low kilovoltage, 50–60 kV, is used and the quality of the radiograph must be such that there is good soft tissue detail. There must be no respiratory blur.

Centre 7·5 cm (3 in) to the right of the spinous processes, 2·5–5 cm (1–2 in) cephalad to the level of the lower costal margin.

If any abnormal opacities are demonstrated on this radiograph, appropriate further views, such as a supine view or a view of the whole abdomen, must be taken.

Technique. The patient lies supine and is made as comfortable as possible because the infusion takes a long time and the patient must not move the arm during it. The infusion need not be given in the X-ray room. The patient may be placed on a stretcher for the infusion in an adjoining room but a nurse must remain with him throughout. Emergency drugs and equipment must be readily available.

As soon as the infusion is completed, the patient is turned into the prone or prone oblique position on the X-ray table as for the preliminary film and a radiograph is taken. Usually, this radiograph demonstrates contrast medium in the biliary ducts and in the pelvi-calyceal system, showing the presence of both protein-bound and non-bound contrast medium. Centering and collimation of the beam should then be adjusted to obtain optimum demonstration of the biliary system.

Further radiographs are taken until the ducts are clearly shown and there is free drainage into the duodenum and opacification of the gall-bladder, if one is present. The ducts are best demonstrated between 45 and 90 minutes after the infusion.

Tomography is important in the demonstration of the ducts (Plate XXXVIII), particularly when gas or faeces overshadow the area or when the ducts are dilated and a calculus is suspected but has not been demonstrated. It is also of advantage in obese patients. Linear tomograms, taken at about 8–12 cm for the average patient in the prone position, are usually sufficient. A multi-layer cassette is not usually found to give good enough detail. If possible, zonography (p. 49) is performed, only one or two exposures being necessary to demonstrate the whole system (Sutherland, 1970).

If the patient has undergone cholecystectomy, the examination is concluded once the ducts have been well demonstrated. Otherwise, further radiographs are taken at half-hourly intervals until the gall-bladder is demonstrated. It should not be assumed that there is cystic duct obstruction unless and until such radiographs have failed to demonstrate the gall-bladder for at least four hours after the end of the infusion. If and when the gall-bladder is demonstrated, further radiographs are taken, as follows:

Prone. To demonstrate the fundus of the gall-bladder.

Supine. To demonstrate the neck of the gall-bladder and Hartmann's pouch.

Erect. To demonstrate floating gall-stones, if present, or 'layering' of contrast medium. In the erect position, the gall-bladder is about 5 cm (2 in) lower than in the prone or supine position and centering must be adjusted accordingly.

Basic trolley setting

Upper (sterile) shelf

Disposable recipient set *or*
One 50 ml syringe and drawing-up cannula (if ampoules of contrast medium are being used)
Gallipot
Gauze swabs
Infusion needle *or* 'Butterfly' needle, size 19

Lower (unsterile) shelf

Skin cleanser (e.g. spirit)
Infusion bottle of contrast medium *or*
Ampoules of contrast medium and infusion bottle of saline
EMERGENCY DRUGS

ENDOSCOPIC RETROGRADE CHOLEDOCHO-PANCREATOGRAPHY

This is the radiographic examination of the pancreatic and biliary systems following intubation of the papilla of Vater by a fibre-optic endoscope and the injection of contrast medium.

The examination is performed (*a*) in the investigation of recurrent jaundice or other biliary tract problems, when simpler techniques have failed or been inadequate (*b*) in the investigation of pancreatic disease (*c*) on patients with ascites or tendency to bleeding when percutaneous choledochography is contra-indicated (Nolan, 1977) and (*d*) on patients who have obstructive jaundice, when the examination (unlike intravenous choledochography) can succeed even if the serum bilirubin is greater than 3 mg per cent (Salmon, 1977).

Contra-indications

The examination is contra-indicated in patients (a) with a positive serological test for Australia antigen, because it is not possible to sterilise the instrument (b) with a history of sensitivity to contrast media or other drugs (c) with pyloric stenosis and in whom, therefore, it would be impossible to pass the endoscope (d) with acute pancreatitis or (e) for whom an anticholinergic drug is inadvisable, e.g. patients with acute glaucoma or with prostatitis. It is also contra-indicated, though less strongly, in patients with acute cholangitis or who are in the recovery phase of acute pancreatitis or are known to have pseudocysts of the pancreas (Cotton, 1974).

Equipment. A fibre-optic endoscope consists basically of a bundle composed of tens of thousands of glass fibres, each of 15 to 25 μ diameter, which are suitably lubricated, bound together and housed in a glass sheath that has a lower refractive index than the fibres so as to prevent loss of light (Schiller, 1972). A xenon light source illuminates the distal end of the endoscope. This is the viewing end and has two apertures, one for direct viewing, the other for attachment of a camera. Down the centre of the bundle is a channel through which can be passed a catheter (for instilling contrast medium or other drugs), biopsy forceps or a cytology brush.

The principle of fibre-optics is that light will pass along the length of a glass fibre and transmit a perfect image, even if the fibre is flexed or twisted.

The examination is performed under fluoroscopic control, using image intensification and television. Both under-couch and over-couch radiographs are taken and, if available, a video-tape recorder is used. During the course of the examination, photographs can be taken, the camera being attached to the viewing end of the endoscope.

Preparation of the patient

1. The patient must have nothing to eat or drink for five hours.
2. Recent radiographs of the abdomen, including prone and left anterior oblique views of the gall-bladder area, must be available.

Premedication. Thirty minutes before the examination the patient is given an Amethocaine lozenge (30 mg) to suck, and ten minutes before the examination he is given 20 mg hyoscine-N-butyl bromide (Buscopan) intramuscularly, to produce duodenal atony.

Contrast media

For the pancreatic duct. Meglumine diatrizoate 65 per cent (e.g. Angiografin) because the contrast medium should have a high iodine content and low toxicity. Meglumine salts are used in preference to sodium salts, as the latter cause pain when injected and may cause pancreatitis.

For the biliary ducts. Meglumine iothalamate 60 per cent (e.g. Conray 280) because the contrast medium must not be too dense as otherwise small opacities, such as those caused by papilloma or radiolucent biliary calculi, may be obscured.

Technique. The patient lies on his left side, on the fluoroscopy table, and is made as comfortable as possible. Diazepam (Valium) is given intravenously at the rate of 5 mg per minute until dysarthria or ptosis occurs (Burwood *et al.*, 1973). The endoscope is then introduced into the oesophagus and passed through the stomach and into the duodenal bulb. Duodenal juice is aspirated and a silicone preparation is instilled to suppress frothing. If there is still motility of the duodenum, a further injection of Buscopan (40 mg) is given intravenously.

The endoscope is positioned in the second part of the duodenum and the papilla of Vater is located. The position of the papilla is variable, as is its shape, and fluoroscopy may occasionally be necessary to assist the endoscopist in locating it.

A polythene catheter is filled with contrast medium and is inserted down the central channel of the endoscope. Care must be taken to ensure that there are no air bubbles in the catheter or in the syringe, as these can simulate calculi. At this stage, bile is usually aspirated as a further safeguard against introducing air into the duct system. Just before the papilla is cannulated, the patient is gently turned into the prone position.

Usually the pancreatic duct fills first and separately, but occasionally both the pancreatic and the common bile ducts fill simultaneously (Plate XXXIXA). To demonstrate the pancreatic duct, 2 to 4 ml of contrast medium are injected under fluoroscopic control. As soon as the larger radicles of the pancreas have been filled, the injection is stopped, as the finer radicles fill without further injection. Under-couch radiographs are taken (*a*) with the patient in the prone position (*b*) in the lateral position and (*c*) sometimes also in both posterior oblique positions (with each side of the body raised 45°). As soon as the cannula is removed from a normal duct, contrast medium flows out of it. If the duct is dilated, further views may be necessary to demonstrate it.

The cannula is then re-positioned, under fluoroscopic control, into the orifice of the common bile duct and contrast medium is injected to fill the biliary ducts (Plate XXXIXB) and gall-bladder (if present). At this stage, the endoscope is usually removed so as to avoid its obscuring the area being examined and to reduce irradiation of the glass fibres as these can eventually be damaged by radiation. Over-couch radiographs are then taken (a) with the patient in the prone position (b) in both anterior oblique positions (with each side of the body raised 45°) and (c) in the lateral position.

After all these radiographs have been seen by the radiologist, a final erect view of the gall-bladder area is usually taken.

If it proves impossible to cannulate the papilla of Vater, hypotonic duodenography (p. 262) is usually performed, so as to take advantage of the fact that there is a catheter in the duodenum, and thus avoiding the necessity for the patient to have further intubation at a later date.

After-care of the patient
1. The patient must have nothing to eat or drink for about an hour after the examination, until full sensation has returned to the pharynx.
2. The serum amylase level should be estimated on the following day and, if indicated clinically, at intervals for about three weeks. Any undue rise may be indicative of pancreatitis. There is always a rise in the level after an injection of contrast medium into the pancreatic duct, but it should return to the patient's usual level within 2 to 7 days.

Basic trolley setting

A sterile trolley is not usually required but the following items are needed:

Endoscope (usually Olympus JF-B) and light source
Catheters for use with endoscope
Aspirator
Two 50 ml disposable syringes
Two 20 ml disposable syringes
Disposable needles
Drawing-up cannulae
Hyoscine-N-butyl bromide (Buscopan) 20 mg ampoules
Anaesthetic lozenge (e.g. Amethocaine, 30 mg)
Diazepam (Valium) ampoules, 10 mg

Contrast media ('Angiografin', 'Conray 280')
Silicone preparation (e.g. 'Darlings powder')
KY jelly
Barium sulphate suspension (for hypotonic duodenography)
Gauze swabs
EMERGENCY DRUGS

PERCUTANEOUS TRANSHEPATIC CHOLEDOCHOGRAPHY

This examination is usually performed for the immediate pre-operative investigation of a patient with jaundice thought to be of obstructive origin. It is used to differentiate between extrahepatic biliary obstruction and intrahepatic cholestasis. When extrahepatic obstruction is present, the nature, size, shape and extent of the obstructing lesion can usually be shown and the ducts proximal to the lesion demonstrated (Nolan, 1977). The injection of contrast medium is made into one of the intrahepatic bile ducts, using a 'Chiba' needle which is a long (15 cm), thin (23F gauge), stainless steel needle with a 30° bevel angle (Ferrucci et al., 1976; Tabrisky et al., 1976).

The examination is carried out under fluoroscopic control, using image intensification and television.

Contra-indications. The examination is contra-indicated in patients (a) who have a tendency to bleeding (b) with biliary tract infection (c) who have a positive serological test for Australia antigen or (d) who have a history of sensitivity to contrast media.

Preparation of the patient
1. The prothrombin time is tested and must be corrected if found to be abnormal.
2. Prophylactic antibiotic cover is given.
3. The patient must have nothing to eat or drink for five hours.

Premedication such as Omnopon and Scopolamine, or Diazepam is given.

Contrast medium. Conray 280 or its equivalent, 20 to 60 ml.

Preliminary film. The patient lies supine on the fluoroscopy table, with his right hand behind his head. An antero-posterior view of the right side of the abdomen is taken, using a 24 × 30 cm (12 × 10 in) cassette, with its lower border at the level of the right iliac crest.

Centre in the mid-clavicular line, 2·5–5 cm (1–2 in) above the level of the lower costal margin.

Technique. The patient lies supine on the fluoroscopy table, with his right hand behind his head. Blood pressure, pulse, temperature and respiration are recorded. Under fluoroscopic control, the puncture site is chosen and marked on the patient's skin. The examination is performed under strict aseptic conditions. The patient's skin is prepared with a suitable antiseptic and draped with sterile towels. Local anaesthetic is injected at the previously determined puncture site, the patient is asked to stop breathing in mid-respiration and the Chiba needle is inserted into the liver. The stylet is removed and the needle is connected, via a flexible polythene connector, to a syringe containing contrast medium. Under fluoroscopic control, the needle is slowly withdrawn while contrast medium is gently injected, until a bile duct is located. Contrast medium is then injected into the bile duct and radiographs are taken using the under-couch tube (Plate XL). If the bile ducts are dilated, bile is aspirated from the ducts before the contrast medium is injected.

If a bile duct is not entered during the first withdrawal of the needle, it can be re-inserted up to 10 times before the examination is abandoned (Fraser *et al.*, 1978).

The quantity of contrast medium injected will vary with the calibre of the ducts. If the ducts are dilated, bile and contrast medium are aspirated from the ducts before the needle is removed. After the needle has been removed, further radiographs are taken with the patient in the supine, oblique, lateral, erect and Trendelenberg (tilted head-down) positions.

If the examination has revealed a dilated or obstructed biliary tree, the patient will go straight to the operating theatre for laparotomy to be performed. If bile was not aspirated from the liver, and therefore no injection was made, the implication may be that the jaundice is not of obstructive origin and the patient is usually returned to the ward.

In suspected extrahepatic biliary obstruction, delayed films—taken two hours after the injection—are of value (Okuda *et al.*, 1974).

After-care of the patient

1. The patient must be under constant observation for 48 hours for any signs of haemorrhage, leakage of bile or peritonitis.
2. Temperature, pulse and blood pressure are recorded every 10 minutes for 1 hour, then 2-hourly for 4 hours, then 4-hourly for 24 hours.

Basic trolley setting

Upper (sterile) shelf

Two Chiba needles
Flexible polythene connector
Two lotion bowls
Two gallipots
One pair dissecting forceps
One pair Spencer Wells forceps
One 5 ml syringe
One 20 ml syringe
Drawing-up cannula
Gloves
Towels
Gauze swabs
Gowns

Lower (unsterile) shelf

Skin cleanser (e.g. Hibitane 0·5% in 70% industrial spirit)
Local anaesthetic (e.g. Lignocaine 1%)
Ampoules of contrast medium in bowl of warm water
Saline
Masks
Disposable needles
EMERGENCY DRUGS

OPERATIVE CHOLEDOCHOGRAPHY

This examination is sometimes performed during cholecystectomy, to demonstrate any gall-stone within the biliary ducts.

Contrast medium. Hypaque 25 per cent or its equivalent, approximately 20 ml depending on the calibre of the ducts.

Preliminary film. An antero-posterior view of the right upper abdomen is taken. Fast films and screens are used so that the exposure time is short. The anaesthetist arrests the patient's respiration while the exposure is made.

Technique. The contrast medium is injected by the surgeon into the biliary tree, usually through the cystic duct. Two radiographs (positioned as for the preliminary film) are taken, one after two-thirds of the contrast medium has been injected and one at the end of the injection, to make sure that any filling defect is constant. Close co-operation between the surgeon, radiographer and anaesthetist is necessary to ensure that there is no respiratory blur and that the contrast medium is injected without bubbles as these may simulate calculi.

When a mobile image intensifier is available, the injection is given under fluoroscopic control. The quantity of contrast medium needed is usually less by this method and the radiographs are centred fluoroscopically.

POST-OPERATIVE CHOLEDOCHOGRAPHY

This examination is usually performed about ten days after operation, just before the drainage tube is removed. It is carried out to ensure that no gall-stone remains in the biliary ducts.

The examination is carried out by the radiologist using fluoroscopy, preferably with image intensification and television.

Preparation of the patient. None is required.

Premedication. No premedication is required.

Contrast medium. Hypaque 25 per cent or its equivalent.

Preliminary film. The patient lies supine on the fluoroscopy table. An antero-posterior view of the right side of the abdomen is taken. A 24 × 30 cm (12 × 10 in) cassette is used, with its lower border at the level of the right iliac crest.

Centre in the right mid-clavicular line, at the level of the lower costal margin.

Technique. The drainage tube is clipped off by means of artery forceps. The tube is wiped with an antiseptic impregnated swab and the injection of contrast medium is made directly into the tube. Care must be taken to ensure that no bubbles are injected (as these may simulate calculi) and that contrast medium does not leak out on to the skin. The injection is watched on the television monitor and continued until the entire biliary tree has been satisfactorily demonstrated. Serial radiographs are taken by the radiologist as required.

When all the necessary radiographs have been taken, the clip is removed from the drainage tube.

Basic trolley setting

Upper (sterile) shelf

    One pair artery forceps *or* adaptor if non-sealing plastic tubing is used

One 20 ml syringe
Drawing-up cannula
Gallipot
Towel
Gauze swabs

Lower (unsterile) shelf

Hibitane in spirit (for wiping tubing)
Ampoules of contrast medium in bowl of warm water
EMERGENCY DRUGS

35

Urinary tract

Anatomy. The two kidneys lie on the upper posterior abdominal wall and are surrounded by peri-renal fat. The left kidney is usually higher than the right and both lie between the levels of the twelfth thoracic and third lumbar vertebral bodies and descend by as much as one and a half vertebrae on full inspiration. They lie obliquely in both planes, their long axes being directed downwards and laterally and their transverse axes forwards and medially.

The renal parenchyma surrounds a variable complex branched collecting system, consisting of minor calyces which join to form major calyces and these in turn unite to form the renal pelvis. The renal pelvis leaves the kidney at its hilum and narrows to join the ureter which descends along the posterior abdominal wall, roughly along the line of the tips of the transverse processes of the lumbar vertebrae. At the pelvic brim it sweeps laterally around the wall of the true bony pelvis and enters the base of the bladder near the mid-line.

The bladder is a distensible, muscular reservoir, situated on the floor of the pelvis anteriorly, extending up the anterior abdominal wall when distended. Its maximum capacity in the adult is usually 700 to 1,000 ml.

In the female, the urethra is about 4 cm long and is directed from the base of the bladder forwards and downwards.

In the male, the urethra is 18 to 20 cm long. The prostatic urethra lies just below the base of the bladder and is surrounded by the prostate gland. It continues as the membranous urethra through the floor of the pelvis and expands into the bulbous urethra which then continues as the penile urethra.

Physiology. The kidneys excrete waste products in aqueous solution and perform a major role in the maintenance of a normal body electrolyte balance. The urine is initially formed by glomerular filtration from the blood and it then passes along a complex nephron where water and some other constituents are re-absorbed and others are actively excreted. Groups of nephrons join to form collecting tubules which drain into the minor calyces.

EXCRETION UROGRAPHY

This is the basic method of examination of the urinary tract and it usually precedes any other radiological examination of this system. Excretion urography depends upon the ability of the kidneys to concentrate and excrete circulating contrast medium. It is better termed excretion urography, rather than intravenous pyelography (I.V.P.) because with modern methods the whole urinary tract, and not just the pelvi-calyceal systems, is demonstrated.

For a female patient, the 10-day rule (p. 19) should be observed if the degree of clinical urgency permits.

Preparation of the patient

1. The patient should take a suitable aperient on each of the two preceding nights.
2. When low dose techniques are employed, the patient should not have more than one pint of fluid during the preceding 24 hours and should have nothing to drink for about 8 hours before the examination. Fluid restriction is contra-indicated in patients who are in renal failure or who have myelomatosis.
3. Whenever possible the patient should be ambulant so as to avoid the accumulation of intestinal gas.
4. The patient must micturate immediately before the examination.

Premedication. None is necessary for adults. For small children, adequate basal narcosis is advisable.

Contrast medium. The sodium or meglumine salts of diatrizoate or iothalamate are used, either separately or as a mixture, i.e.

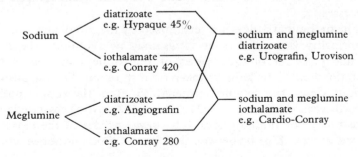

Low, medium or high doses of contrast medium can be used, according to the clinical problem and the radiologist's decision. The dosages (Saxton, 1969) for a 70 kg adult are:

1. *Low*, less than 12 g iodine
    e.g. 20 ml Urografin 76% (7·4 g)
    20 ml Conray 420 (8·4 g)
    40 ml Hypaque 45% (10·8 g)
2. *Medium*, between 12 and 30 g iodine
    e.g. 50 ml Conray 420 (21 g)
    50 ml Urovison (16·25 g)
3. *High*, over 30 g iodine

Preliminary films (K.U.B.). The patient lies supine with the knees flexed over a small pillow. In a child or small adult, the whole urinary tract can be demonstrated on one 35 × 43 cm (17 × 14 in) radiograph but in most cases two radiographs will be necessary to include the whole urinary tract, as follows:

1. A 35 × 43 cm (17 × 14 in) cassette is used, with its lower border at the lower margin of the symphysis pubis, which must be included on the radiograph. The exposure is made on arrested expiration.

Centre in the mid-line, at the level of the middle of the cassette.

2. A 24 × 30 cm (12 × 10 in) cassette—or 30 × 40 cm (15 × 12 in) cassette for a very large patient—placed transversely, is used for the kidney region. The lower border of the cassette is placed 2·5 cm (1 in) below the iliac crests. The aperture is decreased to cover the smaller area included on this view. The exposure is again made on arrested expiration.

Centre in the mid-line, at the level of the middle of the cassette.

It is important to keep the kilovoltage low so as to show optimum soft tissue detail. Rare earth or very fast tungstate screens permit the use of low kilovoltage and short exposure times. A satisfactory exposure will clearly show the renal outlines, the psoas muscle shadows and the trabecular pattern of the lumbar transverse processes.

The preliminary films are scrutinised by the radiologist and if an abnormality is seen, further views may be required; these may include posterior oblique views of the kidneys and an antero-posterior view of the kidneys taken on inspiration. For the posterior oblique views, the patient is rotated 35° from the supine position towards each side in turn. A 24 × 30 cm (12 × 10 in) cassette is used so as to include both kidneys. The lower border of the cassette is placed 2·5 cm (1 in) below the iliac crests. Both posterior oblique views are usually taken. When an exposure is made on arrested full inspiration the kilovoltage required is 5 to 10 more than for the similar view taken on expiration.

Centre to the cassette.

Technique. The contrast medium is injected intravenously. Because the injection may be followed by a minor (or, rarely, a major) reaction the patient must be observed throughout the examination for signs of any adverse effect. The appropriate drugs and apparatus must be readily available (p. 211).

There are variations in detail in the precise timing of the subsequent views and the area to be included on each radiograph. The examination is usually tailored to the presenting diagnostic problem and is then supervised continuously by the radiologist. Usually a radiograph is taken soon after the injection, to record the nephrogram phase and to reveal any difference in function between the two kidneys. Subsequent radiographs are taken to demonstrate the pelvicalyceal systems, ureters and finally the bladder. A commonly used regime will be described.

1. A radiograph of the kidneys—as for the preliminary film—is taken immediately after the injection is completed, to show the nephrogram phase.

2. Five minutes after the injection, a similar view of the kidneys is taken on full arrested inspiration. The level of the kidneys is about 2·5 to 4 cm (1 to 1½ in) lower than on the view taken on expiration and the level of the cassette and the centering point must be adjusted accordingly.

If a large quantity of contrast medium has been injected, the exposure factors must be increased for this and the next views. Depending on the size of the patient and the quantity of contrast medium injected, the mA.s may need to be as much as doubled from that required for the preliminary film.

After this exposure has been made, ureteric compression (see p. 294) is applied.

3. Fifteen and thirty minutes after the injection, views of the kidneys are taken on arrested expiration (Plate XLI), and so the centering point is the same as for the preliminary films but the exposure required is the same as for the 5-minute film. Ureteric compression tends to increase the thickness of the upper abdomen, particularly in an obese patient.

Tomography is used when (*a*) there are confusing overlying shadows or (*b*) the nephrogram or pyelogram is inadequate. The optimum time for tomography is usually 10 minutes after the injection, when the nephrographic density has diminished and pyelographic intensity is best (Dure-Smith and McArdle, 1972) and for an average patient, linear tomography, 9 to 12 cm from the table-top, is usually satisfactory.

4. If the above views have provided adequate visualisation of the kidneys, the compression is released and a view of the lower urinary tract is taken (Plate XLII). A 35 × 43 cm (17 × 14 in) cassette is placed in position (with its lower border at the level of the symphysis pubis) and the tube is centred before the compression is released.

5. A post-micturition view of the bladder is taken. Sometimes the urine passed is collected, to measure quantity and assess density (Benness et al., 1965). The patient lies supine. An 18 × 24 cm (10 × 8 in) cassette is used, with its upper border at the level of the anterior superior iliac spines.

Centre 2·5 cm (1 in) below the anterior superior iliac spines, with the tube angled 15° caudad.

If the radiographs so far taken suggest ureteric obstruction, a full-length post-micturition view is taken to demonstrate renal drainage.

Ureteric compression. The purpose of ureteric compression is to retain within the pelvi-calyceal systems and upper ureters the contrast medium excreted by the kidneys. It is extremely important in low dose techniques where relatively small volumes of contrast medium are excreted. In high dose technique it is not always essential but is employed when pelvi-calyceal filling is inadequate.

There are various methods of compressing the ureters, the most efficient being by means of an inflatable balloon supported by a stiff board usually made of rigid plastic. These are strapped to the patient by means of a belt which encircles him. A band which merely compresses the patient to the table is contra-indicated (Hodson, 1966). The balloon is placed in position mid-way between the anterior superior iliac spines, before the 5-minute radiograph is taken, but the straps are not tightened. After the radiograph has been taken, the straps are tightened as much as possible, care being taken that there are no folds of skin or gown to cause discomfort to the patient. The balloon is then inflated, usually by means of a sphygmo-manometer device. The pressure in the balloon need not be high if the belt has been correctly applied. When the balloon has been inflated sufficiently to become uncomfortable for the patient, he is told to bend his knees and put the soles of his feet on the table, thus reducing the thickness of the abdomen and allowing the belt to be tightened. In this way, though the compression must still be uncomfortably tight, it is more readily bearable by the patient.

At times, compression may impair the venous return from the legs and produce a state of shock in the patient, resulting in cold, clammy skin and low blood pressure. This state usually responds immediately to release of compression and tilt of the patient head-down.

After the 30-minute kidney view has been taken, the compression is released gently, the patient being asked to breathe in and out twice whilst the compression device is being removed. He is then asked to stop breathing and the exposure is made immediately. Using this method of releasing compression, contrast medium is seen in the greater part, if not the whole, of the ureters and also in the bladder (Plate XLII).

Ureteric compression is contra-indicated after recent trauma or operation and in these cases high dose techniques and tomography are invaluable.

Radiation protection. The radiation dose to the gonads is potentially high in examinations of the urinary tract. Gonad protection must be used for all views in male patients. For female patients, gonad protection is not possible when views of the ureters and bladder are being taken. Lead is usually incorporated in the plastic compression device. When views of the kidneys are being taken without the compression device *in situ*, a piece of lead rubber must always be placed over the pelvis, the upper border being placed at the level of the anterior superior iliac spines.

Modifications. There are many modifications which may be required under particular circumstances, the most common being as follows:

Infants and children. Because of the risk of dehydration, fluids must not be restricted for infants. For children, fluid restriction is not usually necessary, especially when high doses of contrast medium are given. A thirsty child is seldom co-operative and hydration may be advantageous in ensuring that the renal pelves and calyces are distended. Adequate bowel preparation is necessary.

The injection is given intravenously if possible. A vein in the elbow or the back of the hand is used but it is often necessary to use a scalp vein for infants. If intravenous injection is not possible, the contrast medium is injected subcutaneously. This will give an adequate, if not optimum, result.

Two ml of contrast medium per kg body weight are injected for babies weighing less than 8 kg, 20 ml between 8 and 30 kg. When renal failure is suspected up to 4 ml per kg are injected.

If intestinal gas obscures the kidneys, the stomach is distended by means of a fizzy drink. The kidneys are then visible against the radiolucent background. A right posterior oblique view may be required to project the gastric gas fully over the right kidney.

Opacities or translucencies. Posterior oblique views are required to demonstrate the exact site of any opacity or translucency seen on the preliminary films, overlying the urinary tract. These views should be taken before contrast medium is injected as this might obscure the opacity or translucency. The positioning is described under 'preliminary films' on page 292.

Intestinal gas. Tomography blurs the obscuring image of intestinal gas. A single exposure using a multi-layer cassette usually provides an excellent demonstration of the kidneys. A small angle (zonography) is usually employed.

Renal failure. To distinguish between obstruction in pre-renal failure (which is not usually conducive to operation) and in post-renal failure (which is operable). There must be no preparatory fluid restriction. A high dose of contrast medium must be given. Delayed radiographs, up to 24 hours or even more, tomography (to show renal size) and additional radiographs of some bones, e.g. hands (p. 143), are needed.

Hypertension. To compare the rate at which the kidneys commence excretion, several radiographs are taken within the first five or six minutes before compression is applied.

Delayed excretion. Views of the kidneys may be required at increasing intervals up to 24 hours after the injection if excretion by the kidneys is delayed.

Ectopia. If no kidney, or only one, is seen to be functioning at five minutes, an antero-posterior view of the whole abdomen must be taken.

Hydronephrosis. The maximum dose of contrast medium is given. Delayed radiographs, up to 48 hours after the injection, may be needed. A prone view of the kidney region is required. As the pelvis of the kidney lies anteriorly, contrast medium pools in it when the patient lies prone. An erect view may also be helpful (Davies *et al.*, 1972).

Bladder abnormalities. These include prostatic hyperplasia, diverticula and bladder carcinoma. Oblique views of the bladder are required. From the supine position, the patient is rotated 35° towards each side in turn. A 24 × 30 cm (12 × 10 in) cassette is used transversely. The knee of the side towards which the patient is turned is flexed and the pelvis is supported on foam pads. A radiograph is taken in each position.

Centre to the anterior superior iliac spine of the raised side.

Patients with haematuria, for which no cause has been demonstrated by radiographs taken at 30 minutes after the injection, should have oblique views taken of the bladder.

Serial renography

When serial observations of the urinary tract are likely to be needed for several months or even years (e.g. in patients with carcinoma of the cervix who have ureteric involvement) renography (p. 68) is often helpful because it is less hazardous for the patient, is tolerated more easily and gives less radiation dose than urography. The timing for the next urogram can be determined by reference to changes shown in the renogram.

NEPHROTOMOGRAPHY

This examination is used to obtain further information regarding a suspected space-occupying lesion demonstrated by excretion urography.

Preparation of the patient. As for excretion urography.

Premedication. None is required.

Contrast medium. 20 ml Hypaque 45 per cent or its equivalent initially, followed by a further injection of 50 ml Hypaque 85 per cent and 5 ml Decholin 20 per cent.

Preliminary films. The patient lies supine on the tomography table. A view of the kidneys is taken as for excretion urography, using a 24×30 cm (12×10 in) cassette. A preliminary tomogram of the kidneys is also taken to check exposure factors and depth of cut. The centering point is marked on the patient's skin.

Technique. A Robb-Steinberg needle or other large cannula is introduced into a vein in the antecubital fossa, 5 ml 20 per cent Decholin is injected and the arm-to-tongue circulation time is measured. This is usually between 10 and 14 seconds. The arm-to-kidney time is practically identical. Twenty ml 45 per cent Hypaque are then injected to produce a pyelogram and 50 ml 85 per cent Hypaque are then injected rapidly. The radiographer must be prepared to expose the first film at the time previously determined by the Decholin test. A second radiograph is taken two to three seconds later. The first radiograph will show the renal arteries and their branches and the second will show opacification of the renal parenchyma (Post and Southwood, 1959).

Two or three tomograms are then taken, a multi-layer cassette being used whenever available. A small arc or circle is used (zonography, p. 49) so as to obtain fairly thick cuts.

The needle or cannula is left *in situ* whilst the films are processed so that a second injection can be given if necessary. When satisfactory radiographs have been obtained it is removed.

RETROGRADE PYELO-URETEROGRAPHY

This examination is usually performed when excretion urography has failed to demonstrate adequately the pelvi-calyceal systems and ureters. Modern high dose techniques have made retrograde studies of the kidney much less common.

Preparation of the patient. A catheter is introduced into the ureter at cystoscopy. No preparation other than for the cystoscopy is required. When general anaesthesia has been employed it is desirable to delay the examination until after the patient is sufficiently conscious to co-operate. It is very important in these circumstances that the patient does not pull out the catheter.

Contrast medium. Usually Hypaque 25 per cent or its equivalent. Up to 10 ml are required for a normal kidney, considerably more in cases of hydronephrosis.

Preliminary film. The patient lies supine with the pelvis positioned symmetrically. A 35 × 43 cm (17 × 14 in) cassette is used, with its lower border at the level of the symphysis pubis. The exposure is made on arrested expiration and a short exposure time is usually employed to ensure that there is no respiratory blur on the radiograph. This is particularly important if the patient is not fully conscious.

Centre in the mid-line, at the level of the middle of the cassette.

A left or right posterior oblique view may be required if an opacity is shown in the line of the catheter. For these views, the patient is rotated 35° towards the side being examined and is supported on foam pads. A 35 × 43 cm (17 × 14 in) cassette is used, with its lower border at the level of the symphysis pubis.

Centre in the mid-clavicular line of the raised side, at the level of the middle of the cassette.

Technique. The examination is usually carried out under fluoroscopic control, preferably with image intensification and television. It is performed under strict aseptic conditions and in particular the end of the catheter must be kept sterile. It is usually immersed in a specimen bottle which is strapped to the inside of the patient's thigh. The catheter is withdrawn until the tip lies within the renal pelvis. Under strict aseptic conditions, urine is aspirated until the pelvis is empty. The specimen bottle, with urine from the syringe added to it if necessary, is sent to the pathology department for analysis. The syringe is then changed and contrast medium is injected under fluoroscopic control by the radiologist.

Appropriate under-couch radiographs are taken. A typical series includes postero-anterior and left and right anterior oblique views, usually taken on 24×30 cm (12×10 in) cassettes divided into two. These radiographs are processed and if they are satisfactory the catheter is withdrawn into the ureter. If there is obstruction at the pelvi-ureteric junction, the contrast medium is first aspirated from the kidney.

More contrast medium is then injected and further under-couch radiographs of the filled ureter are taken. These radiographs are processed and if they are satisfactory the catheter is usually removed.

Modifications
1. When fluoroscopic control is not available, an entirely over-couch technique is used. The general aim of the examination remains the same but it may be necessary to process each radiograph before taking the next or before injecting any further contrast medium. A rapid automatic processor is an advantage.

The position of the kidney is noted from the preliminary film and early views in the series are centred according to this. When the catheter is withdrawn into the ureter, 35×43 cm (17×14 in) cassettes are used, with their lower borders at the level of the symphysis pubis. The whole ureter is then included.

2. If the catheter has been introduced because of acute renal obstruction, it must be left draining the kidney and therefore withdrawal ureterograms are not possible. It is essential to determine whether the catheter is to be left *in situ* before any retrograde pyelo-ureterogram is undertaken.

3. If retrograde catheterisation is found to be impossible, or if ureterograms are required without placing a catheter within the lumen, reflux ureterograms can be produced using a Braasch bulb catheter. This is impacted in the lower ureter at cystoscopy, contrast medium is injected and over-couch radiographs are taken with the cystoscope still *in situ*.

Basic trolley setting

Upper (sterile) shelf

Ureteric catheter connections
Two 20 ml syringes
Drawing-up cannula
Gallipot
Receiver
Dissecting forceps
Towels
Gauze swabs

Lower (unsterile) shelf

Surgical spirit
Ampoules of contrast medium in bowl of warm water
File (for opening ampoules)
EMERGENCY DRUGS

RENAL PUNCTURE

This examination is used to ascertain whether a renal cyst is the cause of a space-occupying lesion which has been previously demonstrated by urography.

It is performed under fluoroscopic control, using image intensification and television. Most of the over-couch radiographs are taken with a horizontal beam.

For a female patient, the 10-day rule should be observed if the degree of clinical urgency permits.

Preparation of the patient

1. The patient should have nothing to drink for six hours unless fluid restriction is contra-indicated, e.g. for a patient in renal failure or with myelomatosis.
2. The patient should have nothing to eat for six hours.
3. The patient should take an aperient for two nights before the examination.
4. The patient should be ambulant if possible, to reduce intestinal gas.

Premedication. Usually none is required but sedation may be needed for an apprehensive patient. Children usually require general anaesthesia.

Preliminary film. The patient will have had an excretion urogram but a view of the kidney area is taken immediately before renal puncture. A 24×30 cm (12×10 in) or 30×40 cm (15×12 in) cassette is used, with its lower border at the level of the iliac crests.

Centre in the mid-line, at the level of the middle of the cassette.

Contrast medium. Hypaque 25 per cent or its equivalent.

Technique. The patient lies supine on the fluoroscopy table. If the position of the kidneys is not clearly demonstrated on fluoroscopy, an injection of a high dose of contrast medium is given (as for excretion urography, p. 291). The patient is then turned into the prone position and is made as comfortable as possible. A radiolucent pad is placed under the abdomen—just caudad to the lower costal margin—to prevent anterior movement of the kidneys. The position of the kidneys is checked by fluoroscopy and a metal marker is placed on the skin to show the optimum site for puncture. The position of this marker is marked on the patient's skin to help in radiographic positioning later.

The examination is performed under strict aseptic conditions. The patient's skin is prepared with a suitable antiseptic and sterile towels are placed in position. Local anaesthetic is injected. Under fluoroscopic control, a long, fine needle (such as a Greenburg exploring needle) is introduced into the cyst. Cyst fluid is aspirated and measured, and a sample is sent to the pathology department for analysis.

Contrast medium is then injected into the cyst until the quantity injected equals half the original volume of the fluid aspirated. Air is then injected to give double contrast. The quantity of air injected should be a little less than would fill the remainder of the cyst because air expands as it warms to body temperature (Kerr and Roylance, 1977). When the contrast media have been injected, the needle is removed and a series of radiographs is taken, all but the supine antero-posterior view being taken with a horizontal beam and vertically-placed grid cassette. All the views are taken on arrested respiration and the X-ray tube is centred to the cyst, using the mark made on the patient's skin at initial fluoroscopy.

Prone lateral. The patient remains in the prone position, with his hands on the pillow. The grid cassette is supported vertically against the side under examination.

Right and left lateral decubitus. The patient lies on each side in turn, with the vertically-placed cassette supported behind him, so that an antero-posterior view is obtained each time.

Supine lateral. The patient lies supine, raised from the table on foam pads. His hands are placed on the pillow. The cassette is supported vertically against the side under examination.

Antero-posterior. The patient remains supine. A vertical beam is used.

Erect antero-posterior. Either the fluoroscopy table is tilted into the vertical position, or the patient sits or stands against a vertical cassette stand.

Modifications

1. If blood-stained fluid is aspirated, the space-occupying lesion is probably a carcinoma, but it could be a haematoma or a haemorrhage into a simple cyst (Watt and Penry, 1973). Fluid aspirated is sent to the pathology department for differentiation. Often the examination is terminated at this point but some authorities advocate the injection of 1 to 2 ml of contrast medium to show the typical coarse irregularly-arranged stroma of carcinoma (Wright, 1972). Antero-posterior, lateral and both oblique views are then taken.

2. When image intensification is not available, an entirely over-couch method can be used (Gordon, 1958). The injection of contrast medium is given as previously described and the patient is turned into the prone position. A marker, consisting of lead shot embedded in perspex at 1 cm intervals, is attached to the patient's back, so as to lie approximately over the pelvis of the kidney which is being examined.

Postero-anterior and lateral views are taken. The lateral is taken using a horizontal beam and with a grid cassette supported vertically. Whilst these films are being processed, the patient must remain in the same position, with the marker *in situ*.

The puncture site is selected so that it is immediately above the centre of the suspected lesion. The depth of the lesion is determined from the lateral view, using the magnified image of the marker as a scale. A stop, or collar, is fixed to the puncture needle at the measured depth of the lesion. The needle is then inserted. Postero-anterior and lateral views are taken as before, to check the position of the needle. When the needle has been correctly sited, fluid is collected and contrast medium is injected and the same series of views is then taken as previously described.

3. Demonstration of the kidney in (*a*) prograde pyelography (which is performed to fill an obstructed hydronephrotic kidney when excretion and retrograde urography have failed) or (*b*) percutaneous needle biopsy, is undertaken in a similar manner using either the fluoroscopic or the radiographic method.

4. Renal puncture can be performed also under computed tomographic control (Haaga *et al.*, 1977) or under ultrasonic control.

After-care of the patient

1. A radiograph of the chest is taken following the examination, because a pneumothorax sometimes, though rarely, occurs (Jeans *et al.*, 1972).

2. The patient must stay in hospital for the night following the examination and should be observed for signs of haemorrhage.

PERCUTANEOUS NEPHROSTOMY

This is the percutaneous drainage of an obstructed kidney. The examination consists of two parts (*a*) antegrade (or prograde) pyelography to locate and fill with contrast medium a kidney about which insufficient information has been obtained by excretion or retrograde urography and (*b*) the draining of the kidney. It is performed on patients with obstruction of the ureters due to malignant disease, or with obstruction of the pelvi-calyceal junction (Saxton *et al.*, 1972).

The examination is carried out under local anaesthesia except on infants, for whom ketamine sedation is recommended (Sherwood and Stevenson, 1972).

Preparation of the patient. As for excretion urography (p. 291).

Premedication. Uraemic patients are often slightly drowsy, so sedation is not usually needed.

Contrast medium. 60 ml Conray 420 or its equivalent.

Preliminary film. Usually this is not necessary, as the patient will have had a recent urogram. If no recent radiographs are available, an antero-posterior view of the abdomen and kidney area is taken as for excretion urography.

Technique. An intravenous injection of contrast medium is given. The patient is turned into the prone position and is made as comfortable as possible. Using image intensification and television, the renal area is examined fluoroscopically. If the pelvi-calyceal system is not well demonstrated, it may be necessary to take a radiograph of the abdomen, with a metal marker on the probable site of the kidney.

The skin is infiltrated with local anaesthetic and, under fluoroscopic control, a long exploring needle (at least 15 cm) is advanced into the pelvi-calyceal system. When the needle is in place, urine is withdrawn and contrast medium is injected so as to outline the system clearly. Under fluoroscopic control, the needle is replaced by a large-bore renal biopsy needle (e.g. Vim-Silverman) or a catheter-over-needle assembly. The catheter is secured in place by a skin stitch and by adhesive strapping and is attached to a disposable plastic drainage bag.

The time which drainage takes varies between about 9 to 65 days depending on the condition of the patient (Saxton *et al.*, 1972).

After-care of the patient. The sudden relief of obstruction in a uraemic patient may cause a sudden diuresis, so fluid must be maintained. Apart from this, no special after-care is needed.

MICTURATING CYSTOGRAPHY

This examination is used mainly to demonstrate vesico-ureteric reflux, especially in children. It is also used in the investigation of stress incontinence and of outflow tract obstruction. It is performed under fluoroscopic control, preferably with image intensification and television. Ciné-fluorography is of advantage if micturition is to be studied at length.

The examination is contra-indicated if there is acute infection of the bladder or urethra.

Preparation of the patient. The patient micturates immediately before the examination.

Premedication. None is necessary. Occasionally a short general anaesthetic may be required for children, but premedication should be avoided as it may make the child resent any disturbance (Edwards, 1973).

Contrast medium. Dilute water-soluble contrast medium is used, such as Hypaque 10 to 25 per cent or its equivalent.

Preliminary films. Plain films of the urinary tract (K.U.B.) are required (p. 292) unless recently taken.

Technique. The patient lies supine on the fluoroscopy table. Under strict aseptic conditions, a catheter is introduced into the bladder. Catheterisation inevitably carries a high risk of introducing infection and this risk is reduced if (*a*) the catheter is lubricated with a cream containing Hibitane (*b*) rigid asepsis is observed and (*c*) the time during which the catheter is in position is kept to the minimum possible.

Any residual urine is drained, measured and sent to the pathology department for examination. The contrast medium is run into the bladder using a drip technique. A relatively slow infusion is necessary, usually with the bottle about 90 cm (36 in) above the table and with the tap in the full 'on' position. The infusion is controlled by intermittent fluoroscopy of the abdomen. If reflux is seen, appropriate radiographs are taken, usually on 35×43 cm (17×14 in) cassettes, using the over-couch tube. When the bladder is full (for which usually 700 to 1,000 ml are required in the adult) the catheter is withdrawn. The table is then tilted to the vertical position and the patient stands firmly on the step. Under-couch films are taken during micturition (Plate XLIII). Some form of receiver is required during the micturition series. Usually a plastic urine bottle held by the patient is used for male patients and a suitable rubber and plastic urinal for female patients. This must be secured in position before the patient stands up, in case micturition begins immediately.

Difficulty may be experienced by the patient in emptying the bladder at this time. This can be overcome by (a) affording the patient as much privacy as possible (b) ensuring that the bladder is filled to its maximum capacity and (c) reducing to a minimum the time interval between removing the catheter and being ready to examine micturition.

Modifications

Children. For small children, the examination is best conducted in the supine oblique position. It is useful to continue the infusion until micturition is initiated, before the catheter is removed. It is sometimes advocated that the contrast medium be introduced into the bladder through a supra-pubic needle.

When the examination is for the investigation of reflux, the whole renal tract must be included on the radiographs taken during micturition, so that any reflux occurring is demonstrated.

Stress incontinence. Lateral views in the erect position are taken of the bladder (a) at rest (b) straining, with the catheter *in situ* and (c) with the patient micturating. These must be true lateral views of the pelvis and must include the whole of the sacrum and coccyx and the symphysis pubis.

A suitable receiver is placed in position and the patient sits or stands in the lateral position against the erect Bucky. The radiographer must be ready to change the cassette rapidly between the exposures, particularly between (2) and (3); 24×30 cm (12×10 in) cassettes are used.

Centre to the head of the femur.

Additional examination

Radionuclide cystography, using $^{99}Tc^m$ pertechnetate, can be used as a complementary technique for dynamic studies of the bladder in children (Rothwell *et al.*, 1977). Visual monitoring and photography are carried out during micturition. The radiation dose is considerably lower than with the routine examination described above.

Basic trolley setting

Upper (sterile) shelf

Disposable catheters
Catheter connection
Two lotion bowls
Gallipot
Receiver
Disposable recipient set

Lower (unsterile) shelf

Cleanser (e.g. Cetavlon 1%)
Lubricating agent (e.g. Hibitane 0·05% in glycerine)
Contrast medium
Adhesive strapping
Suitable receiver

EXCRETORY MICTURITION CYSTO-URETHROGRAPHY

This examination is sometimes performed, on an adult patient, at the end of a high dose excretion urography examination, to demonstrate the bladder and urethra and is of particular use in the diagnosis of prostatic hyperplasia and carcinoma, prostatitis, urethral stenosis and obstruction, vesical and urethral diverticula, or vesical descent and herniation. It may avoid the need for further investigation of the bladder and urethra by other methods.

High dose urography is performed as already described (p. 291) and when contrast medium has filled the bladder, the patient is placed in the erect position, with a suitable receptacle (p. 305). Undercouch radiographs are taken during micturition.

DOUBLE CONTRAST CYSTOGRAPHY

This examination is usually carried out to localise and grade a bladder tumour before radiotherapy. It is of particular value when the neoplasm lies in a diverticulum (Doyle, 1961).

Preparation of the patient
1. The patient should have not more than one pint of fluid during the preceding 24 hours and nothing to drink for eight hours.
2. The patient micturates immediately before the examination.

Premedication. None is usually required.

Contrast medium. Sterile barium sulphate, such as Steripaque, 120 ml.

Technique. The patient lies supine on a foam mattress on the X-ray table. Under strict aseptic conditions the bladder is catheterised and emptied and the Steripaque is run in under fluoroscopic control, preferably with image intensification and television. The catheter is left in position and three over-couch views are taken:

Antero-posterior. The patient lies supine. A 24 × 30 cm (12 × 10 in) cassette is used with its upper border at the level of the anterior superior iliac spines.

Centre 2·5 cm (1 in) below the anterior iliac spines, with the tube angled 15° caudad.

Posterior obliques. From the supine position the patient is rotated 35° to each side in turn. The raised side of the pelvis is supported by foam pads. A 24 × 30 cm (12 × 10 in) cassette is placed transversely, with its upper border at the level of the iliac crests. A radiograph is taken in each position.

Centre 2·5 cm (1 in) below the anterior superior iliac spine of the raised side.

After these radiographs have been inspected, most of the contrast medium is drained off, leaving only about 20 ml. Under fluoroscopic control the bladder is then distended with 60 to 80 ml carbon dioxide. The barium remaining in the bladder will coat any tumour or ulcer but will not adhere to normal mucosa. A series of views is taken using a horizontal beam, as follows:

Antero-posterior I. The patient lies on his side, facing the tube, with the knees extended. A grid cassette is supported vertically behind the pelvis with its caudal border at the level of the symphysis pubis.

Supine lateral. The patient lies supine, with the hands on the chest. The cassette is supported vertically at the side of the pelvis.

Prone lateral. The patient lies prone, with the hands under the chin. The cassette is supported vertically at the side of the pelvis.

Antero-posterior II. The position of the patient is reversed so that he can lie on the opposite side from that in the first antero-posterior view. The cassette is supported vertically behind the pelvis.

Erect antero-posterior. From the horizontal position the table is tilted until the patient is erect and standing comfortably on the foot-rest. The Bucky is used for this view. The lower border of the cassette is again placed at the level of the symphysis pubis and the tube is directed horizontally.

Modification

Simple cystography. This is rarely employed except for radio-therapy planning. After the bladder has been filled the catheter is removed. Strips of radiopaque markers are placed on the front, back and both sides of the patient.

If available, the examination is performed using a simulator. If not, antero-posterior, postero-anterior and both lateral views of the pelvis are taken. A standard focus-film distance, usually 100 cm (40 in), must always be used. The markers must remain *in situ* at the end of the examination or their positions must be accurately marked on the patient's skin.

URETHROGRAPHY

This examination is used mainly in the investigation of strictures, diverticula or false passages in the male urethra (Spackman, 1977).

Preparation of the patient. The patient should micturate immediately before the examination.

Premedication. None is required.

Contrast medium. Usually 30 to 40 ml of viscous contrast medium such as Umbradil viscous is used. But in cases of suspected urethral rupture, a water-soluble contrast medium, such as Urografin 60 per cent or its equivalent, may be preferred (Edwards, 1972).

Equipment. One method of introducing the contrast medium is by means of a Knutsson clamp, but some authorities recommend the use of a Foley catheter (de Lacey and Wignall, 1977). The examination is performed under fluoroscopic control by the radiologist preferably using image intensification and television.

Preliminary film. The patient lies supine on the X-ray table and an antero-posterior view of the bladder base and lower urethra is taken. A 24 × 30 cm (12 × 10 in) cassette is used, with its upper border at the level of the anterior superior iliac spines.

Centre in the mid-line 2·5 cm (1 in) below the anterior superior iliac spines, with the tube angled 15° caudad.

Technique. The catheter or cannula is inserted into the urethra under strict aseptic conditions (p. 304). If a cannula is used, it is firmly fixed in position by adjustment of the arms of the clamp. If a catheter is used, the balloon is inflated.

The patient is rotated into the right posterior oblique position with the right hip and knee flexed and with the raised side of the pelvis supported on foam pads. The contrast medium is injected under fluoroscopic control and serial films are taken as required. A typical series of films would be postero-anterior and both oblique views of the posterior urethra and bladder neck. The injection is continued until the base of the bladder is outlined by the contrast medium. At the end of the injection, an over-couch antero-posterior view is taken, as for the preliminary film. The cannula or catheter is then removed and the patient allowed to empty the bladder.

Modifications

1. The bladder may be distended with 10 to 25 per cent Hypaque before the viscous contrast medium is injected and views during micturition are then obtained after the standard views previously described.

2. An entirely over-couch technique can be used (de Lacey and Wignall, 1977). After infusion of approximately 200 ml of contrast medium (e.g. Urografin 30 per cent), three radiographs are taken with the patient lying in the right posterior oblique position (*a*) at the end of the infusion when the patient urgently requires to void the bladder (*b*) during micturition and (*c*) after abruptly arresting micturition.

3. Double contrast technique is sometimes used—with air as the negative contrast medium—in the investigation of urethral diverticula (Spackman, 1977).

Basic trolley setting

Upper (sterile) shelf

Knutsson penile clamp (*or* Foley catheter)

One 50 ml syringe
Gallipot
Towels
Gauze swabs
Lotion bowl
Gloves

Lower (unsterile) shelf

Cleanser (e.g. Cetavlon 1%)
Lubricating agent (e.g. Hibitane 0·05% in glycerine)
Contrast medium
Receiver

VESICULOGRAPHY

Vesiculography is the radiographic demonstration of the vasa deferentia, seminal vesicles and ejaculatory ducts following the injection of contrast medium into the ducts. It is usually performed to differentiate between prostatic hyperplasia and carcinoma. It is also valuable in the investigation of epididymo-orchiditis (Presland, 1968). The examination is carried out during operation, following vasectomy.

The radiographs usually have to be taken in the operating theatre, using mobile equipment, but sometimes the patient can be transferred, with the catheters *in situ*, to the radiology department.

Preparation of the patient. No preparation, other than that for vasectomy, is required.

Contrast medium. Hypaque 45 per cent, Conray 280 or their equivalent, 1·5 to 2 ml per side per injection.

Preliminary film. The patient lies supine. An antero-posterior view of the bladder is taken, using a 30 × 40 cm (15 × 12 in) cassette, with its upper border at the level of the anterior superior iliac spines.

Centre in the mid-line, at the level of the anterior superior iliac spines, with the tube angled 15° caudad.

Technique. Catheters are inserted into the ducts at operation and they must be long enough to avoid the surgeon's (or radiologist's) hands being irradiated when the exposures are made. Contrast medium is injected into each duct simultaneously for the antero-posterior view and into each duct separately for the oblique views. Oblique views are of value when the ducts are obscured by over-flow of contrast medium into the prostatic urethra on the first injection.

The success of the examination depends on the exposures being made during the injection, when there is maximum filling of the ducts.

Antero-posterior. As for the preliminary film.

Posterior obliques. From the supine position, the patient is rotated about 30° to each side in turn and an exposure is made in each position. The right posterior oblique view is taken to demonstrate the left duct, and the left posterior oblique view to demonstrate the right duct.

Centre 2·5 cm (1 in) medially to the anterior superior iliac spine of the raised side.

36

Female genital tract

1. GYNAECOLOGICAL EXAMINATIONS

Radiographic examination of the non-pregnant patient by means of plain films is performed to exclude or confirm the presence of lesions such as ovarian or uterine tumours and cysts, and fibroids, any of which may show calcification. Usually only an antero-posterior view of the abdomen (p. 195) is required.

Radiological examination in the investigation of infertility comprises hystero-salpingography (below) and gynaecography (p. 331). Before gynaecography, radiography of the pituitary fossa is carried out to exclude abnormalities of the pituitary gland which may cause amenorrhoea and infertility. Radiography of the chest is always included in the investigation of infertility to exclude tuberculosis and hence the possibility of conditions such as tuberculous salpingitis. Chest radiographs are also taken in the case of patients with carcinoma of the uterus, chorion epithelioma or hydatidiform mole, to demonstrate possible metastatic involvement of the lungs.

A full bladder may simulate pathology or make diagnosis difficult and it is therefore important that the patient should micturate immediately before the examination.

HYSTERO-SALPINGOGRAPHY

Hystero-salpingography is the radiographic examination of the uterus and uterine tubes, following injection of contrast medium. It is usually employed in the investigation of infertility.

In most departments, the gynaecologist and radiologist carry out the examination jointly, the gynaecologist giving the injection and the radiologist controlling the examination by fluoroscopy.

Timing of the examination is very important. It must not be performed during the week before or after menstruation, when the endometrium is either engorged or denuded. It is best carried out mid-cycle, when the possibility of irradiating an unrecognised pregnancy is minimal.

The examination is usually performed on out-patients but occasionally a patient may need to be admitted for antibiotic cover to be given. On rare occasions, sedation or a general anaesthetic may be necessary for an excessively apprehensive patient but usually no anaesthetic is given.

Preparation of the patient

1. The patient should take a suitable aperient on each of the preceding two nights.
2. She should micturate immediately before the examination.

Premedication. Usually no premedication is required but an apprehensive patient or one on whom the examination has been previously undertaken without success may require sedation.

Preliminary film. A preliminary film is usually taken but this may be omitted as a routine and taken only if abnormality is suspected on initial fluoroscopy. If a preliminary film is required, the patient lies supine on the X-ray table, with the pelvis positioned symmetrically. An 18 × 24 cm (10 × 8 in) cassette, placed transversely, is used.

Centre in the mid-line, 2·5 cm (1 in) below the anterior superior iliac spines.

Radiation protection. Strict attention must be paid to keeping the radiation dose to the minimum because it is impossible to protect the gonads. For this reason rare earth or very fast tungstate screens and high kilovoltage are used. Image intensification should be employed and the screening current kept as low as possible consistent with good visualisation.

Some method of protecting the hands of the gynaecologist giving the injection must be provided as the injection is given during fluoroscopy. Such protection may consist simply of a large sheet of lead rubber placed under the patient's legs with its upper border just below the symphysis pubis. Alternatively, a lead-lined box may be placed between the patient's thighs and the instruments inserted through it, a lid being placed over the top when the instruments are in position (Barnett, 1972).

Contrast medium. Oily and water-soluble contrast media have each been used for hystero-salpingography. No ideal medium has yet been discovered, the main disadvantages of those presently used being pain when peritoneal spill occurs. Oily medium, usually in the form of Neo-hydriol fluid, adheres well to the mucosa and does not cause much pain but it takes 24 hours for peritoneal spill to occur and there is also the danger of oil embolism if the medium enters a vein. This is more likely to occur if the examination is carried out near menstruation. Therefore, water-soluble contrast medium (e.g. Diaginol viscous, Urografin 60 per cent) is the more frequently used, the exact quantity varying with different patients but usually being approximately 10 ml.

Technique. The position of the patient depends on the routine of the gynaecologist. The patient lies either on her side or, more usually, on her back, with the knees and hips flexed or the buttocks raised on a sandbag. She should be covered with dressing towels and given as much privacy as possible so as to promote relaxation which is an important part of the examination.

Following examination, for which a cold-light speculum is used, the anterior lip of the cervix is gripped by vulsellum forceps, a uterine sound is inserted to show the length and direction of the uterus and the injection cannula is inserted into the cervical canal and the speculum is removed. If a sandbag has been used it is removed and the patient's legs are extended and separated slightly. The sheet of lead rubber or protective box is adjusted in position to protect the gynaecologist's hands. Fluoroscopy, preferably using television, is commenced and the injection of contrast medium observed. The patient is often able to relax better if she is able to watch the procedure on the television screen. If spasm occurs, preventing tubal filling, inhalation of an antispasmodic drug such as octyl nitrite may be required. This is contained in a glass phial which is crushed and held near the patient's nose while she breathes deeply in and out. A phial of octyl nitrite and a gauze swab must be readily available in case required.

After tubal filling has been observed, the injection is continued until free peritoneal spill is observed. An under-couch radiograph is taken, the injection being continued while the exposure is made (Plate XLIV). If necessary, an oblique or lateral view is also taken, the injection being continued while each exposure is made. After the injection, the instruments are removed and either the patient is provided with a pad and bandage, or the gynaecologist will insert a tampon. If a pad is used, it must be removed when the follow-up radiograph is taken as otherwise any contrast medium on it will be superimposed on the area of interest on the radiograph.

Fifteen minutes after the injection, a follow-up radiograph is taken to demonstrate whether the contrast medium has been absorbed or whether residual contrast medium has pooled in loculated areas of adhesions, or is contained in an abnormal tube. Occasionally a further radiograph is taken 45 minutes after the injection, to confirm pooling of contrast medium.

After-care of the patient. The patient must not leave the department until a check has established that there is no haemorrhage and that she has fully recovered.

Some patients may feel upset or be in pain or be ill after this examination and the radiographer must make sure that a recovery room is available. This must be arranged before the examination is commenced, even if a room not normally available for this purpose has to be used.

Basic trolley setting

Upper (sterile) shelf

Vulsellum forceps
Vaginal speculum
Uterine sound
Uterine cannula
Sponge-holding forceps
Tissue forceps
One 10 ml syringe (usually with finger grips and screw cap)
Lotion bowl
Gallipot
Towels
Gauze swabs
Gown
Rubber gloves

Lower (unsterile) shelf

Cleansing lotion (e.g. Bradosol, 1 in 2,000)
Obstetric cream (e.g. Hibitane 1%)
Ampoules of contrast medium in bowl of warm water
File (for opening ampoules)
Masks
Pad and bandage *or* tampon
Octyl nitrite
EMERGENCY DRUGS

2. OBSTETRIC EXAMINATIONS

Radiography during pregnancy is avoided whenever possible so as not to irradiate the foetus but occasionally examination of the foetus or of the maternal pelvis is required. Great care must then be taken to ensure that the required information is obtained with the minimum number of exposures.

Ultrasonography (p. 70 and Plate IX) has become established as the procedure of choice for many obstetric investigations, particularly in early pregnancy. Often radiography and ultrasonography are carried out as complementary investigations. In late pregnancy, radiography may be more reliable, e.g. to confirm suspected foetal abnormality or death, or to determine foetal maturity.

The main radiographic examinations carried out on obstetric patients are (a) plain films of the abdomen (for foetal presentation, maturity, multiplicity, abnormality or death) (b) pelvimetry and (c) placentography.

PLAIN FILMS OF THE ABDOMEN

Prone oblique. This view is usually taken in preference to a postero-anterior or antero-posterior view because (a) it avoids overshadowing of the foetal skeleton by the maternal spine and (b) the dose to the foetus is lower than in other views.

If the foetal spine lies to the left of the maternal spine, a left anterior oblique view is taken. If the foetal spine lies to the right of the maternal spine, a right anterior oblique view is taken. Thus, the foetal spine will be nearer the film and the foetal limbs will usually be projected away from the maternal spine. Therefore it is necessary to know in advance which way the foetus is lying. This information is usually given by the referring clinician, or it can be ascertained by ultrasonography if this is available.

Rare earth or very fast tungstate screens are used which permit short exposure times—to avoid blurring due to movement of the foetus—and keep the radiation dose as low as possible.

Before the patient is positioned, the X-ray beam is collimated to within the limits of a 35×43 cm (17×14 in) cassette in the Bucky tray. The patient lies in the appropriate oblique position, the side raised 45° and with a pillow under the head and chest. Her hands are placed on the pillow and the knee of the raised side is flexed slightly to aid balance. A wide (e.g. 40 cm) compression band is applied firmly but gently over the whole abdomen. The exposure is made on deep, arrested inspiration as this is when the least foetal movement is possible.

Centre 2·5 cm (1 in) cephalad to the iliac crest, mid-way between the maternal spinous processes and the anterior edge of the abdominal curve.

Supplementary views

Antero-posterior or postero-anterior. One of these views may be taken (*a*) in preference to the oblique view if multiple pregnancy is suspected or if the pelvic measurements are required or (*b*) in addition to an oblique view if extra information is required in a case of suspected foetal abnormality or death.

The prone position is usually preferable to the supine, provided sufficient pillows are placed under the patient's chest and thighs for her comfort and support. In this position, the patient herself provides compression and may avoid the use of a compression band which is always needed in the supine position. Also, the foetal head is nearer the film and thus there is less distortion of the cephalic dimensions. A 35 × 43 cm (17 × 14 in) cassette is used, with its lower border 1 cm ($\frac{1}{2}$ in) below the symphysis pubis. The exposure is made on deep, arrested inspiration. A very short exposure time is essential to avoid movement blur.

Centre in the mid-line at the level of the iliac crests.

PELVIMETRY

This examination is performed when doubt exists as to the relative sizes of the maternal pelvis and the foetal head. It has been carried out less frequently in recent years because the number of patients presenting with disproportion has decreased with the lower incidence of rachitic diseases and tuberculosis. It is now usually required for patients who have suffered trauma to the pelvis, or who have congenital abnormality of the pelvis or who have had poliomyelitis.

The obstetrician needs to know the shape of the sacrum and the exact measurements of the true conjugate and pelvic outlet. The true conjugate is the distance between the upper inner border of the symphysis pubis and the sacral promontory. The pelvic outlet is the distance between the lower inner border of the symphysis pubis and the tip of the sacrum.

Initially it is standard practice to take only a lateral view of the pelvis followed by an antero-posterior orthodiagraphic view if clinically necessary. Full pelvimetry, consisting of lateral, inlet and outlet views, is no longer undertaken because of the high radiation dose to the foetus. Inlet and outlet views may sometimes be taken following a difficult delivery or Caesarean section in case the patient has a further pregnancy. Details of these views may be found in long-established books such as those by Clarke (1964) and Sterling Fisher and Russell (1975) in which can also be found details of the necessary corrections for magnification.

The measurement must be absolutely accurate and the method employed should be as simple as possible, so that the examination can be carried out in any department and at any time. Usually every department carrying out pelvimetry, even if only occasionally, has a routine method. The degree of magnification and the actual measurements of the pelvic diameters are sometimes determined by sophisticated methods but the simplest and most reliable method is by the use of a metal ruler with holes at centimetre spaces. This ruler is held between the patient's thighs when the lateral radiograph is taken. Thus, the image of the ruler, which has the same magnification as the mid-line structures of the pelvis, appears on the radiograph. Measurements of the conjugate and pelvic outlet can then be made.

Films and screens. To keep radiation dose to the minimum, rare earth or very fast tungstate screens are used.

Exposure factors. A very short exposure time is essential to prevent blurring due to movement of the foetus. The machine with the highest output in the department should always be used for pelvimetry.

Filtration. Although total filtration (inherent plus added) of 2 mm of aluminium for voltages between 70 and 100 kV, and 2·5 mm for voltages above 100 kV, is required for all tubes (Code of Practice, 1972), extra filtration is often used in pelvimetry, e.g. 1 mm aluminium and 0·2 mm copper are added. For a lateral view of the pelvis, a wedge filter of aluminium and an insert of 2 mm of lead are sometimes used to shield the foetus from the primary beam (Sterling Fisher and Russell, 1975).

Basic view

Lateral. The patient stands in the lateral position against the erect Bucky. If labour is imminent or has commenced, the patient will need help and encouragement to stand. The feet should be slightly apart and the arms folded across the chest. The pelvis must be positioned symmetrically. If the patient is examined in the lying position, her legs must be extended so that the symphysis pubis is not obscured. A radiopaque ruler is placed between the thighs and held firmly in position. A 35×43 cm (17×14 in) cassette is used and the patient is positioned so that the anterior abdominal wall, maternal spine and symphysis pubis are all included on the radiograph.

Centre 6·5 cm ($2\frac{1}{2}$ in) above the greater trochanter.

This radiograph, from which the diameters of the pelvic inlet and outlet can be determined, is scrutinised by the radiologist or obstetrician before any other view is taken.

Antero-posterior orthodiagraphic view. The patient lies supine with the pelvis positioned symmetrically. This view can be taken without a grid, in which case the patient lies directly on the cassette instead of its being placed in the Bucky tray (Robson, 1975). The X-ray beam is collimated to cover a film area approximately 5 cm (2 in) wide by 12 cm (5 in) long. The tube is first angled 15° cephalad and is then centred to the mid-line of the patient at the level of the anterior superior iliac spines. The cassette is then adjusted so that the beam is centred to it. The tube is then moved 5 cm (2 in) to one side of the mid-line and an exposure is made. It is then moved 10 cm (4 in)—i.e. 5 cm to the other side of the mid-line—and a second exposure (on the same film) is made. The patient must not move at all between these exposures.

From this radiograph can be determined the transverse diameter of the pelvic inlet (intertuberous distance) and the bi-ischial distance (interspinous distance) which forms part of the pelvic outlet (Sterling Fisher and Russell, 1975).

PLACENTOGRAPHY

Placentography is the radiographic localisation of the placental site and is usually undertaken in an attempt to demonstrate placenta praevia. If available, ultrasonography (p. 70 and Plate IX) is the examination of choice for placentography as it entails no radiation hazard. If ultrasonography is not available, scintigraphy (p. 63) can be used. If neither of these methods is available, conventional placentography is performed.

To be of value, all placentography must provide a high degree of accuracy. With conventional placentography, the radiation dose to the mother and the foetus must at the same time be kept to the minimum.

Placentography must be used in selected cases only and not as a routine investigation. The radiation dose must be kept to the minimum in view of possible genetic effects.

Apart from ultrasound and scintigraphy, the main methods of placentography are soft tissue radiography and arteriography (angio-placentography).

Soft tissue placentography

The uterine wall, placenta and amniotic fluid are of the same radiographic density but the placental site is distinguishable if calcification is present. Placentography by this method is most reliable near full term when there is demonstrable calcification in about 30 per cent of cases examined, but the upper segment of the placenta can often be demonstrated even when it is not calcified.

Preparation of the patient

1. A suitable aperient should be taken by the patient as the rectum must be empty.
2. The patient must micturate immediately before the examination.

The bladder and rectum must be empty because distension of either may simulate displacement of the presenting part.

Accessory apparatus. Rare earth or very fast tungstate screens should be used. Sometimes a cassette containing two or more pairs of screens, graduated in speed, is used. Several films of different density are then produced without extra radiation to the foetus (for multiple radiography see page 35).

Exposure factors. Low kilovoltage (usually about 65 kV) is employed for optimum soft tissue differentiation and to show any calcification that may be present.

Filtration. Additional filtration (as for Pelvimetry, p. 318) is often used. A wedge filter of aluminium, graduated in thickness from about 0 to 2 cm, is used to avoid over-exposure of the anterior part of the abdomen and so allow the maternal spine, foetal soft tissues and any calcification to be demonstrated on one exposure.

Views

Supine lateral. The patient lies on her side, with the legs extended and with a pad between the knees so that the pelvis is positioned symmetrically. If necessary, a compression band is used for support. A 35 × 43 cm (17 × 14 in) cassette is used, with its lower border at the level of the symphysis pubis. The patient is adjusted so that all the abdomen is included on the radiograph. The symphysis pubis, sacral promontory and the foetal parts must all be clearly shown. This is best achieved by the use of a multi-layer cassette as already mentioned.

Centre to the cassette.

This film is processed and viewed by the radiologist. If the space between the foetal head and the sacral promontory is wider than normal, a semi-reclining lateral view is taken to see if the gap can be narrowed by postural means (Sutton, 1975). For this view, the patient lies supine on a tilting table, raised from the table-top on a thick foam mattress. The legs must be extended and the feet must rest firmly on the foot-rest so that the pelvis is positioned symmetrically. The table is then tilted 45° feet downwards. If a tilting table is not available, the patient should sit on the X-ray table, with the legs extended, leaning backwards 45° and supported on pillows. A 35 × 43 cm (17 × 14 in) grid-cassette is supported vertically by the side of the patient.

Centre to the upper border of the head of the femur with the X-ray tube directed horizontally.

One of the following views may sometimes be needed but, because of the radiation dose, it is never justifiable to take them all.

Prone. As for plain films of the abdomen (p. 317).

Oblique. As for plain films of the abdomen (p. 316).

Erect lateral (to confirm the presence of a low-lying placenta). As for Pelvimetry (p. 318).

Angio-placentography

The femoral artery is catheterised using the Seldinger technique (p. 224).

Preparation of the patient

1. The patient must have nothing to eat or drink for five hours.
2. Local preparation of the injection site, including shaving of the groins, is carried out.
3. The patient should micturate immediately before the examination.

Premedication. Premedication such as Omnopon and Scopolamine, is given.

Contrast medium. 25 ml meglumine diatrizoate or iothalamate (e.g. Angiografin or Conray 280).

Preliminary film. *No* preliminary film is taken. This is to minimise the radiation dose to the foetus.

Technique. Seldinger catheterisation of the femoral artery is performed and the tip of the catheter is advanced 10 to 12 cm so that it is positioned just above the aortic bifurcation.

When only one film is to be taken, the right posterior oblique position is usually preferred to the antero-posterior position as with the former it is possible to determine whether any low-sited sinuses are on the anterior or the posterior wall of the uterus. A lateral view gives the most information but the increased radiation dose usually precludes its use as a routine method and the posterior oblique view is usually the best compromise when only one film is taken.

For the right posterior oblique view the patient is positioned with the right knee flexed and with the left side of the abdomen raised from the table and supported on foam pads. A 35 × 43 cm (17 × 14 in) cassette is used, with its lower border at the level of the symphysis pubis. The patient is positioned so that the whole abdomen is included on the film and the X-ray tube is directed vertically to the centre of the cassette.

Some authorities (e.g. Sutton, 1975) recommend that a vaginal speculum be left *in situ* to localise the position of the cervix.

The contrast medium is injected by hand or by a pressure pump. The exposure is made 2 to 4 seconds after the injection.

Only one radiograph is taken, again to minimise the radiation dose received by the foetus.

After-care of the patient

1. Pulse and respiration are recorded every half-hour for 4 hours, then pulse, respiration, blood pressure and temperature every 4 hours for 24 hours.
2. The site of the puncture must be observed at regular intervals.
3. The patient should avoid flexing the leg on the side which was examined.
4. She should remain in bed for 24 hours.

Another method of carrying out this examination is by inclined angio-placentography (Herlinger, 1968) in which the X-ray tube is angled cephalad so that the central ray is aligned through the plane that separates the two segments of the uterus. A simple device is employed which measures the angle of the inter-segmental plane to the table-top and this angle is used as the angulation of the tube for the subsequent angiogram.

The advantages of this method are the increased accuracy of diagnosis of placenta praevia and the reduction of radiation dose. In this method, the patient lies supine instead of in the right posterior oblique position but otherwise the procedure is similar to that previously described.

37

Mammography

Mammography, the radiographic examination of the breast, is undertaken mainly in the assessment of a palpable lump in the breast before biopsy is performed (Egan, 1972). It is used also as a screening procedure for pre-clinical diagnosis of carcinoma of the breast.

Radiographic examination may be carried out by conventional soft tissue mammography, by 70 mm mammography, by xeroradiography (p. 77), or by contrast medium injection. The breast can be examined also by thermography (p. 80) and by ultrasonography (p. 70). The most usual radiographic method is still by soft tissue mammography and this method only will be described in this chapter.

Principles. The tissues making up the breast have very low inherent contrast. Soft tissue mammography depends on the fact that tumour tissue is denser than breast tissue, particularly in the post-menopausal breast where glandular tissue has been replaced by fat. To obtain maximum soft tissue differentiation, kilovoltages of between 25 and 35 are employed. Carcinoma of the breast may display punctate calcification of approximately 0·2 mm diameter, and a meticulous technique is necessary to show this.

Apparatus. Equipment specially designed for mammography is now widely available and this makes the procedure simpler and gives consistently good results. Such apparatus (e.g. Senograph) has a water-cooled tube with a molybdenum anode and beryllium window. It produces 25–35 kV at 30–40 mA. A variety of cones is available, contoured to suit all sizes and shapes of breast. The cone also compresses the breast and so tends to spread it over the film holder, thus making the tissue of more even density.

If this type of equipment is not available, standard equipment can be used but it must have been modified to obtain the necessary low kilovoltage. To increase contrast further, all additional filtration is removed, leaving only the inherent filtration of the tube. A long, specially shaped cone, often made of copper, is usually employed to provide accurate collimation.

Film. The main essentials for mammograms are (*a*) maximum soft tissue detail and (*b*) maximum sharpness. In the past, non-screen film was considered to give the best detail. A pack of films of differing speeds was often used, producing, with one exposure, radiographs of different densities to show both the thinner and the denser parts of the breast. Xeroradiography was introduced for examination of the breast, approximately halving the dose from that for non-screen film mammography (Gilbe, 1973).

But radiation dose to the skin during mammography has caused concern, especially when carried out as a screening procedure, or if repeated examinations are needed for women at risk (Rothenberg *et al.*, 1975; Lester, 1977). For this reason special X-ray films for mammography have been introduced. These are used with a single rare earth screen, packed together in a vacuum bag (Chang *et al.*, 1976). This type of film/screen combination is now used widely and provides excellent detail, with significantly lower dose to the patient and as an added advantage can be processed in a rapid automatic film processor.

Markers. Accurate marking of the films is very important. Unless a mastectomy has been performed, views of both breasts are taken for comparison and it is essential to know which quadrant of which breast is being viewed. A routine method of placing markers should be used, the 'L' or 'R' marker being placed towards the axilla. The use of lead markers along the site of a clinical lesion or biopsy scar is sometimes recommended.

Immobilisation. Immobilisation of the patient is important because the soft tissue technique requires long exposure times. The patient must therefore be made as comfortable as possible so that she can co-operate in keeping absolutely still while the exposures are being made.

Viewing. Mammograms are viewed under optimum normal viewing conditions and with a bright light and magnifying lens. Good quality mammograms should look over-exposed by normal standards and a bright light is of advantage in detailed viewing of the over-exposed part of the film.

Basic views

Supero-inferior (Plate XLVA). If specially designed equipment is being used, the patient sits at its adjustable film support. If modified standard equipment is being used, she sits at a small adjustable table. The breast is positioned on the film which is placed on the support (or table), the height of which is adjusted until the under-surface of the breast is as flat as possible and the nipple is in profile. The shoulder is relaxed in order to move the clavicle and supra-clavicular tissues away from the X-ray beam. With small breasts it is advisable to bend the film slightly over the edge of the table. Large breasts may require a further film to ensure that all the breast tissue is included. Care must be taken to ensure that there are no skin folds.

Centre to the thoracic aspect of the breast.

Lateral (Plate XLVB). If specially designed equipment is being used, the patient usually sits up for this view—the film being placed at either the lateral or the medial side of the breast, according to the type of apparatus being used. If modified standard equipment is being used, the patient lies on her back on the X-ray table. She then rolls over towards the side under examination. The hand on that side is placed under the back of the head. The film is supported on a foam pad and is placed under the breast. The patient is adjusted until the nipple is in profile, an almost true lateral view of the breast being thus obtained. The foam pad supporting the film allows it to bend slightly and to adopt the shape of the chest wall. If necessary, the patient should be asked to draw the other breast clear of the X-ray beam. Skin folds must again be avoided. The chest wall must be included on the film to ensure that all the breast tissue has been included.

Centre to the centre of the breast.

Supplementary view

Axillary. If specially designed equipment is being used, the patient usually sits up for this view, but if modified equipment is being used, the patient lies on her back on the X-ray table. She is then rotated 30° towards the side under examination so that the breast falls away from the chest wall. The arm is abducted 90° so that the axillary region is seen clearly without superimposition of the scapula. An 18×24 cm (10×8 in) film is used for each side. It is placed with its long axis in the cranio-caudal direction so as to include the axilla and breast.

Centre 5 cm (2 in) below the apex of the axilla.

CYST PUNCTURE

This examination is used to ascertain whether a mass in the breast is a cyst (Hébert and Ouimet-Oliva, 1972).

Under aseptic conditions and local anaesthesia, a 21 gauge needle is introduced into the mass. If the mass is a cyst, fluid should come freely into the syringe, especially if it is under pressure. If no fluid is aspirated, the position of the needle is checked by moving the mass to see if the needle moves as well. If it does, the mass is a solid and not a cyst.

If it is a cyst, it is aspirated. The aspiration must be complete, if possible, because a small amount of residual fluid can simulate a thick wall which is usually indicative of neoplasm. Therefore, if complete aspiration is not possible, additional radiographs are taken in varying degrees of obliquity so that the whole of the inner wall can be demonstrated.

After the cyst has been aspirated, air with or without a drop of contrast medium, is then introduced into it. The volume of air introduced should be a little less than the volume of fluid withdrawn because the heat of the body causes expansion of the air. If too much air is introduced, it may diffuse into the interstitial tissue of the breast and this could prevent adequate visualisation.

Supero-inferior and lateral mammograms (pp. 325 and 326) are then taken, after which the air is withdrawn.

MAMMARY DUCT INJECTION

This examination is performed in the investigation of nipple discharge, to demonstrate lesions such as intraduct papilloma, duct ectasia and intraduct carcinoma (Nunnerly and Field, 1972).

After a clinical examination of the breasts and local lymph glands, the orifice from which the discharge emanates is identified. It is dilated and cannulated, using a silver lachrymal dilator and lachrymal cannula. Contrast medium (sodium diatrizoate, 45 per cent, or its equivalent) is injected until the patient feels mild discomfort or there is leak around the cannula. Usually about 0·4 ml is sufficient but up to 4 ml may be needed. The cannula is then removed and supero-inferior and lateral mammograms (pp. 325 and 326) are taken.

38

Pneumography

Pneumography is a method of radiographic examination in which air or other gas is used as the contrast medium. It is undertaken in the examination of peritoneal or retro-peritoneal structures, by silhouetting them against a radiolucent background. The anterior mediastinum may also be examined by pneumography. The examination of the ventricular cisterns of the brain by pneumography is usually termed air encephalography.

The contrast medium usually employed for these examinations is carbon dioxide or nitrous oxide because of the risk of gas embolism when air or oxygen is employed. The procedures are then virtually without risk (Lumsden and Truelove, 1957). However, both carbon dioxide and nitrous oxide are rapidly absorbed, usually within about 45 minutes, and when tomography is required, as in pre-sacral and mediastinal pneumography, it is difficult to obtain all the necessary radiographs before the gas begins to disappear. Some authorities (Saxton and Strickland, 1972) recommend that the pneumoperitoneum be induced with carbon dioxide and completed with air or oxygen once the pneumoperitoneum has been safely established. The same authorities recommend that a cannula or catheter be used for pre-sacral pneumography so that repeated injections of carbon dioxide can be given if required.

Although various methods of obtaining the gas for pneumography are available, probably the most convenient is via a Maxwell pneumothorax machine which is charged from time to time with a sparklet cylinder of carbon dioxide. Another is by the use of an automatic gas dispenser (McCallum, 1971) which permits a slow, steady infusion.

If gas embolism occurs, treatment is very urgent and the routine (Ansell and Ansell, 1964) is as follows:
1. The patient is placed in the left lateral position.
2. The head is lowered to prevent air travelling up into the brain.

3. The patient is given oxygen under positive pressure. This should be continued for one or two hours after the episode.
4. If cardiac arrest occurs, intra-cardiac air must be aspirated before cardiac massage is commenced. External cardiac massage is therefore contra-indicated in air embolism.
5. The patient must not be allowed to sit up for several hours.

PRE-SACRAL PNEUMOGRAPHY

Pre-sacral pneumography is used to demonstrate retro-peritoneal structures, particularly the supra-renal glands.

Preparation of the patient

1. The patient should take a suitable aperient on each of the preceding two nights.
2. The patient should have nothing to eat or drink for five hours.
3. Local preparation of the injection site, including shaving of the perianal area, should be carried out.
4. The patient should micturate immediately before the examination.

Premedication. Premedication such as Omnopon is given.

Contrast medium. Usually 300 to 400 ml of carbon dioxide each side.

Apparatus. A tilting table is required, preferably equipped for tomography. An image intensifier and television are desirable.

Preliminary film. The patient lies supine on a tilting fluoroscopy table. A 35×43 cm (17×14 in) cassette is used, with its lower border at the level of the iliac crests. The diaphragm must be included on the radiograph. The centering point is marked on the patient's skin for easy positioning later. This radiograph is used to assess bowel clearance and to establish exposure factors.

Centre to the cassette.

Technique. The patient lies on his left side on the tilting table. The perianal area is cleansed with a mild antiseptic and local anaesthetic is infiltrated between the anus and the coccyx. A needle-catheter or needle-cannula is then introduced. When the needle is correctly positioned, 20 ml of saline are injected to expand the pre-sacral space and to render it relatively more avascular (Saxton and Strickland, 1972). The needle is then withdrawn so that the injection of gas can be given through the catheter or cannula, thus diminishing the risk of gas embolism. The catheter is attached to the patient by adhesive tape and remains *in situ* until the examination is completed.

The injection of carbon dioxide is given, half the gas being injected on each side. This is usually carried out under fluoroscopic control by the radiologist, using image intensification and television. The patient is gently turned into the prone position, and the foot of the couch is lowered about 15°. Antero-posterior and oblique views are then taken using the under-couch tube. The patient is then turned into the supine position and an antero-posterior view is taken using the over-couch tube. A 30×40 cm (15×12 in) cassette is placed transversely, with its lower border at the level of the iliac crests.

Owing to the rapid absorption of carbon dioxide, radiography must be completed as quickly as possible after instillation of the gas, though when a catheter is used, a further injection of gas may be given if necessary. Lateral tomograms of both renal areas are taken, usually employing a multi-layer cassette to reduce the time required to complete the examination.

After-care of the patient. The patient remains in bed for 24 hours.

Basic trolley setting

Upper (sterile) shelf

Needle-cannula *or* needle-catheter
Polythene connection
Two lengths of rubber tubing
Longer length of rubber tubing to connect to carbon dioxide
  supply
Two-way tap
Two gallipots
One 10 ml syringe
One 50 ml syringe
Towels
Gauze swabs
Gown
Rubber gloves

Lower (unsterile) shelf

Skin cleanser (e.g. Hibitane 1 in 5,000)

Local anaesthetic (e.g. Lignocaine 0·5% or 1%)
Disposable needles
Masks
EMERGENCY DRUGS

GYNAECOGRAPHY

Gynaecography (pelvic pneumography) is the radiographic examination of the uterus and ovaries by silhouetting them against a radiolucent background, following instillation of carbon dioxide into the peritoneal cavity (Plate XLVI).

The examination is performed in (*inter alia*) the investigation of primary or secondary amenorrhoea or infertility, in the diagnosis of the Stein-Lowenthal syndrome (Edwards and Evans, 1963), ovarian agenesis and certain kinds of ovarian neoplasm and cysts (Stevens *et al.*, 1966).

Preparation of the patient

1. Routine examination of the chest and skull is carried out to exclude abnormalities of the pituitary gland.
2. The patient should take a suitable aperient on each of the preceding two nights. Bowel preparation must be satisfactory, as otherwise the examination cannot be performed. A colonic washout may be required.
3. She should have nothing to eat or drink for at least four hours.
4. She is admitted to a ward for about four hours, both before and after the examination.
5. She *must* micturate immediately before the examination. In some departments, the patient is catheterised to ensure that the bladder is completely empty.

Premedication. Premedication such as Omnopon and Scopolamine is given.

Contrast medium. 1,000 to 1,500 ml carbon dioxide.

Apparatus. A tilting table is required. An efficient method of support for the patient must be provided because she is tilted 45° head downwards. A myelography-type harness is preferable but shoulder and hand-grips may be used instead. A pneumothorax machine or anaesthetic bag and a supply of carbon dioxide are required.

Preliminary film. A preliminary film is taken about three or four hours before the examination (which will usually be when the patient is admitted) to see if bowel preparation has been adequate, as otherwise an enema may be necessary. The patient lies on the tilting table and is firmly secured. The table is then tilted 45° head downwards (Fig. 37). A 30 × 40 cm (15 × 12 in) cassette is used with its lower border at the level of the symphysis pubis. The focus-film distance should be at least 100 cm (40 in) to reduce magnification. For optimum soft tissue detail, 60 to 70 kV is used.

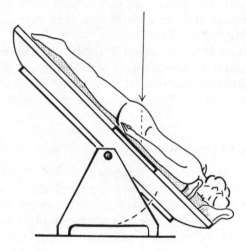

Fig. 37

Centre to the coccyx, about 2·5 cm (1 in) below the natal cleft, with the tube at right angles to the floor.

The centering point and exposure factors must be noted so that later films can be taken without delay. If a tilting table is not available when the preliminary film is taken, a view may be taken with the tube angled instead of tilting the patient. For this, the patient lies prone on the X-ray table. The tube is angled 45° cephalad and centred to the coccyx. The resulting film gives a similarly elongated view of the pelvic cavity.

Technique. Once instillation of the gas has been completed, radiography must be carried out without delay. The X-ray tube is therefore centred to the table, the cassette placed in the Bucky tray and the exposure set before the surgical procedure begins. If at this stage there is still any doubt about the bowel preparation having been satisfactory, a film is taken to confirm this.

The patient lies comfortably on her back on the X-ray table with her arms folded across her chest or by her sides. After injection of local anaesthetic, a long needle is inserted into the abdomen usually on the left side of the umbilicus or in the mid-line mid-way between the symphysis pubis and the umbilicus. When the needle has been correctly sited, 1,000 to 1,500 ml of carbon dioxide are injected. The patient usually complains of abdominal discomfort and shoulder pain (the latter being referred from pressure on the under-surface of the diaphragm) and to relieve this the table is tilted slightly head down-wards.

When the required amount of gas has been injected, the patient is turned into the prone position and the harness or shoulder grips are adjusted and fixed securely. The table is tilted gently until it is at 45° (Fig. 37). The cassette and X-ray tube are then centred as for the preliminary film and the exposure is made. A short exposure time is normally used. Further views with the tube angled 10° caudad or with the patient rotated to the left or right, may be necessary. The radiographs are processed and viewed as soon as possible so that any further views may be taken before the gas has been absorbed. Usually carbon dioxide is completely absorbed within 30 minutes.

After-care of the patient. The patient usually remains in bed for about four hours before going home.

Basic trolley setting

Upper (sterile) shelf

Saugmann needle
Two-way tap
Glass connector (containing sterile wool)
Two lengths of tubing
Longer length of tubing to connect to carbon dioxide supply
One 10 ml syringe
Two gallipots
Towels
Gauze swabs
Gown
Rubber gloves

Lower (unsterile) shelf

Skin cleanser (e.g. Hibitane 0·5% in 70% industrial spirit, blue stain)

Local anaesthetic (e.g. Lignocaine 0·5% or 1%)
Disposable needles
Masks
EMERGENCY DRUGS

UPPER ABDOMINAL PNEUMOGRAPHY

This examination is used to demonstrate the inferior surface of the diaphragm and thus to evaluate masses in the upper abdomen or chest base. It is also used to distinguish between intrinsic and extrinsic filling defects in the stomach and between benign and malignant gastric ulcers.

Preparation of the patient

1. The patient should take a suitable aperient on each of the two nights preceding the examination.
2. The patient must have nothing to eat or drink for at least four hours.
3. The patient should micturate immediately before the examination.

Premedication. Premedication such as Omnopon and Scopolamine is given.

Contrast medium. 1,000 to 1,500 ml carbon dioxide are used.

Preliminary film. The bowel should be free from faecal shadows and the bladder must be empty but as this preparation is not as critical as in pelvic pneumography, the preliminary film is taken immediately before the start of the surgical procedure.

The patient lies supine on the tilting table. A 35 × 43 cm (17 × 14 in) cassette is used, with its lower border at the level of the anterior superior iliac spines. A short exposure time is used.

Centre to the cassette.

Technique. The procedure is the same as for the examination of the pelvic viscera except that the patient is not tilted head-downwards and therefore a myelography harness is not necessary. After instillation of the gas, the patient is placed in whatever position will manoeuvre the gas into the appropriate region. For example, if the diaphragm is being examined the table is brought slowly into the vertical position so that the gas will rise under the diaphragm; if one side of the abdomen is being examined, the patient lies on the opposite side for a few minutes. The following views are then taken:

VIEWS

Prone. The patient is turned into the prone position. The lower border of a 35×43 cm (17×14 in) cassette is placed at the level of the anterior superior iliac spines.

Centre to the cassette.

Lateral decubitus. The patient lies on the side not under examination. A grid cassette, supported vertically, is positioned so as to include the area under examination. The tube is directed horizontally.

Centre to the cassette.

Supine lateral. The patient lies supine on foam pads to raise him from the table-top. A grid cassette, supported vertically at the side of the patient, is positioned so as to include the area under examination. The tube is again directed horizontally.

Centre to the cassette.

Erect or supine oblique views may also be required and in some cases the radiologist may wish to use fluoroscopy.

Basic trolley setting

The basic trolley setting is the same as for gynaecography (p. 333).

MEDIASTINAL PNEUMOGRAPHY

Mediastinal pneumography is performed (*a*) in cases of myasthenia gravis or of primary or tertiary hyperparathyroidism where a suspected tumour has not been demonstrated on plain films or by tomography (*b*) in cases of oesophageal carcinoma where the examination can be used to assess the extent and operability of the tumour (Kreel, 1972) and (*c*) in the demonstration of mediastinal lymph nodes.

Mediastinal pneumography is contra-indicated in patients with impaired respiratory function.

The examination is carried out on an X-ray table equipped for tomography. Some authorities recommend the use of fluoroscopy as well, but this is usually impracticable unless the fluoroscopy table is equipped for tomography.

Preparation of the patient

1. Recent plain films of the chest including penetrated views

and lateral tomograms of the anterior mediastinum are taken, usually the day before (Kreel and James, 1965).
2.   The patient must have nothing to eat or drink for five hours.
3.   If the patient is on anti-cholinergic drugs, these must come to the department with him and must be given at the set times even if this is during the examination.
4.   The patient should micturate immediately before the examination.

Premedication such as sodium amytal is given, but respiratory depressants such as morphine or pethidine must be avoided.

Contrast medium. Oxygen or air is the contrast medium usually employed despite the risk of gas embolism. This is because, in the examination of the mediastinum, tomography is required and carbon dioxide and nitrous oxide are absorbed too rapidly.

Air may give better definition (Mahaffey, 1969). If air is used, 350 ml are injected over a period of not less than 30 minutes.

Preliminary film. A preliminary tomogram is taken to determine exposure factors and depth of 'cut' required. The patient is placed in the lateral position, with the arms over the head, and a mid-line tomogram of the anterior mediastinum is taken.

Centre over the anterior mediastinum at the level of the manubrio-sternal angle, 5 cm (2 in) posterior to the anterior surface of the sternum.

Technique. The procedure is explained to the patient. The patient lies supine on the tomography table, with the neck extended. The skin and tissues immediately behind the manubrium sterni are infiltrated with local anaesthetic. A puncture is made above the suprasternal notch and the needle, with stilette, is inserted in the mid-line, in line with the manubrio-sternal joint. Sometimes a lateral view of the anterior mediastinum is taken at this stage to check the position of the needle, or this is done by fluoroscopy if available.

The gas is then injected, the quantity (usually between 100 ml and 500 ml) depends on the technique of the radiologist. A further check radiograph is taken or, if fluoroscopy is available, the anterior mediastinum is screened instead.

When the gas has been injected, the patient sits up for one or two minutes, and is then placed in the lateral position and tomograms are taken in the mid-line and at 1 cm intervals up to 4 cm on either side of the mid-line (Plate XLVII). A multi-section cassette is of advantage. Sometimes tomograms with the patient in the prone position are also required, extending from the sternum to 9 cm behind it.

After-care of the patient

1. Pulse, temperature, respiration and blood pressure are recorded every 15 minutes for 2 hours and then 4-hourly for the next 24 hours.
2. The patient remains in bed for 24 hours and must remain under observation in the ward for a further 24 hours.

Basic trolley setting

Upper (sterile) shelf

Needle with short bevel and stilette, Luer-lok (e.g. Howard Jones needle)
One 50 ml syringe
One 10 ml syringe
One three-way tap, Luer-lok
Gallipot
Towels
Gauze swabs
Gown

Lower (unsterile) shelf

Skin cleanser (e.g. Chlorhexidine 0·5% in 70% industrial spirit)
Local anaesthetic
Disposable needles
EMERGENCY DRUGS

AIR ENCEPHALOGRAPHY

Air encephalography is the radiographic demonstration of the cerebral ventricular system using air as a contrast medium. The air is injected into the subarachnoid space via a lumbar puncture. The examination is most informative in the investigation of intracranial space-occupying lesions and in the investigation of cerebral atrophy and hydrocephalus.

The examination should be performed only on in-patients. It is usually carried out under local anaesthesia but if the patient is under 17 years of age or is unable or unwilling to co-operate, general anaesthesia is necessary and some departments carry out all such examinations under general anaesthesia. The patient may experience severe headache for the ensuing 24 hours or even longer. Nausea and vomiting occur occasionally. Efficient premedication helps to mitigate these complications. Because the examination is an unpleasant one for the patient, C.T. scanning—if available—is the examination of choice for preliminary investigations and may avoid the necessity for air encephalography.

Preparation of the patient

1.   Routine views of the skull and chest are taken.
2.   The patient must have nothing to eat or drink for five hours.
3.   All radiopaque objects (e.g. dentures, hair-pins) must be removed.
4.   The patient should micturate before the examination.
5.   The patient should wear an open-backed gown.

Premedication such as Nembutal and Omnopon is given. Some radiologists prescribe an anti-emetic, such as Phenergan, to be taken the night before the examination.

Contrast medium. 20 to 30 ml of air.

Preliminary film. A preliminary lateral film is sometimes taken but this is not routine in all departments.

Technique. The pinnae of the ears are pushed forward and downwards and secured by adhesive strapping. The patient sits on a special hydraulic encephalography chair or, if the apparatus is available, is strapped into a motor-driven rotatable chair. The patient must be made as comfortable as possible, with the back arched and the forehead resting on a foam block secured to the skull table. The chin is tucked in so that the radiographic base line is at 20° to the horizontal. An 18×24 cm (10×8 in) cassette and grid are adjusted to the side of the patient's head. The X-ray tube is directed horizontally and centred just superior to the external auditory meatus, over the region of the fourth ventricle.

A lumbar puncture is performed and 10 ml of air are injected. An automatic gas dispenser permits a slow, steady infusion which reduces the severity of the side effects (McCallum, 1971; Ashley, 1973). A lateral view is taken and the film is processed and viewed as soon as possible, to ascertain whether the air has entered the ventricular system. If so, more air is injected and a further lateral view is taken. Autotomography, or tomography, may be carried out at this stage. Autotomography involves the taking of a further lateral film with the patient slowly shaking the head from side to side throughout the exposure of one to two seconds. A reverse Townes view is then taken with the tube angled 25° cephalad to the radiographic base line and centred on the external occipital protuberance. If the radiographs are satisfactory, a specimen of cerebro-spinal fluid is taken for pathological analysis. The lumbar puncture needle is then removed and the patient is placed horizontal for the routine supine and prone radiographs to be taken.

Supine views (Fig. 38)

Fronto-occipital. The patient is positioned with the top of the head near the top of the skull table, so that there will be no need to move him between views. The tube is off-centred towards the top of the patient's head and then directed vertically. The cassette is placed at the top of the Bucky tray.

Centre to the glabella.

Townes. The tube is re-centred and angled 30° caudad. If the patient was correctly positioned at the top of the skull table, there will be no need to move him again for this view. The cassette is placed in the centre of the Bucky tray.

Centre 5 cm (2 in) above the glabella.

Lateral. The patient's head is supported and the skull table is lowered slightly and a foam block is placed under the occiput. A

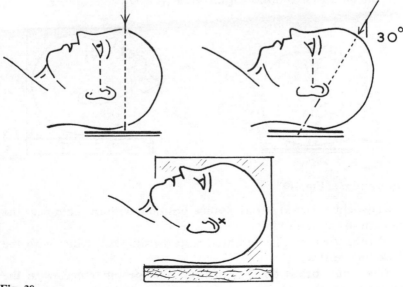

Fig. 38

cassette and grid are placed at the side of the patient's head and the X-ray tube is directed horizontally.

Centre 5 cm (2 in) above the external auditory meatus.

'*Hanging head*' *lateral*. This view may be required at this stage to show air in the anterior part of the third ventricle. The skull table is lowered and the patient's head adjusted until the base line is parallel with the skull table.

Centre 5 cm (2 in) above the external auditory meatus with the tube directed horizontally.

Views for temporal horns (Fig. 39)

To demonstrate lesions in the temporal region, the temporal horns are filled, usually one at a time. The patient is turned on to the side not being filled, the head being supported firmly throughout the manœuvre. The head is kept on the side, lowered and then rotated so that the patient is looking towards the floor. This brings the air into the occipital region. The head is then rotated back to face the ceiling, with the chin extended, and the patient is turned on to his back, all in a continuous movement. This allows the air to ascend into the uppermost temporal horn.

Fronto-occipital. The chin is raised so that the base line is 20° from the vertical.

Centre in the mid-line at the level of the interpupillary line.

Lateral. As for routine supine view (p. 339).

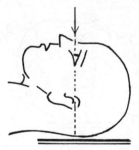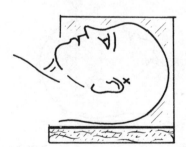

Fig. 39

Prone views (Fig. 40)

The patient is turned into the prone position, with the chin near the bottom of the skull table.

Reverse Townes. The forehead rests on the skull table, with the base line vertical.

Centre just below the external occipital protuberance, with the tube angled 25° cephalad.

Occipito-frontal. The patient remains in the same position and the X-ray tube is off-centred towards the occiput. The cassette is placed at the bottom of the Bucky tray. The X-ray tube is directed vertically.

Centre to the glabella.

Lateral. The patient's head is supported and the skull table is lowered. A foam block is placed under the patient's forehead. A cassette and grid are placed at the side of the patient's head. The X-ray tube is directed horizontally.

Centre 2·5 cm (1 in) above the external auditory meatus.

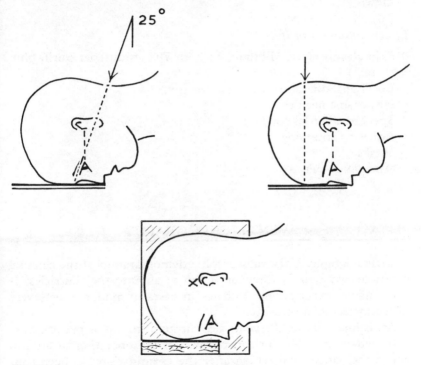

Fig. 40

After-care of the patient

1. Pulse and blood pressure are recorded every 15 minutes for 4 hours. Temperature, pulse, respiration and blood pressure are then recorded 4-hourly for 24 hours.
2. The patient remains in bed for 24 hours.

Basic trolley setting

Upper (sterile) shelf

Two lumbar puncture needles (e.g. Harris's or Pitkin's)
One 2 ml syringe
One 10 ml syringe
Gallipot
Sponge-holding forceps
Towels
Gauze swabs
Gown

Lower (unsterile) shelf

Skin cleanser (e.g. Hibitane 0·5% in 70% industrial spirit, blue stain)
Local anaesthetic (e.g. Lignocaine 2%)
Disposable needles
Specimen bottles for c.s.f.
Adhesive strapping
Masks
EMERGENCY DRUGS

VENTRICULOGRAPHY

Ventriculography is the radiographic demonstration of the cerebral ventricular system by direct injection of air into the ventricles. It is the usual investigation of choice in cases of moderate or severe raised intracranial pressure.

Air is injected into the ventricles through frontal or parietal burr holes which are made for this purpose in the operating theatre, to which the patient will return after the examination has been concluded, if craniotomy is to be performed.

Routine supine and prone views are taken as for encephalography (pp. 339 to 341).

MYODIL VENTRICULOGRAPHY

Myodil ventriculography is carried out in cases where the outline of the third and fourth ventricles is particularly required.

Frontal burr holes having been made, the patient comes from the operating theatre to the X-ray department where 2 ml of Myodil are injected into the frontal horn. Using fluoroscopy, preferably with image intensification and television, the radiologist guides the Myodil through the foramen of Munro and into the third ventricle.

Erect lateral and postero-anterior views are taken with the neck flexed in order to visualise the anterior end of the third ventricle and to demonstrate any lateral shift (Jennett, 1969).

The patient is placed in the supine position and Townes and lateral views are taken immediately, and as rapidly as possible, to demonstrate the Myodil in the aqueduct.

MYODIL CISTERNOGRAPHY
(Basal cisternography)

Myodil cisternography is carried out to demonstrate the region of the petrous angles, in the investigation of a possible acoustic neuroma. A lumbar puncture is performed and 5–6 ml of Myodil, or similar, are injected. The patient is then turned into the prone position and the table is tilted head-down so that the contrast medium travels along the spinal subarachnoid space into the head.

The head is then placed in the lateral position, first on one side and then on the other, so that the contrast medium flows across the posterior aspect of the petrous bone. The examination is carried out under fluoroscopic control, with image intensification and television. Any space-occupying lesion, such as an acoustic neuroma, will be demonstrated by the presence of a filling defect.

Under-couch and over-couch radiographs are taken. The most important over-couch view is usually a submento-vertical, using a horizontal beam. For this the patient lies with the side of the head under examination on the table, so that the contrast medium travels to that side.

39

Myelography

Myelography is the radiographic examination of the spinal canal following the injection of contrast medium into the subarachnoid space. The contrast medium used is normally radiopaque but sometimes a gas is used instead. The injection is usually given via a lumbar puncture but if this is not possible or if a complete block of the canal is present and the upper level of the block has to be demonstrated, a cisternal puncture is used instead.

The examination is performed to demonstrate the spinal cord and nerve roots and to show any blockage of the canal by tumour or any encroachment by prolapsed discs into the canal.

A tilting table (preferably with a 90°–90° tilt) is used. The positioning of the contrast medium is controlled by the radiologist, using fluoroscopy, with image intensification and television. If possible, a 'C' arm or bi-plane intensifier is used.

The patient must be warned *in advance* that he will be tilted head-downwards during the examination, so that he will not be alarmed when this happens. He should be reassured that he will not fall.

Preparation of the patient

1. The patient must have had recent radiographic examination of the whole spine.
2. The patient must have nothing to eat or drink for about five hours.

Premedication. Premedication is not usually necessary except for very apprehensive patients or for children. When indicated, premedication such as Omnopon and Scopolamine is given.

Contrast medium. 5 to 6 ml Myodil, or similar. Larger quantities can be used but, if so, the contrast medium should be removed after the examination is completed.

Preliminary films. As the patient will have had recent radiographs of the spine, preliminary films are not usually necessary, but antero-posterior and lateral views of the lumbar spine are often taken to check exposure factors. Exposure factors for the rest of the spine can usually be adjusted from these.

Technique. A lumbar puncture is performed and the contrast medium is injected into the subarachnoid space. A specimen of cerebro-spinal fluid is usually taken and is sent to the pathology department for analysis. The patient is placed prone on the fluoroscopy table and firmly supported. This support may be provided by means of shoulder and foot-rests but the use of a harness similar to a parachute harness is more satisfactory. The patient must be absolutely secure, as he will be tilted head-downwards during the examination. The head is kept straight, with the chin resting on a pad to prevent contrast medium from entering the head. In this position, the contrast medium will pool in the cervical region, and subsequent manœuvring of the neck with the patient horizontal will allow the full extent of the cervical spine to be demonstrated. Some of the contrast medium may be run through the foramen magnum at some stage of the examination, to exclude an obstruction at this level; most of such contrast medium will be retrieved when the patient is finally tilted feet-downwards.

Myodil is heavier than cerebro-spinal fluid and so sinks to the lowest level of the spinal canal. By tilting the patient first of all feet-downwards and then slowly head-downwards, contrast medium will travel from one end of the spinal canal to the other, unless it is obstructed. For a complete examination of the canal, the patient may have to be examined in the supine as well as in the prone position.

Antero-posterior views are taken with the patient prone, using the under-couch tube. Usually two, sometimes three, exposures are made on a 24×30 cm (12×10 in) film divided vertically. As more than one region of the spine may be radiographed on one film, the radiographer must know which region is being examined on each exposure so that the exposure factors can be adjusted. A small 'L' or 'R' is placed on the fluorescent screen so that it will appear on each radiograph to indicate the side. This is particularly important when the patient is examined in both the prone and supine positions. Lateral views are taken, either of each region of the spine or at the site of a suspected lesion. These are taken with the X-ray tube directed horizontally, using a grid cassette supported vertically by the side of the patient. The patient's arm on the side nearer the tube must be raised above the head so that it does not obscure the spine. The other arm can often be used to help support the cassette.

Myodil is absorbed gradually at the rate of about 1 ml per year. Some radiologists routinely remove as much as possible of the Myodil at the conclusion of the myelogram, usually by leaving the lumbar puncture needle *in situ*. Alternatively, a second lumbar puncture may be made for this purpose, usually on a subsequent day, but as it is unlikely that any damage will be caused by leaving the Myodil, many radiologists do not attempt to remove it. Myodil is visible on radiographs of the lumbar spine taken up to several years afterwards.

After-care of the patient

1. Pulse and blood pressure are recorded every half-hour for 4 hours, then 4-hourly for 24 hours.
2. The patient remains in bed for 24 hours.

Basic trolley setting

Upper (sterile) shelf

Two lumbar pucture needles (e.g. Harris's or Pitkin's)
One 2 ml syringe
One 10 ml syringe
Gallipot
Sponge-holding forceps
Towels
Gauze swabs
Gown

Lower (unsterile) shelf

Skin cleanser (e.g. Hibitane 0·5% in 70% industrial spirit, blue stain)
Local anaesthetic (e.g. Lignocaine 2%)
Disposable needles
Contrast medium in bowl of warm water
Specimen bottles for c.s.f.
Adhesive strapping
Masks
EMERGENCY DRUGS

40

Radiculography

Radiculography is the radiographic examination of the cauda equina and the lumbar and sacral nerve roots following the injection of water-soluble contrast medium into the lumbar subarachnoid space (Plate XLVIII).

The contrast medium now used, meglumine iocarmate (Dimer X), gives good visualisation of the nerve roots and sheaths. Being water-soluble, it diffuses with cerebro-spinal fluid and demonstrates the root sheaths in much greater detail and to a greater distance than can an oil-based contrast medium (Grainger *et al.*, 1971). However, because of possible toxic effects on the spinal cord, it must not be allowed to travel further cephalad than L1 and the quantity injected must not exceed 5 ml (Gonsette, 1971).

Water-soluble contrast medium is completely absorbed in 6 to 12 hours, unlike the oil-based contrast medium used in myelography which takes several years to do this.

A tilting table is used and the examination is controlled by fluoroscopy, with image intensification and television. The tilting table should be equipped with a foot-rest and hand-grips.

Preparation of the patient

1. The patient must have had recent radiographs of the lumbar spine.
2. The patient should have nothing to eat or drink for five hours.
3. The patient should micturate immediately before the examination.

Premedication. Usually none is required, but if the examination is carried out on a child, suitable sedation is required. However, radiculography is not usually performed on children under about 12 years of age.

Contrast medium. Meglumine iocarmate (Dimer X), not more than 5 ml.

Technique. The patient is seated on the X-ray table and a lumbar puncture is performed. The contrast medium, mixed with 2 ml cerebro-spinal fluid, is injected fairly slowly (over about 20 seconds) into the subarachnoid space, using a fine lumbar puncture needle, via one of the lower inter-spinous spaces. The needle is then withdrawn, the patient is placed prone and the table is tilted 15° feet-down. The patient must *never* be tilted head-down and therefore a harness is not necessary.

Antero-posterior and oblique views are taken using the under-couch tube. Usually two, sometimes three, exposures are made on a 24 × 30 cm (12 × 10 in) cassette divided vertically. A small 'L' or 'R' is placed on the fluorescent screen so that it will appear on each radiograph to indicate the side. This is particularly important when the patient is examined in both the prone and supine positions. Lateral views are taken with the tube directed horizontally, using a grid cassette supported vertically by the side of the patient. The table is tilted from 0° to 45° feet-down to enable the whole of the lumbar spine to be demonstrated.

The radiographic contrast of meglumine iocarmate is less than that of the contrast medium used in myelography, because it contains less iodine. To obtain maximum radiographic contrast, the kilovoltage should be kept fairly low, 70–75 kV (Grainger *et al.*, 1971).

Care of the patient

For at least eight hours after the injection the patient must not be allowed to lie flat. His trunk must be raised and supported on at least two pillows and this support *must* be maintained even if the patient develops a 'lumbar-puncture headache' (in contrast with the usual treatment for this condition which is for the patient to lie flat).

After the examination is completed, the patient returns to the ward, propped up on a stretcher and also supported by two pillows. Instructions to the ward must emphasise that the patient must not lie flat for at least eight hours. The patient should remain in bed for 24 hours after the examination. Thereafter, a slow return to normal ambulation over the next two to three days is advised.

Basic trolley setting

Upper (sterile) shelf

Two lumbar puncture needles
One 2 ml syringe

One 10 ml syringe
Gallipot
Sponge-holding forceps
Towels
Gauze swabs
Gown

Lower (unsterile) shelf

Skin cleanser (e.g. Hibitane 0·5% in 70% industrial spirit, blue stain)
Local anaesthetic (e.g. Lignocaine 2%)
Disposable needles
Contrast medium
Specimen bottle for c.s.f.
Adhesive strapping
Masks
EMERGENCY DRUGS (including Diazepam)

41

Dacryocystography

Dacryocystography is the radiographic investigation of the lacrimal system following the injection of contrast medium.

The lacrimal system (Fig. 41) is composed of two lacrimal glands situated in the supero-lateral part of the orbit, and the ducts by which tears pass to the nose. Tears are secreted by the glands and pass into the lacrimal ducts via minute orifices called puncta lacrimalia (one on each eye-lid at the medial canthus) and thence into the canaliculi. The ducts open into lacrimal sacs and are connected to the nasal cavity by the naso-lacrimal ducts.

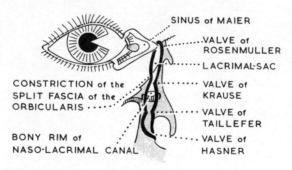

Fig. 41

Dacryocystography is usually employed to demonstrate the site and degree of obstruction in cases of obstructive epiphora, a condition in which the lacrimal passages are inadequate or blocked, causing tears to overflow. With adults the investigation is usually carried out under local anaesthesia, although it is not essential. Children may require general anaesthesia.

Preparation of the patient. None is required.

Premedication. Usually no premedication is required, but children may require sedation.

Contrast medium. 0·5 to 2 ml Lipiodol fluid, according to the quantity necessary to fill the available space. The injection is continued until reflux occurs from the upper punctum and the patient tastes the contrast medium in the pharynx.

Preliminary films. The patient can be examined in either the erect or the horizontal position. Macroradiography (p. 38) is performed if a 0·3 mm² or 0·6 mm² focus tube is available. Cassettes large enough, e.g. 24 × 30 cm (12 × 10 in), are used so as to include the orbits and the floor of the nose and also, in the lateral view, the nasopharynx. Subtraction (p. 41) may also be performed in conjunction with macroradiography (Bunce, 1972).

Occipito-mental. The patient faces the table, with the chin raised and the base line at 35°, this angle being reduced from that in the routine occipito-mental position to avoid distortion as the lacrimal duct is then parallel with the film. The median sagittal plane must be at right angles to the film. The head is immobilised.

Centre to the lower orbital margin.

Lateral. The head is placed in the lateral position with the median sagittal plane parallel with the film and the interpupillary line at right angles to the film. The head is immobilised.

Centre to the lower orbital margin.

Technique. The procedure is explained to the patient and he is warned that the local anaesthetic may sting and that he should not blink during the insertion of the cannula or catheter. A local anaesthetic such as Ophthaine is put into the lacrimal lake. The punctum is dilated.

Using a cannula. A silver lacrimal cannula is inserted through the lower punctum into the canaliculus. When the cannula is in the required position, contrast medium is injected. Radiography must be completed as quickly as possible after the injection because the contrast medium remains in the system for only 15 to 30 seconds.

Occipito-mental and lateral views are taken, as for the preliminary films.

Using catheters. The use of nylon catheters instead of cannulae (Sutton, 1975; Bunce, 1972) has the advantage that radiographs can be taken during the injection and the lacrimal duct and canaliculi are shown filled. If catheters are used, both eyes can be examined at the same time. Each catheter is attached to a 2 ml syringe and the catheter is taped to the pinna of the respective ear. The patient is then turned into the prone position, the head is positioned for the occipito-mental view, as for the preliminary film, and immobilised.

Three exposures are made: (*a*) the first before the injection is commenced, to serve as the plain film for subtraction (*b*) the second when 1 ml of contrast medium has been injected and (c) the third when the injection has been completed. The radiographs are then processed and subtracted.

If only one side has been injected, a lateral view is taken, as for the preliminary film, but if both sides have been injected, a lateral view is not taken, as the contrast medium in one side would be superimposed over that in the other.

After-care of the patient. The patient is usually kept in the department for about half an hour after the examination until the effects of the local anaesthetic have worn off. If not, he must be warned not to allow dust to get into the eye whilst the anaesthetic is still active as it tends to reduce blinking and prevents the eye watering.

Basic trolley setting

Upper (sterile) shelf

Nettleship dilator (blunt)
Silver lacrimal cannula *or* two nylon catheters
Two 2 ml syringes with suitable lock to fit cannula or catheter
Adaptor
Drawing-up cannula
Gauze swabs
Towels
Receiver

Lower (unsterile) shelf

Ampoule of contrast medium in bowl of warm water
Local anaesthetic (e.g. Ophthaine or Amethocaine 1%)
File for opening ampoules

42

Sialography

Sialography is the radiographic examination of the salivary glands and ducts, following the injection of contrast medium. The parotid and submandibular glands can be examined in this way but the anatomy of the sublingual ducts precludes sialography. One or both sides may be examined at one time. Macroradiography (p. 38) is often employed in this examination. An outline of the anatomy of the salivary glands and ducts is given on page 172. The secretions from the parotid glands enter the mouth, via Stenson's ducts, at orifices opposite the second upper molar teeth. The secretions from the submandibular glands enter the mouth, via Wharton's ducts, at orifices on either side of the frenulum of the tongue.

Preparation of the patient. No preparation is required.

Premedication. Premedication is not usually required but children may require sedation.

Contrast medium. Usually Lipiodol Fluid or its equivalent. Sometimes Hypaque 85 per cent or its equivalent is used instead. Because of the narrow calibre of the ducts it is essential to have a dense contrast medium. If water-soluble contrast medium (e.g. Hypaque) is used, the examination can if necessary be repeated after 15 minutes. An oily medium is gradually absorbed but it obscures the area for a repeat examination if this proves to be necessary. The amount of contrast medium required varies with different patients. Usually the patient's symptoms are used as a guide; when he experiences slight pain the injection is stopped. Overfilling must be avoided, so as not to obscure branches of the ducts within the glands.

Preliminary films. The views taken vary according to the gland and duct being examined.

Parotid gland and duct

Antero-posterior. The patient faces the X-ray tube, with the base line at right angles to the table. The head is then rotated about 5° away from the side being examined so that the gland is in profile.

Centre in the mid-line, at the level of the lower lip.

Lateral. The head is placed in the lateral position, with the median sagittal plane parallel with the table, and the interpupillary line at right angles to it.

Centre to the angle of the mandible.

Lateral oblique. From the lateral position, the head is rotated slightly so that the chin is in contact with the table.

Centre to the angle of the mandible, with the tube angled 20° cephalad.

Submandibular gland and duct (Plate XLIX)

Lateral oblique. As for parotid gland (above).

Lateral. The head is placed in the lateral position. Using a pad of swabs, or a swab wrapped round a wooden tongue-depressor, the patient depresses the floor of the mouth. This may enable a calculus otherwise hidden by the mandible to be demonstrated.

Centre to the angle of the mandible.

Infero-superior. The patient sits with the chin raised and head tilted backwards. An occlusal film is placed as far back as possible in the mouth and over to the side under examination.

Centre from below the mandible, at right angles to the film.

Technique. If the orifice of the duct is not visible, the patient is given a slice of lemon (or lime) to suck. This stimulates the secretions from the glands and makes the orifice visible. When the orifice has been located, a salivary duct dilator is inserted into it to facilitate entry of a cannula or catheter.

If a cannula is used, the exposure is made immediately after the contrast medium has been injected. If a catheter is used, the exposure can be made while the contrast medium is being injected or, alternatively, the 'drip-feed' method can be employed.

With the 'drip-feed' method, water-soluble contrast medium is used. A tap-adaptor is fitted between the catheter and the syringe and after insertion of the catheter into the duct, the syringe is suspended on a drip-stand or attached by adhesive tape to the X-ray tube. The tap is turned on and the contrast medium is run in until the patient feels slight pain. The tap is then turned off and the exposure is made.

The catheter is left *in situ* until the end of the examination.

Views. After injection of contrast medium into the parotid duct, antero-posterior, lateral and lateral oblique views are taken, as for the preliminary films. After injection of contrast medium into the submandibular duct, lateral and lateral oblique views are taken.

The infero-superior view is not usually taken routinely at this stage but it is invaluable in the detection of calculi and this is why it is always taken as one of the preliminary films.

After the contrast medium has been given and all the views necessary have been taken, the patient is given a slice of lemon or lime to suck. Post-secretory radiographs, lateral and lateral oblique, are taken five minutes later to show emptying of the duct.

After-care of the patient. Usually no special after-care is necessary.

Basic trolley setting

Upper (sterile) shelf

Salivary duct dilators
Lacrimal duct cannula *or* polythene catheter and adaptor
One 2 ml syringe
One 5 ml syringe
Drawing-up cannula
Towels
Gauze swabs

Lower (unsterile) shelf

Ampoules of contrast medium in bowl of warm water
Slices of lemon (or lime)
Adhesive strapping
Receiver
Mouth wash
Disposable cup
File (for opening ampoule)
Angle-poise lamp

43

Nasopharyngography

Nasopharyngography is the radiographic demonstration of the naso-pharynx following instillation of contrast medium. The examination is performed in the investigation of carcinoma, lymphosarcoma or angiofibroma of the nasopharynx and to demonstrate the position and extent of the lesion. The examination is sometimes repeated after radiotherapy, to study the progress and response of the lesion (Morgan and Evison, 1966). The eustachian tubes may also be demonstrated by this technique.

Whenever possible, a skull unit is used because positioning of the patient for the submento-vertical view (p. 93) is much easier with this apparatus. Ciné-fluorography has been recommended for studies of the eustachian tubes (Khamapirad and Khamapirad, 1973).

Preparation of the patient. None is required except for the removal of radiopaque objects such as dentures and hair-pins. Recent plain films, including a soft tissue lateral, occipito-mental and submento-vertical views, must be available.

Premedication. Atropine, or similar, is given 30 minutes before the examination, to suppress nasopharyngeal and buccal secretions.

Contrast medium. Dionosil aqueous, 8 to 10 ml.

Preliminary films. If recent plain films have been taken, pre-liminary films are not usually needed but, if a skull unit is not avail-able, it is helpful to take a submento-vertical view before the examin-ation, to obtain a convenient method of positioning the patient for the same view when this is taken after the instillation of contrast medium.

Technique. The procedure is explained to the patient. The patient lies supine with the neck hyper-extended and with a foam pad under the head. Topical anaesthetic, e.g. Lignocaine 4 per cent, is sprayed into each nostril. Contrast medium is then instilled into each nostril via fine polythene catheters. The patient is instructed not to swallow during the instillation but to indicate, by raising the hand, when he feels the need to swallow. This is taken as an indica-tion that the nasopharynx is filled with contrast medium (Morgan and Evison, 1966). It has been recommended (Ryan, 1973) that the patient should gargle with the contrast medium (as well as having it instilled into the nostrils) so as to get the contrast medium well up into the nasopharynx.

As soon as the contrast medium has been instilled, the series of radiographs is taken. 24 × 30 cm (12 × 10 in) cassettes are used. The submento-vertical view is taken first as this is the most important view (Plate L).

Views

Submento-vertical (p. 93). The patient faces the X-ray tube, with the chin raised and the neck hyper-extended. The skull table, or grid cassette, is angled so that it is parallel with the base line.

Centre in the mid-line, between the angles of the jaw, and at right angles to the cassette.

Reverse occipito-mental (p. 95). The patient remains in the same position but the head is adjusted so that the base line is at 45° to the cassette.

Centre in the mid-line, at the level of the tip of the nose.

Lateral. The patient remains supine, with the head resting on a foam block. A horizontal beam is used and a grid cassette is supported vertically by the side of the patient's face.

Centre to the lower border of the zygoma.

After-care of the patient. Usually no special after-care is necessary.

Basic trolley setting

Upper (*sterile*) *shelf*

Two fine polythene catheters
Two 10 ml syringes
Drawing-up cannula
Towels
Gauze swabs

Lower (*unsterile*) *shelf*

Throat spray
Topical anaesthetic (e.g. Lignocaine 4%)
Contrast medium
Receiver
EMERGENCY DRUGS

44

Laryngography

Laryngography is the radiographic demonstration of the larynx following the instillation of contrast medium. The examination is performed mainly in the investigation of carcinoma of the larynx. It is also of value in the investigation of paresis, oedema or fibrosis of the larynx. It is carried out under local anaesthesia except for small children or infants who require general anaesthesia.

The examination is performed using fluoroscopy and image intensification. Tomography is also used. Ciné-radiography is of value for infants and it also enables the motility of the structures to be assessed. Subtraction may occasionally be useful (Hemmingsson, 1972).

Preparation of the patient. The patient must have nothing to eat or drink for five hours.

Premedication. Atropine is given 30 minutes before the examination, to suppress nasopharyngeal and buccal secretions and prevent laryngospasm. Omnopon or Nembutal may be given as sedation but the patient must not be too heavily sedated as his co-operation is required. If the examination is being performed under general anaesthesia, the premedication will be prescribed by the anaesthetist.

Contrast medium. Dionosil, 10 to 15 ml.

Preliminary films
Lateral. The patient lies supine on the X-ray table with the head and shoulders supported on foam pads. A horizontal beam is used and the cassette is supported vertically at the side of the patient's shoulder. Low kV (55–60) is used. Two exposures are made, one taken on arrested deep inspiration and the other with the patient performing the Valsalva manœuvre (p. 178).

Centre 2·5 cm (1 in) caudal to the angle of the jaw.

Antero-posterior. The foam pads are removed and the patient lies with the chin raised slightly. The exposure is made on arrested deep inspiration.

Centre in the mid-line of the neck, at the level of the cricoid cartilage.

Technique. The patient sits on the side of the X-ray table. The pharynx and larynx are sprayed with topical anaesthetic (e.g. Lignocaine, 4 per cent) which is also instilled into the larynx via a curved laryngeal syringe. The contrast medium is dripped slowly, also via a curved laryngeal syringe, over the back of the tongue during inspiration. The contrast medium fills the vallecula and piriform fossa and coats the larynx. The patient is instructed not to swallow or cough, and is then positioned on his back as for the preliminary films.

Lateral and antero-posterior views are taken as for the preliminary films. Alternatively, fluoroscopy may be used and 'spot' films taken (*a*) with the patient performing the Valsalva manœuvre (*b*) on deep inspiration and (*c*) on phonation. Antero-posterior tomography is performed with the patient phonating (saying 'eeee'). The centering point is the same as for the preliminary films.

These radiographs are viewed by the radiologist who may require a second series of tomograms taken on deep inspiration. For a full assessment, views in inspiratory and expiratory phonation and in quiet respiration should be taken to show movement of the vocal cords and the ventricular bands (Ryan, 1970).

After-care of the patient. The patient must have nothing to eat or drink for at least four hours or until after the effects of the local anaesthetic have worn off, whichever is the longer.

Basic trolley setting

Upper (sterile) shelf

Two curved laryngeal syringes
Drawing-up cannula
Towels
Gauze swabs

Lower (unsterile) shelf

Throat spray
Topical anaesthetic (e.g. Lignocaine Hyd. 4%)
Contrast medium
Receiver
EMERGENCY DRUGS

45

Bronchography

Bronchography is the radiographic investigation of the bronchial tree following the administration of contrast medium. The examination is performed mainly in the investigation of bronchiectasis (Plate LI) but may also be of value in the investigation of peripheral tumours of the lung.

It is usually carried out under local anaesthesia but children under about 12 years of age require general anaesthesia. Sometimes bronchography is performed immediately after bronchoscopy, in which case the patient will still be under general anaesthesia. Usually both lungs are examined.

Preparation of the patient

1. A patient who has bronchiectasis or who produces copious sputum should have physiotherapy (postural drainage and percussion) for at least three days before the examination. Such patients are usually given antibiotics for about the same period.
2. The patient must have nothing to eat or drink for at least five hours before the examination and only a light diet for the previous 24 hours.

Premedication. When the examination is being performed under local anaesthesia, premedication such as Atropine (to dry up the bronchial, nasopharyngeal and buccal secretions) and Omnopon (for sedation) are given, but the patient must not be heavily sedated because his co-operation is needed. When the examination is being performed under general anaesthesia, the anaesthetist will prescribe the premedication. Atropine is still needed to dry up the secretions.

Contrast medium. Dionosil, aqueous or oily, 12 to 16 ml per side for adults, 1 ml per side for each year of age for children. In cases of bronchiectasis, 1 to 3 ml extra may be needed.

Preliminary films. Usually, after the administration of the contrast medium radiographs are taken with the patient lying on the X-ray table. Occasionally the erect position may be preferred, in which case postero-anterior and lateral views are taken as for the basic views of the chest (p. 184). In either case the kilovoltage required is 5 to 10 more than for the basic views. A grid is used for all the views throughout the examination.

Antero-posterior. The patient lies supine. The elbows are flexed and the arms are abducted so as to prevent superimposition of the scapulae on the lung fields. The upper border of the cassette is placed 2·5 cm (1 in) above the level of the shoulders. The exposure is made on arrested full inspiration.

Centre to the cassette.

Lateral. The patient lies on the side, with the hands on the pillow and the knees flexed to aid balance. The upper border of the cassette is placed 2·5 cm (1 in) above the level of the shoulders. The exposure is again made on arrested full inspiration.

Centre in the mid-axillary line to the centre of the cassette.

Radiation protection. If the radiographs are taken with the patient in the horizontal position, the pelvis must be covered with lead rubber. If the radiographs are taken with the patient in the erect position, normal protective measures for chest radiography must be taken (p. 180). If a nurse holds the patient, she must wear a lead apron.

Technique. There are several methods of introducing the contrast medium into the bronchi. The most usual methods are the trans-nasal method and the crico-thyroid method.

Trans-nasal method. If the examination is being performed under local anaesthesia, the patient is given an anaesthetic lozenge to suck. The nose, throat, nasopharynx and trachea are sprayed with topical anaesthetic. A catheter is passed through the nose into the nasopharynx and into the trachea. The proximal end of the catheter is attached to the cheek by means of adhesive tape.

Some radiologists prefer to pass the catheter into the trachea through the mouth, using indirect laryngoscopy. In this case, the nose need not be anaesthetised. When the examination is performed under general anaesthesia, the catheter is passed down the endo-tracheal tube which is already *in situ.*

Contrast medium is injected down the catheter, usually in three or four equal amounts, the first two or three portions being used to demonstrate the lower and middle lobes and the lingula, the last portion being used to fill the upper lobe. The direction the contrast medium takes is dependent on gravity. To fill the middle and lower lobes, the patient leans towards the side being examined, then bends forwards, then sideways, then backwards, contrast medium being injected in each position. To fill the upper lobe, the patient lies on the side being examined, with the head raised and the feet lowered. Following injection of the contrast medium, he is then turned half-way on to the face and then half-way on to the back, and during these manœuvres, the head of the table is lowered slightly (Saxton and Strickland, 1972).

In each position, the contrast medium is injected quite quickly. The patient is held in position for about five seconds during which he is asked to take in a deep breath slowly, so as to draw contrast medium out to the periphery of the lung. He is then moved into the next position. All breathing should be calm and slow, so as to prevent coughing.

If both sides are being examined at one time, the right lung is usually filled first but some radiologists prefer to fill the side of the suspected lesion first.

Crico-thyroid method. The patient lies supine or sits on a chair. Local anaesthetic is injected into the skin over the crico-thyroid area and into the trachea through the crico-thyroid membrane. The patient leans towards the side being examined and is supported by a nurse. A crico-thyroid needle is inserted into the trachea and when it is correctly sited contrast medium is injected. The needle is then withdrawn and the patient is placed in the positions previously described for the trans-nasal method of filling the various parts of the lung.

Views. A series of radiographs is taken as soon as the contrast medium has been given. After the first side has been filled, antero-posterior and lateral views are taken, as for the preliminary films. After the other side has been filled, antero-posterior and right and left posterior oblique views are taken. For the posterior oblique views, the patient is rotated 45° from the supine position towards each side in turn. The upper border of the cassette should be 2·5 cm (1 in) above the level of the shoulders and the whole chest must be included. Each exposure is made on arrested inspiration. Satisfactory views of the first side must be obtained before the second side is filled.

After-care of the patient

1. As soon as the examination is completed, the patient is encouraged to cough in order to remove as much of the contrast medium as possible.

2. The patient must have nothing to eat or drink for at least three hours until the effects of the anaesthetic have worn off. This is to avoid accidental aspiration of food or drink.

3. Physiotherapy (postural coughing and percussion) is required to remove further contrast medium.

4. If the examination has been performed on an out-patient, the patient must not be allowed to leave the department before he has completely recovered from the sedation and local anaesthetic. This is particularly important if he is driving home.

5. Radiography of the chest is often carried out 24 hours after the examination, to see how much contrast medium remains.

Basic trolley setting

Upper (sterile) shelf

Catheters (Jacques' and Tiemann's)
Two short 1 in (2·5 cm) needles, short bevel
Dissecting forceps
Gallipot
Lotion bowl
Two 20 ml syringes
One 2 ml syringe
Towels
Gauze swabs

Lower (unsterile) shelf

Skin cleanser (e.g. Hibitane 0·5% in 70% spirit)
Local anaesthetic (e.g. Lignocaine 2%) for crico-thyroid method
Topical anaesthetic (e.g. Lignocaine Hyd. 4%) for trans-nasal method
Throat spray with topical anaesthetic for trans-nasal method
Contrast medium
Bowl with antiseptic (e.g. Domittol) for expectoration
Masks
EMERGENCY DRUGS

SELECTIVE BRONCHOGRAPHY

Selective bronchography may be carried out during bronchoscopy if a fibre-optic bronchoscope is being used. Samples of lung tissue are obtained by cytology forceps which are introduced down one of the channels of the endoscope. The same channel is used for injecting contrast medium (Dionosil oily) via a 100 cm long dispos- able catheter to the part of the lung being examined (Higginbottom, 1977). The contrast medium is injected under fluoroscopic control. Antero-posterior and oblique views of the chest are taken.

PERCUTANEOUS LUNG BIOPSY

The purpose of this examination is to obtain specimens of lung tissue for bacteriological and histological analysis. It is performed under fluoroscopic control using image intensification and television. If possible, a 'C' arm intensifier is used.

The examination is contra-indicated in patients (a) with severe generalised lung disease (b) with pulmonary hypertension or (c) on artificial ventilators (Howatt, 1976).

Full resuscitation facilities must be immediately available. The examination is carried out only on an 'in-patient' so that he can be closely observed afterwards.

Preparation of the patient

1. Full radiographic examination of the chest, including tomography to localise the lesion, must have been carried out within the previous 24–48 hours.
2. The patient must have nothing to eat or drink for 4–6 hours.

Premedication. Premedication such as Diazepam is given.
Preliminary films. None are required.
Technique. The patient lies supine on the fluoroscopy table and is made as comfortable as possible. Under fluoroscopic control, the optimum site for puncture is located and its position marked on the patient's skin. The skin is cleansed and local anaesthetic is infiltrated. The biopsy needle is inserted through the skin and pleura and into the lung tissue. While the needle is being inserted through the lung tissue, the patient is asked to stop breathing, so as to minimise the risk of air embolism. Specimens of lung tissue are sent to the pathology department for analysis.

A radiograph of the chest, on expiration, is taken 30 minutes to one hour after the end of the examination, to demonstrate whether a pneumothorax is present.

After-care of the patient

1. The patient must stay in bed for six hours and be observed frequently for signs of pneumothorax.
2. Radiographs of the chest may be required during this time but a pneumothorax is unlikely to occur later than five hours after the examination (Higginbottom, 1977).
3. The patient must remain in the ward, under observation, for 24 hours.

Basic trolley setting

Upper (sterile) shelf

Biopsy needle
5 ml syringe
Gallipot
Lotion bowl
Scalpel blade
Gauze swabs
Towels

Lower (unsterile) shelf

Skin cleanser (e.g. Chlorhexidine 0·5% in 70% spirit)
Local anaesthetic (e.g. Lignocaine 1%)
Disposable needles
Specimen bottles and slides
Plastic dressing spray
Masks
EMERGENCY DRUGS

46

Arthrography

Arthrography is the radiographic demonstration of the internal anatomy of a joint, following injection of contrast medium. Either single or double contrast technique can be used. Sometimes a negative contrast medium only is used and the examination is then called pneumo-arthrography.

Although arthrography can be performed on any synovial joint, the most usual sites are the shoulder, the hip and the knee. These only will be described.

Arthrography is contra-indicated if there is (a) acute infection of the joint or of the over-lying skin or (b) known sensitivity to contrast media.

SHOULDER

Arthrography of the shoulder is performed mainly to demonstrate injury to the musculo-tendinous (rotator) cuff. It is also used in the investigation of recurrent dislocation, capsulitis and loose bodies in the joint.

Either single or double contrast technique can be used. Double contrast gives additional information as to the width of a tear, presence of degenerative changes in the cuff, conditions of the articular surfaces and state of injured tendons (Ghelman and Goldman, 1977).

The examination is carried out under fluoroscopic control. Most of the radiographs are taken using the over-couch tube.

A method using double contrast will be described.

Preparation of the patient. Usually none is required.

Premedication. Usually no premedication is required.

Contrast medium. 4 ml of the meglumine salts of diatrizoate or iothalamate are used. 10 ml of air are used for double contrast.

Preliminary films. A grid should be used for all but the axial view which is usually taken using a curved cassette. If a curved cassette is not available, a grid is used for this view also. The radiographs should be well penetrated, the kilovoltage required is 5 more than for the basic views.

Antero-posterior. From the supine position, the patient is rotated about 60°, the side not under examination being raised and supported on foam pads and sandbags. The arm of the side under examination should rest by the side, with the palm facing upwards.

Centre to the coracoid process.

Axial. The patient sits beside the X-ray table, with the arm abducted and the elbow flexed. A curved cassette is placed under the axilla. The shoulder is flattened as much as possible over the cassette (Fig. 16, p. 128).

Centre to the head of the humerus.

Technique. The patient lies supine on the fluoroscopy table, with the arm held in minimal external rotation and abduction. The examination is performed under strict aseptic conditions. Local anaesthetic is infiltrated. Under fluoroscopic control, a needle—usually a child's lumbar puncture needle with a short bevel—is inserted into the joint-space. To confirm the position of the tip of the needle, 1 ml of contrast medium is injected under fluoroscopic control. If the position of the needle is satisfactory, the contrast media are injected under fluoroscopic control. If the patient experiences pain, the quantity of contrast media injected is decreased. The size of a rotator cuff tear can be estimated by noting the rate of leakage of contrast medium into the subacromial bursa (Preston and Jackson, 1977).

When the contrast media have been injected, the needle is removed and the shoulder is gently exercised. The patient then sits up and two radiographs are taken, using the vertical Bucky or vertically-supported grid cassette. The air will have risen to the superior portion of the joint and the inferior surface of the rotator cuff, coated with contrast medium, will be outlined.

Erect antero-posterior in internal and external rotation. The patient is rotated about 60°, the side not under examination being supported by foam pads. Two radiographs are taken, one on internal and one on external rotation (see p. 129 and Fig. 18).

Centre to the coracoid process.

Supine antero-posterior. As for the preliminary film.

'Stryker's view'—taken mainly in the investigation of recurrent dislocation. The patient lies supine with the hand placed on top of the head and the elbow directed forwards.

Centre to the axilla, with the tube angled 25° cephalad.
Axial. As for the preliminary film.
After-care of the patient. Usually none is required.

HIP

When arthrography of the hip is performed on a child, it is usually in the investigation of irreducible or unstable congenital dislocation (dysplasia) of the hip, Perthé's disease, capsular lesions or loose bodies in the joint. When performed on an adult it is usually in the assessment of a prosthesis (i.e. whether it is loose, infected, etc.) and to investigate a painful, 'clicking' hip, or loose bodies in the joint.

As the technique for a child differs from that required for an adult, each will be described separately.

CHILDREN

The examination is performed under general anaesthesia.

Preparation of the patient. The child must have nothing to eat or drink for about five hours.

Premedication. As the examination is performed under general anaesthesia, the anaesthetist will prescribe the premedication.

Contrast medium. Hypaque 25 per cent or its equivalent is used for the investigation of congenital dislocation of the hip, Hypaque 12·5 per cent or its equivalent is used for the investigation of Perthé's disease. 1 ml per year of age.

Preliminary films. Usually the child will have had recent radiographs of the hips in which case, to avoid excess irradiation, preliminary films are not taken.

If recent radiographs are not available, antero-posterior and 'Von Rosen' views are taken, for which the child's pelvis is positioned symmetrically and immobilised by means of a plastic jig (Grech, 1972) or foam pads and sandbags.

Antero-posterior. The child lies supine with the legs extended.

Centre in the mid-line, at the level of the femoral pulse.

'Von Rosen'. The child lies supine with each leg abducted 45° (producing a mutual angle of 90°) and internally rotated (p. 150 and Fig. 24).

Centre in the mid-line, at the level of the femoral pulse.

Radiation protection. Strict attention must be paid to protecting the gonads by means of lead rubber and by accurate coning so that they are never directly irradiated. The jig, previously mentioned, incorporates lead protection in its design. If this is not available, radiolucent adhesive tape should be used to secure lead protection in position and prevent it from slipping off the child's pelvis and obscuring essential detail.

Technique. The examination is performed under strict aseptic conditions. Under fluoroscopic control, a needle (usually a child's lumbar puncture needle with a short bevel) is inserted into the joint capsule. When the needle has been correctly sited, the contrast medium is injected and the needle is then withdrawn.

Under fluoroscopic control, the child's hips are manipulated through the full range of movements including neutral, abduction (with internal and external rotation) and adduction positions. An occasional 'spot' film (Plate LII) is taken using the under-couch tube. For these under-couch radiographs, the screen must always be at the same distance from the patient so that the magnification is the same for each radiograph.

After-care of the patient. When the effects of the anaesthetic have worn off, no special after-care is needed.

ADULTS

Preparation of the patient. None is required.

Premedication. No premedication is required.

Contrast medium. 10 to 15 ml of the meglumine salts of iothalamate or diatrizoate.

Radiation protection. Patients undergoing arthrography of the hip for investigation of a prosthesis are often elderly, but when the examination is performed on a younger adult, careful attention must be paid to lead shielding of the gonads, for both under-couch and over-couch radiographs. The X-ray beam should be collimated accurately so that the gonads are not directly irradiated.

Preliminary films. Antero-posterior and lateral views of the hip are taken. These radiographs also serve as the plain films for later subtraction. The centering points should be marked on the patient's skin and the positioning used should be easily repeatable for successful subtraction.

Antero-posterior. The patient lies supine with the leg slightly internally rotated.

Centre to the femoral pulse.

Lateral. From the supine position, the patient is rotated towards the side being examined, the knee is flexed and the leg is abducted and allowed to rest on the table, or is supported on a sandbag or foam pad.

Centre to the femoral pulse.

Alternatively, a lateral view as for the neck of the femur may be preferred by the radiologist, with the patient either supine (Fig. 23) or seated (p. 150).

Technique. The patient lies supine on the fluoroscopy table. The examination is performed under strict aseptic conditions. Local anaesthetic is infiltrated and a long—7·5 cm (3 in)—lumbar puncture needle with a short bevel, is inserted into the joint capsule or towards the neck of the prosthesis if one is present. Fluid in the joint is aspirated and sent to the pathology department for culture. If no fluid can be aspirated from the joint, a little saline is injected and this is aspirated and sent for culture.

Contrast medium is injected slowly, under fluoroscopic control.

Traction is applied to the hip, to open up the joint space. When the contrast medium has been injected, the needle is removed. The following radiographs are taken, the positioning and centering being the same as for the preliminary films but with rotation and abduction of the limb:

Antero-posterior with the leg internally rotated as far as possible.
Antero-posterior with the leg externally rotated as far as possible.
Antero-posterior in abduction.
Antero-posterior with traction applied to the hip.
Lateral.

Subtraction (p. 41) is carried out. Because of the various positions of the limb in which the contrast films are taken, it may be necessary to make more than one subtracted image for each view to obtain a complete demonstration.

After-care of the patient. No special after-care is needed.

KNEE

Arthrography of the knee will demonstrate (*a*) derangement of the capsule or intra-articular structures, e.g. damaged cruciate ligaments or tears of the menisci (*b*) defects in the articular surfaces of the femoral condyles, e.g. in osteochondritis dissecans (*c*) synovial diseases, e.g. benign pigmented villonodular synovitis of the knee or (*d*) joint rupture, which may or may not have associated Baker's cysts.

Usually the examination is performed to localise meniscus injuries and assess their extent (Ringertz, 1976). In some cases of rheumatoid arthritis, the full extent of the synovial proliferation of the joint space can be visualised (Taylor, 1969).

Either single or double contrast method can be used, depending on the choice of the radiologist, but usually double contrast is the method of choice to demonstrate tears in the menisci, and single contrast to demonstrate ruptures of the capsule and Baker's cysts. Double contrast arthrography will be described.

The examination is performed using fluoroscopy, with image intensification and television. Over-couch and under-couch radiographs are taken. The fine focus should be used (Stoker, 1975) and the beam should be collimated to include just the meniscus being examined. A small circular lead diaphragm on the under-couch tube helps to reduce scattered radiation and improve image detail. A grid is not usually needed. Low kilovoltage (50–60 kV) is used. During the examination, radiographs are taken with the knee in stress varus and valgus positions and a method of maintaining the joint in these positions is required (Levinsohn, 1977).

Preparation of the patient. Usually none is required.

Premedication. No premedication is usually required.

Contrast medium. 4 to 5 ml of meglumine iocarmate (Dimer X) or the meglumine salts of iothalamate or diatrizoate (Conray 280 or Angiografin). The sodium salts are not used because they cause more pain. Double contrast is provided by air or carbon dioxide, or both. If both are used, the negative contrast medium remains in the joint long enough for further views to be taken after initial viewing.

Radiation protection. Often patients undergoing arthrography of the knee are young and careful attention must be paid to lead shielding of the gonads, for both under-couch and over-couch radiography.

Preliminary films

Antero-posterior. The knee is extended and the leg is supported on suitable foam pads so that the tibial plateau is vertical.

Centre just below the apex of the patella.

Inter-condylar. The knee is flexed over a curved cassette which is supported on pads so that the angle at the knee is approximately 135°.

Centre to the lower border of the patella, with the tube angled so that it is at right angles to the leg and therefore parallel with the tibial plateau (Fig. 26, p. 155).

Lateral. The patient is turned towards the side being examined. The knee is flexed at right angles. A pad is placed under the heel. The tibial plateau must be at right angles to the cassette, the patella must be vertical and the femoral condyles superimposed.

Centre to the medial tibial condyle.

Technique. The patient lies supine on the fluoroscopy table and is made comfortable. The examination is performed under strict aseptic conditions. The skin is cleansed and sterile towels are draped round the knee. The skin is infiltrated with local anaesthetic and a thin-walled needle—18 or 19 gauge, 3·75 cm (1½ in) long, with a short bevel—is inserted into the joint. Fluid from the joint space is aspirated. 0·3 mg of adrenaline is injected into the joint, thereby reducing the rate of absorption of contrast media. This is particularly useful if there is an effusion or active sinovitis.

Under fluoroscopic control, the positive contrast medium is injected followed by the air and/or carbon dioxide (50–70 ml) until the supra-patellar pouch is tense (like a balloon). The needle is then removed and the knee is either flexed and extended several times or the patient exercises it for a few moments. Movement of the knee helps to distribute the contrast media throughout the joint.

The patient is then turned into the prone position and the knee is rotated under fluoroscopic control, varus and valgus stress being applied until each meniscus is separated by gas from the contiguous hyaline cartilages and plateaux and can therefore be demonstrated. Radiographs are taken using the under-couch tube (Plate LIII), usually about eight views being taken of each meniscus.

When the menisci have been demonstrated satisfactorily, over-couch views of the whole joint are taken, as follows:

Lateral. As for the preliminary film but the knee is flexed at an angle of about 135°. This view demonstrates the cruciate ligaments and any degenerative cysts that are present.

Antero-posterior. As for the preliminary film.

'*Skyline*' view of patella (p. 156 and Fig. 27). This view is taken to demonstrate chondromalacia patellae.

Lateral, using a horizontal beam.

Intercondylar. As for the preliminary film.

If suspected joint rupture or a Baker's cyst is being investigated, after the above views have been taken, the patient is asked to walk about a little and then another lateral view is taken.

After-care of the patient. No special after-care is required.

Basic trolley setting

Upper (sterile) shelf

Two lumbar puncture needles (short bevel)
One 2 ml syringe
One 10 ml syringe
One 50 ml syringe
Two-way tap
Drawing-up cannula
Sponge-holding forceps
Gallipot
Towels
Gauze swabs
Gown

Lower (unsterile) shelf

Skin cleanser (e.g. Hibitane 0·5% in 70% industrial spirit)
Local anaesthetic (e.g. Lignocaine 1%)
Ampoule of contrast medium
Ampoule of adrenaline
Disposable needles
Adhesive strapping

47

Discography

Discography is the radiographic examination of an intervertebral disc, following the injection of contrast medium. The examination is performed to demonstrate disc herniation or degeneration. It is usually performed in the lumbo-sacral region, less often in the cervical region.

Preparation of the patient

1. The patient must have had recent radiographic examination of the whole spine.
2. The patient must have nothing to eat or drink for five hours.

   Premedication. Adequate sedation is essential so that the patient is relaxed and drowsy but he must be able to co-operate and describe the pattern and distribution of any pain induced. A combination of 10 mg droperidol (e.g. Droleptan) and 0·15 mg phenoperidine (e.g. Operidine) has been found very effective (Park, 1973).

   Contrast medium. The meglumine salts of iothalamate or diatrizoate (e.g. Angiografin or Conray 280) are used. The sodium salts are not used because they can have a direct irritant effect on the dura and cause a pain pattern not reproduced by saline or a sodium-free contrast medium.

   Usually 0·5 ml is required for a normal lumbar disc and less for a cervical disc but up to 2 ml may be needed if there is rupture of the annulus fibrosus (Sutton, 1975).

   Preliminary films. Localised antero-posterior and lateral views are taken of the disc or discs to be examined, as determined from the previous films. The centering points are marked on the patient's skin.

   Technique. The patient lies on his side, with the back arched and the knees flexed. Foam pads should be placed where necessary to maintain the spine parallel with the table. The patient is immobilised in this position with foam pads and sandbags.

The skin, subcutaneous tissues and bone periosteum are in-filtrated with local anaesthetic. Under fluoroscopic control, with image intensification and television, a 12·5 cm (5 in) 20 gauge needle is passed, as a guide, into the interspinous space and directed to the annulus of the disc being examined. The point of the needle should just penetrate the annulus. A 25 gauge needle is passed through the guide needle, the former being 1 cm longer than the latter and so lying within the nucleus pulposus.

The contrast medium is injected with a tuberculin syringe. In some normal discs there is such resistance to injection that it is impossible to introduce any contrast medium. The resistance to injection may be markedly reduced in disc degeneration or disc prolapse.

Antero-posterior and lateral (Plate LIV) views are taken as for the preliminary films. Occasionally, oblique views may also be required. Radiography must be completed without delay because the contrast medium diffuses rapidly from the disc.

The examination is considered positive when the patient volun-teers the information that his symptoms have been reproduced but this information is not of value if he has been told beforehand to expect these symptoms. The radiographer and nurse must therefore avoid mentioning that this may happen.

After-care of the patient

1. Pulse and respiration are recorded every half-hour for 4 hours and then 4-hourly for 24 hours.
2. The patient must remain in bed for 24 hours.

Basic trolley setting

Upper (sterile) shelf

One exploring needle, 20 gauge, 12·5 cm (5 in) long, with stilette
One exploring needle, 25 gauge, 13·5 cm long
Sponge-holding forceps
One 10 ml syringe
One 2 ml tuberculin syringe
Drawing-up cannula
Gallipot
Gauze swabs
Towels
Gown

Lower (unsterile) shelf

Skin cleanser (e.g. Hibitane 0·5% in 70% industrial spirit)
Local anaesthetic (e.g. Lignocaine 1%)
Ampoule of contrast medium in bowl of warm water
Disposable needles
EMERGENCY DRUGS

References

Abel, M. S. & Smith, G. R. (1977) Visualization of the postero-lateral elements of the lumbar vetebrae in the antero-posterior projection. *Radiology*, **122**, 824–825.

Adrian Report (1960) Radiological hazards to patients. The second report of the committee. London: H.M. Stationery Office.

Ahlberg, N. E., Bartley, O. & Chidekel, N. (1968) Venous arteriography—a modified technique and indications for its use. *Acta Radiologica*, **N.S.7**, 321.

Ansell, G. & Ansell, A. (1964) Medical emergencies in the X-ray department: prevention and treatment. *British Journal of Radiology*, **37**, 881.

Ansell, G. & Faux, P. A. (1973) Low-dose infusion cholangiography. *Clinical Radiology*, **24**, 95.

Anthonsen, W. (1943) An oblique projection for roentgen examination of the talo-calcanean joint, particularly regarding intra-articular fracture of the calcaneus. *Acta Radiologica*, **24**, 306.

Ardran, G. M. & Crooks, H. E. (1976) Chest Symposium: Radiography of the chest. *X-ray Focus*, **15**, No. 2.

Ardran, G. M. & Kemp, F. H. (1975) The larynx. In *Recent Advances in Radiology*, 5, pp. 89–98, ed. Lodge, T. & Steiner, R. E. Edinburgh: Churchill Livingstone.

Ashley, A. J. (1973) Air encephalography using the McCallum automatic gas dispenser. *Radiography*, **39**, 171.

Axelsson, A. & Jensen, C. (1975) The roentgenologic demonstration of sinusitis. *American Journal of Roentgenology*, **122**, 621–627.

Ayre-Smith, G. (1976) Hyoscine-N-Butylbromide (Buscopan) as a duodenal relaxant in tubeless duodenography. *Acta Radiologica*, **17**, Fasc. 5, 701–713.

Barnett, E. (1972) Hysterosalpingography. In *Practical Procedures in Diagnostic Radiology*, ed. Saxton, H. M. & Strickland, B. 2nd edition. London: Lewis.

Beeson, B. B. (1978) Personal communication.

Benness, G. T., Bullen, A. & Barker, A. (1965) Double-dose urography—renal function test. *Journal of the College of Radiologists of Australasia*, **9**, 234.

Berdon, W. E., Baker, D. H. & Leonidas, J. (1968) Advantages of prone positioning in gastro-intestinal and genito-urinary roentgenologic studies in infants and children. *American Journal of Roentgenology, Radium Therapy and Nuclear Medicine*, **103**, 444.

Boag, J. W., Stacey, A. J. & Davis, R. (1972) Xerographic recording of mammograms. *British Journal of Radiology*, **45**, 633–640.

Boag, J. W., Stacey, A. J. & Davis, R. (1976) Radiation exposure to the patient in xeroradiography. *British Journal of Radiology*, **49**, 253–261.

Brewerton, D. A. (1967) A tangential radiographic projection for demonstrating involvement of the metacarpal heads in rheumatoid arthritis. *British Journal of Radiology*, **40**, 233.

Bryan, G. J. (1971) Infusion choledochography. *X-ray Focus*, **11**, No. 1, 15.

Bull, J. W. D. & Zilkha, K. J. (1968) Rationalising requests for X-ray films in neurology. *British Medical Journal*, **4**, 569.

Bunce, A. H. (1972) Macrodacryocystography. *Radiography*, **38**, 335.

Burwood, R. J., Davies, G. T., Lawrie, B. W., Blumgart, L. H. & Salmon, P. R. (1973) Endoscopic retrograde choledocho-pancreatography. *Clinical Radiology*, **24**, 397.

Butterman, G. & Dressler, J. (1973) Simultaneous double nuclide subtraction scintigraphy of the pancreas using two-channel scanners and magnetic tape recorder. *Electromedica*, 1/1973, 13.

Campbell, W. (1964) Radiology of the lacrimal system. *British Journal of Radiology*, **37**, 1.

Canigiani, G. & Wickenhauser, J. (1972) The contribution of panoramic radiography in the diagnosis of fractures of the facial skull. *Electromedica*, 3/1972, 90.

Chang, C. H., Sibala, J. L., Martin, N. L. & Riley, R. C. (1976) Film mammography, new low radiation technology. *Radiology*, **121**, 215–217.

Chehata, O. & du Boulay, G. H. (1975) The value of colour subtraction in cerebro-vascular disease. *British Journal of Radiology*, **48**, 360–365.

Chesney, D. N. (1967) Radiography of the acute abdomen. *Radiography*, **33**, 141.

Chesney, D. N. & Chesney, M. O. (1978) *Care of the Patient in Diagnostic Radiography*. 5th edition. Oxford: Blackwell.

Chuang, V. P., Reuter, S. R., Kyung, J. C. & Schmidt, R. W. (1976) Alterations in gastric physiology caused by selective embolization and vasopressin infusion of the left gastric artery. *Radiology*, **120**, 533–536.

Clarke, K. C. (1964) *Positioning in Radiography*. 8th edition. London: Heinemann.

Code of Practice for the Protection of Persons against Ionising Radiations arising from Medical and Dental Use (1972) London: H.M. Stationery Office.

Cotton, P. B. (1974) In *Topics in Gastroenterology*, 2, p. 53, ed. Truelove, S. C. & Trowell, J. Oxford: Blackwell Scientific Publications.

Cotton, P. B., Salmon, P. R., Blumgart, L. H., Burwood, R. J., Davies, G. T., Lawrie, B. W., Pierce, J. W. & Read, A. E. (1972) Cannulation of papilla of Vater via fiber-duodenoscope. Assessment of retrograde cholangio-pancreatography in 60 patients. *The Lancet*, Jan. 8th, 53.

Couch, R. S. J. & Brodie, V. (1966) Close layer multi-section tomography. *British Journal of Radiology*, **39**, 358.

Cowley, E. J. (1975) New concepts in radiography. *Radiography*, **41**, 153–164.

Cremin, B. J. (1972) Investigation of neo-natal heart disease. *British Journal of Radiology*, **45**, 75.

Crooks, H. E. & Ardran, G. M. (1977) An air gap technique for nasal sinus radiography. *Radiography*, **43**, 195–202.

Davies, E. R. (1975) Radio-isotope scanning. In *Textbook of Radiology*, ed. Sutton, D. 2nd edition. Edinburgh: Churchill Livingstone.

Davies, P., Roylance, J. & Gordon, I. R. S. (1972) Hydronephrosis. *Clinical Radiology*, **23**, 312.

Davies, P., Roberts, M. B. & Roylance, J. (1975) Acute reactions to urographic contrast media. *British Medical Journal*, **2**, 434–437.

Davis, R. (1977) High-kilovoltage technique and the choice of optimal filtration in xeroradiography. *British Journal of Radiology*, **50**, 234.

Dawson, J., Phillips, G. M. & Wilcox, B. A. M. (1966) Computation of X-ray diagnostic exposure factors. *British Journal of Radiology*, **39**, 117.

Deichgraber, E. & Olsson, B. (1975) Soft tissue radiography in painful shoulder. *Acta Radiologica*, **16**, 393–400.

de Lacey, G. (1977a) The double contrast barium meal. *X-ray Focus*, **15**, No. 2, 43–49.

de Lacey, G. (1977b) The double contrast barium enema. *X-ray Focus*, **15**, No. 3, 59–66.

de Lacey, G. & Wignall, B. K. (1977) Urethrography simplified: the drip infusion technique. *British Journal of Radiology*, **50**, 138–140.

Dodds, W. J., Lydon, S. B., Stewart, E. T. & Binder, G. A. (1975) Value of the tilt upside down maneuver for roentgen examination of the pelvic small bowel loops. *American Journal of Roentgenology*, 123, No. 2, 412–414.

Doi, K. & Imhof, H. (1977) Noise reduction by radiographic magnification. *Radiology*, 122, 479–487.

Dombrowski, H. (1968) Zonography with linear blurring in the diagnostic routine. *Electromedica*, 2/1968, 35.

Doyle, F. H. (1961) Cystography in bladder tumours, a technique using Steripaque and carbon dioxide. *British Journal of Radiology*, 34, 205.

Doyle, F. H. (1972) Radiological patterns of bone disease associated with renal glomerular failure in adults. *British Medical Bulletin*, 28, No. 3, 220.

du Boulay, G. & Bostick, T. (1969) Linear tomography in congenital abnormalities of the ear. *British Journal of Radiology*, 42, 161.

Dure-Smith, P. & McArdle, G. H. (1972) Tomography during excretory urography. Technical aspects. *British Journal of Radiology*, 45, 896.

Edwards, D. (1972) Injection urethrography in the male. In *Practical Procedures in Diagnostic Radiology*, ed. Saxton, H. M. & Strickland, B. 2nd edition. London: Lewis.

Edwards, E. M. & Evans, K. T. (1963) Pelvic pneumography in the Stein Lowenthal syndrome. *British Journal of Radiology*, 36, 46.

Egan, R. L. (1972) *Mammography*. Springfield, Illinois: Thomas.

Esberg, H. & Haverling, M. (1977) Orthopantomography of the mandible. *Acta Radiologica*, 18, Fasc. 3, 357–359.

Ferrucci, J. T., Wittenberg, J., Sarno, R. A. & Dreyfus, J. R. (1976) Fine needle transhepatic cholangiography. A new approach to obstructive jaundice. *American Journal of Roentgenology*, 127, 403–407.

Fraser, G. M., Cruikshank, J. G. & Sumerling, M. D. (1978) Percutaneous transhepatic cholangiography with the Chiba needle. *Clinical Radiology*, 29, 101–112.

Genant, H. K., Doi, K., Mall, J. C. & Sickles, E. A. (1977) Direct radiographic magnification for skeletal radiology. *Radiology*, 123, 47–55.

Ghelman, B. & Goldman, A. B. (1977) The double contrast shoulder arthrogram: evaluation of rotary cuff tears. *Radiology*, 124, 251–254.

Gilbe, P. (1973) Xeroradiography of the breast. *Radiography*, 39, 127.

Goergen, T. G. & Resnick, D. (1975) Evaluation of acetabular anteversion following total hip arthroplasty: necessity of proper centring. *British Journal of Radiology*, 48, 259–260.

Goldsmith, M. R., Paul, R. E., Poplack, W. E., Moore, J. P., Matsue, H. & Bloom, S. (1976) Evaluation of routine double contrast views of the anterior wall of the stomach. *American Journal of Roentgenology*, 126, 1159–1163.

Goldstein, H. M., Wallace, S., Anderson, J. H., Bree, R. L. & Gianturce, C. (1976) Transcatheter occlusion of abdominal tumours. *Radiology*, 120, 539–545.

Gonsette, R. (1971) An experimental assessment of water-soluble contrast medium in neuroradiology: a new medium—Dimer-X. *Clinical Radiology*, 22, 44.

Gordon, I. R. S. (1958) Renal puncture. *Journal of the Faculty of Radiologists*, 9, 108.

Gordon, I. R. S. & Ross, F. G. M. (1977) *Diagnostic Radiology in Paediatrics*. London: Butterworth.

Graham, D. (1973) *The Use of X-ray Techniques in Forensic Investigations*, Edinburgh: Churchill Livingstone.

Graham, D. & Butler, O. H. (1969) The value of radiography in forensic pathology. *X-ray Focus*, 9, No. 2, 24.

Grainger, R. G. (1970) Radiological contrast media. In *Modern Trends in Diagnostic Radiology*, 4th series, ed. McLaren, J. W. London: Butterworth.

Grainger, R. G. (1972) Renal toxicity of radiological contrast media. *British Medical Bulletin*, 28, No. 2, 191.

Grainger, R. G., Gumpert, J., Sharpe, D. M. & Carson, J. (1971) Water-soluble lumbar radiculography. A clinical trial of Dimer X—A new contrast medium. *Clinical Radiology*, 22, 57.

Grech, P. (1972) Arthrography in hip dysplasia in infants. *Radiography*, 38, 172.

Greulich, W. W. & Pyle, S. I. (1959) *Radiographic Atlas of Skeletal Development of the Hand and Wrist*. 2nd edition. Stanford, California: Stanford University Press.

Gupta, S. K., Gupta, O. P., Samani, H. C. & Varma, D. N. (1973) Roentgen diagnosis of nasopharyngeal masses. *Australasian Radiology*, 17, 14.

Gyll, K. (1977) *A Handbook of Paediatric Radiography*. Oxford: Blackwell.

Haaga, J. R., Zelch, M. G., Alfidi, R. J., Stewart, B. H. & Daughert, J. D. (1977) CT guided antegrade pyelography and percutaneous nephrostomy. *American Journal of Roentgenology*, 128, 621–624.

Habel, J. (1970) *Electromedica*, 6, 330–336.

Halliwell, M. (1978) Personal communication.

Hårdstedt, C., Rundelius, B. & Welander, V. (1976) Photographic subtraction. II Technical aspects and method. *Acta Radiologica*, 17, 101–106.

Harned, R. K., Steeling, G. B., Williams, S. & Wolf, G. L. (1976) Glucogon and barium enema examinations. A controlled clinical trial. *American Journal of Roentgenology*, 126, 981–984.

Harris, L. (1975) Improved techniques for hilar tomography. *Radiography*, 41, 209.

Hébert, G. & Ouimet-Oliva, D. (1972) Diagnosis and management of breast cysts. *American Journal of Roentgenology, Radium Therapy and Nuclear Medicine*, 115, No. 4, 801–807.

Hemmingsson, A. (1972) Roentgenologic examination of the larynx—a clinical comparison. *Acta Radiologica*, 12, Fasc. 4, 433–451.

Herlinger, H. (1968) Single film inclined angio-placentography in the diagnosis of placenta praevia. *Clinical Radiology*, 19, 59–64.

Higginbottom, E. (1977) 'Chest a minute'. *Radiography*, 43, 73–81.

Hill, C. R. (1977) Biological effects of ultrasound. In *Ultrasonics in Clinical Diagnosis*, ed. Wells, P. N. T. Edinburgh: Churchill Livingstone.

Hodson, C. J. (1966) Excretion pyelography as a technique. *Radiography*, 32, 15.

Horton, R. E., Ross, F. G. M. & Darling, G. H. (1965) Determination of the emptying-time of the stomach by use of enteric-coated barium granules. *British Medical Journal*, 1, 1537.

Hounsfield, G. N. (1973) Computerised transverse axial scanning (tomography): Part 1. Description of system. *British Journal of Radiology*, 46, 1016–1022.

Howatt, J. (1976) Percutaneous lung biopsy. *Radiography*, 42, 70–72.

Hungerford, G. D. (1975) Cerebral magnification angiography. *Electromedica*, 2–3/1975, 78–85.

Hunter, R., Simpson, W. & Young, J. R. (1973) An evaluation of supine and erect chest films in children. *Radiography*, 39, 27.

Isard, H. J., Ostrum, B. J. & Cullinan, J. E. (1962) Magnification roentgenography. *Medical Radiography and Photography*, 38, 92.

Isherwood, I. (1961) A radiological approach to the sub-talar joint. *Journal of Bone and Joint Surgery*, 43B, 566.

Isherwood, I. (1972) Intra-osseous venography. In *Practical Procedures in Diagnostic Radiology*, ed. Saxton, H. M. & Strickland, B. 2nd edition. London: Lewis.

Jackson, B. T. & Kinmonth, J. B. (1974) Lumbar lymphatic cross-over. *Clinical Radiology*, 25, 187–203.

James, P., Boag, J. W., Baddeley, H., Johns, H. E. & Stacey, A. J. (1973) Xeroradiography—its uses in peripheral contrast medium angiography. *Clinical Radiology*, 24, 67.

Jeans, W. D., Penry, J. B. & Roylance, J. (1972) Renal puncture. *Clinical Radiology*, 23, 298–311.

Jenkins, D. J. (1976) The subtraction mask in single-order radiographic image subtraction. *Radiography*, 42, 105–110.

Jennett, W. B. (1969) Contrast radiology of the brain—Myodil ventriculography. *Ilford X-ray Focus*, **9**, No. 2, 15.

Jing, B-S, Villanueva, R. & Dodd, G. D. (1977) A new radiological technique in evaluation of prosthetic fitting. *Radiology*, **122**, 534–535.

Kamdar, K. N. & Oza, R. K. (1973) Palatography. A study of velo-pharyngeal closure. *Australasian Radiology*, **17**, 26–31.

Kerr, R. A. & Roylance, J. (1977) Renal puncture. *Radiography*, **43**, 15–22.

Khamapirad, T. & Khamapirad, B. (1973) Cine eustachiography. *Australasian Radiology*, **17**, 8–13.

Kimber, P. M. (1967) Routine photographic subtraction. *Radiography*, **33**, 255.

Kimber, P. M. (1969) A thin-layer cassette for precision neuroradiography. *Radiography*, **35**, 183.

Kinmonth, J. B. (1972) *The Lymphatics. Diseases, lymphography and surgery.* London: Arnold.

Kinmonth, J. B. & Taylor, G. W. (1954) The lymphatic circulation in lymphedema. *Annals of Surgery*, **139**, 129.

Köhler, R. (1965) Parietography of the stomach. *Acta Radiologica*, **3**, 393.

Kreel, L. (1972) Mediastinal pneumography. In *Practical Procedures in Diagnostic Radiology*, ed. Saxton, H. M. & Strickland, B. 2nd edition. London: Lewis.

Kreel, L. (1973) Radiology of the biliary system. In *Clinics in Gastroenterology*. Vol. 2, No. 1. London: Saunders.

Kreel, L. (1976) The EMI whole body scanner in the demonstration of lymph node enlargement. *Clinical Radiology*, **27**, 421–429.

Kreel, L. & James, V. (1965) Pneumo-mediastinography by the transternal method. A technique for radiographic visualisation of the thymus gland. *Radiography*, **31**, 133–137.

Kreel, L., Herlinger, H. & Glanville, J. (1973) Technique of the double contrast barium meal with examples of correlation with endoscopy. *Clinical Radiology*, **24**, 307–314.

Lang, E. K. (1965) Clinical evaluation of side-effects of radiopaque contrast media administered via intravenous and intra-arterial routes in the same patient. *Radiology*, **85**, 666.

Laws, J. W., Spencer, J. & Neale, G. (1967) Radiology in the diagnosis of disaccharidase deficiency. *British Journal of Radiology*, **40**, 594.

Lederman, M. (1971) Cancer of the larynx. 1—Natural history in relation to treatment. *British Journal of Radiology*, **44**, 569–578.

Lester, R. G. (1977) Risk benefit in mammography. *Radiology*, **124**, 1–6.

Levinsohn, E. M. (1977) A new simple device for fluoroscopically monitored knee arthrography. *Radiology*, **122**, 827.

Lewin, W. (1966) Radiology in acute head injury. *British Journal of Radiology*, **39**, 168.

Linsman, J. F. (1965) Gastroesophageal reflux elicited while drinking water. *American Journal of Roentgenology, Radium Therapy and Nuclear Medicine*, **94**, 325.

Lloyd, G. A. S. (1970) The radiological investigation of proptosis. *British Journal of Radiology*, **43**, 1.

Lloyd, G. A. S. (1972) The localisation of lesions in the orbital apex and cavernous sinus by frontal venography. *British Journal of Radiology*, **45**, 405–414.

Lloyd, G. A. S. (1973) Multisection tomography as an aid in the localisation of intra-ocular foreign bodies, *British Journal of Radiology*, **46**, 34–37.

Lloyd, G. A. S. (1975) Axial hypocycloidal tomography of the orbits. *British Journal of Radiology*, **48**, 460–464.

Lloyd, G. A. S. & Ardagh, J. (1972) Adaptation of a standard skull table for enlargement angiography and dacryocystography. *X-ray Focus*, **12**, No. 1, 16.

Lloyd, G. A. S., Bartram, C. I. & Stanley, P. (1974) Ethmoid mucocoeles. *British Journal of Radiology*, **47**, 646–651.

Lloyd Williams, K., Lloyd Williams, F. J. & Handley, R. S. (1960) Infrared radiation thermometry in clinical practice. *Lancet*, 2, 958.

Lodge, T. & Higginbottom, E. (1966) Fractures and dislocations of the cervical spine. *Ilford X-ray Focus*, 7, No. 2, 2.

Lumsden, K. & Truelove, S. C. (1957) Diagnostic pneumoperitoneum. *British Journal of Radiology*, 30, 516.

Lysholm, E. (1963) *Lysholm Precision Apparatus for Skull and Skeletal Radiography*. Stockholm: Zetterstrom & Person.

Mahaffy, R. G. (1969) An assessment of thymic tissue in autoimmune disease. *Clinical Radiology*, 20, 213.

Mansong-Hing, L. R. (1976) *Panoral Dental Radiography*. Springfield, Illinois: Thomas.

Mayall, G. F. (1965) Inclined frontal tomography using the polytome. *Clinical Radiology*, 16, 390.

McCall, I. W., Davies, E. R. & Delahunty, J. E. (1973) The acid-barium test. *British Journal of Radiology*, 46, 578.

McCall, I. W., Park, W. M. & MacSweeney, T. (1973) The radiological demonstration of acute lower cervical injury. *Clinical Radiology*, 24, 235.

McCallum, A. H. (1971) A simple automatic gas dispenser for encephalography and myelography. *British Journal of Radiology*, 44, 396.

McInroy, J. R., Stewart, M. W. & Moss, W. D. (1976) *Studies of Plutonium in Human Tracheobronchial Lymph Nodes*. US Energy Research and Development Administration Symposium, Series 37. Springfield, Virginia: US Department of Commerce, National Technical Information Service.

McLaughlin, A. I. G. (1965) Macroradiography in the diagnosis of pneumoconiosis. *Radiography*, 41, 2.

Meeroff, J. G., Jorgens, J. & Isenberg, J. I. (1975) The effect of glucogon on barium enema examinations. *Radiology*, 115, 4–7.

Meredith, W. J. & Massey, J. B. (1977) *Fundamental Physics of Radiology*. 3rd edition. Bristol: Wright.

Miller, R. E. (1965) Complete reflux small bowel examination. *Radiology*, 84, 457.

Miller, R. E. & Skucas, J. (1977) *Radiographic Contrast Agents*. Baltimore: University Park Press.

Morag, B. & Shahin, N. (1975) The value of tomography of the sterno-clavicular region. *Clinical Radiology*, 26, 57–62.

Morgan, N. V. & Evison, G. (1966) Contrast radiography in the follow-up of naso-pharyngeal tumours. *Journal of Laryngology*, 80, 690.

Nolan, D. J. (1977) In *Topics in Gastroenterology*. Vol. 5, ed. Truelove, S. C. & Lee, E. Oxford: Blackwell.

Nolan, D. J. (1978) Personal communication.

Nolan, D. J. & Gibson, M. J. (1970) Improvements in intravenous cholangiography. *British Journal of Radiology*, 43, 652.

Nunnerley, H. B. & Field, S. (1972) Mammary duct injection in patients with nipple discharge. *British Journal of Radiology*, 45, 717.

Okuda, K., Kyuichi, T., Emura, T., Kuratomi, S., Jinnouch, S., Urabe, K., Sumikoshi, T., Kanda, Y., Fukuyana, Y., Musha, H., Mori, H., Shimokawa, Y., Yakushiji, F. & Matsuuiza, Y. (1974) Nonsurgical percutaneous transhepatic cholangiography—diagnostic significance in medical problems of the liver. *American Journal of Digestive Diseases*, 19, 1, 21–36.

Ottoe, R. C., Poulliadis, G. P. & Kumpe, D. A. (1976) The evaluation of pathologic alterations of juxtaosseous soft tissue by xeroradiography. *Radiology*, 120, 297–302.

Park, W. M. (1973) Personal communication.

Patil, K. D., Williams, J. R. & Lloyd Williams, K. (1970) Thermographic localisation of incompetent perforating veins in the leg. *British Medical Journal*, 24th Jan., 1970.

Pigott, R. W. & Makepeace, A. P. W. (1975) Technique of recording nasal pharyngoscopy. *British Journal of Plastic Surgery*, 28, 26–33.

Pim, H. P. (1972) The technique of lower limb phlebography. *X-ray Focus*, 12, No. 1, 2.

Pitt, M. & Ingram, T. T. S. (1975) Radiology of speech disorders in childhood. Part 2. Radiology in the diagnosis of speech disorders. *Radiography*, 41, 90–104.

Pochaczevsky, R., Leonidas, J. C., Feldman, F., Naysan, P. & Ratner, H. (1975) Aspirated and ingested teeth in children. *Clinical Radiology*, 24, 349–353.

Post, H. W. A. & Southwood, W. F. M. (1959) The technique and interpretation of nephrotomograms. *British Journal of Radiology*, 32, 734.

Presland, L. W. (1968) An operative vesiculogram. *Radiography*, 34, 239.

Preston, B. J. & Jackson, J. P. (1977) Investigation of shoulder disability by arthrography. *Clinical Radiology*, 28, 259–266.

Reichmann, S., Astrand, K., Deichgraber, E. & Olsson, B. (1975) Soft tissue xeroradiography of the shoulder joint. *Acta Radiologica*, 16, 572–576.

Richardson, P. J. (1977) Soft tissue xeroradiography. *Radiography*, 43, 117–125.

Ringertz, H. G. (1976) Arthrography of the knee. II. Isolated and combined lesions. *Acta Radiologica*, 17, 235–248.

Robson, N. (1975) Orthodiagraphic pelvimetry technique as used at Rikshospital, Oslo. *Radiography*, 41, 145–146.

Ross, F. G. M. (1975) Ultrasound in diagnosis. In *Medical Annual 1975*. Bristol: Wright.

Rothenberg, L. N., Kirch, R. L. A. & Snyder, R. E. (1975) Patient exposures from film and xeroradiographic mammographic techniques. *Radiology*, 117, 701–703.

Rothwell, D. L., Constable, A. R. & Albrecht, M. (1977) Radionuclide cystography. *Lancet*, 1/1977, 1072–1075.

Royal College of Radiologists (1976) Recommendations on the implementation of the 10-day rule. *British Journal of Radiology*, 49, 201–202.

Ryan, J. F. (1969) Thermography. *Australasian Radiology*, 13, 23.

Ryan, J. F. (1970) Carcinoma of the larynx—Radiology. *Australasian Radiology*, 14, 173.

Ryan, J. F. (1973) Personal communication.

Salmon, P. R. (1977) Diagnostic aspects—endoscopy. In *Principles of Surgical Oncology*, ed. Raven, R. W. New York: Plenum.

Samuel, E. (1970) Thermography. In *Modern Trends in Diagnostic Radiology*. 4th series, ed. McLaren, J. W. London: Butterworth.

Sanders, D. E. & Ho, C. S. (1976) The small bowel enema: experience with 150 examinations. *American Journal of Roentgenology*, 127, 743–751.

Sandin, B., Kreel, L. & Slavin, G. (1973) The pancreas—radiographic demonstration of pancreatic morphology at autopsy. *Radiography*, 39, 151.

Sandin, I. R. G. (1966) A new technique for examining the ankle in forced inversion. *Radiography*, 32, 255.

Saxton, H. M. (1977) Radiology now. Starting the double contrast barium meal. *British Journal of Radiology*, 50, 610–612.

Saxton, H. M. (1969) Urography. *British Journal of Radiology*, 42, 321.

Saxton, H. M. & Strickland, B. (1972) *Practical Procedures in Diagnostic Radiology*. 2nd edition. London: Lewis.

Saxton, H. M., Ogg, C. S. & Cameron, J. S. (1972) Needle nephrostomy. *British Medical Bulletin*, 28, No. 3, 210.

Scher, A. & Vambeck, V. (1977) An approach to the radiological examination of the cervico-dorsal junction following injury. *Clinical Radiology*, 28, 243–246.

Schiller, K. F. R. (1972) Fibre-endoscopy of the stomach (Part 1). *Teach-In*, 1, No. 4, 307.

Schobinger, R. A. (1960) *Intra-osseous Venography*. New York: Grune and Stratton.

Schwarz, G. S. (1961) *Unit-step Radiography*. Springfield, Illinois: Thomas.

Scott-Harden, W. C. (1960) Examination of the small bowel. In *Modern Trends in Radiology*. 3rd series, ed. McLaren, J. W. London: Butterworth.

Sellink, J. L. (1976) *Radiological Atlas of Common Diseases of the Small Bowel*. Leiden: Stenfert Kroese.

Sheldon, J. J., Sersland, T. & Leborgne, J. (1977) Computed tomography of the lower lumbar vertebrae. *Radiology*, 124, 113–118.

Sherwood, T. & Stevenson, J. J. (1972) Antegrade pyelography—a further look at an old technique. *British Journal of Radiology*, 45, 812.

Sidaway, M. E. (1972) Small vessel changes in renal disease. *British Medical Bulletin*, 28, No. 3, 247.

Smith, P. B. & Robinson, A. W. (1969) A radiographic jig for the von Rosen view. *Radiography*, 35, 166.

Spackman, T. J. (1977) Double contrast urethrography—to demonstrate urethral diverticulum. *Radiology*, 124, 259.

Stafne, E. C. & Gibilisco, J. A. (1975) *Oral Roentgenographic Diagnosis*. Philadelphia: Saunders.

Sterling Fisher, A. & Russell, J. G. B. (1975) *Radiography in Obstetrics*. London: Butterworth.

Stevens, G. M., Weigen, J. F. & Lee, R. S. (1966) Pelvic pneumography. *Medical Radiography and Photography*, 42, 82.

Stoker, D. (1975) Double contrast arthrography of the knee in the diagnosis of meniscus injury. *X-ray Focus*, 14, 26–34.

Stripp, W. J. (1963) Radiography of the scapulo-thoracic region. *X-ray Focus*, 4, No. 2, 8.

Stripp, W. J. (1964) Radiography of the shoulder joint. *X-ray Focus*, 5, No. 2, 23.

Stripp, W. J. (1966) The knee joint: exacting radiographic demands. *X-ray Focus*, 7, 7.

Sutherland, G. R. (1970) Inclined plane zonography. *British Journal of Radiology*, 43, 492.

Sutton, D. (1962) *Arteriography*. Edinburgh: Livingstone.

Sutton, D. (1975) *Textbook of Radiology*. 2nd edition. Edinburgh: Churchill Livingstone.

Tabrisky, J., Lindstrom, R. L., Hanelin, L. G. & Pfisterer, W. F. (1976) Chiba percutaneous transhepatic cholangiography—a valuable method for visualizing the non-dilated biliary tract. *American Journal of Roentgenology*, 126, 755–760.

Tanner, J. M., Whitehouse, R. H. & Marshall, W. A. (1975) *Assessment of Skeletal Maturity and Prediction of Adult Height (TW2 method)*. London: Academic Press.

Taylor, A. R. (1969) Arthrography of the knee in rheumatoid arthritis. *British Journal of Radiology*, 42, 493.

Templeton, F. E. & Addington, E. A. (1951) Roentgenologic examination of the colon using drainage and negative pressure. *Journal of the American Medical Association*, 145, 702.

Tolman, D. E. (1975) Roentgenographic technique. Appendix Part 1. In *Oral Roentgenographic Diagnosis*. Stafne, E. C. & Gibilisco, J. A. 4th edition. Philadelphia: Saunders.

Trapnell, D. H. (1977) The 'magnification sign' of triple mandibular fracture. *British Journal of Radiology*, 50, 97–100.

Tucker, A. K. (1967) Subtraction in radiology. *Radiography*, 33, 125.

Von Rosen, S. (1962) Diagnosis and treatment of congenital dislocations of the hip in newborn. *Journal of Bone and Joint Surgery*, 44B, 284.

Walker, T. M., Davies, E. R. & Roylance, J. (1977) The value of urography following lymphography in malignant disease. *British Journal of Radiology*, 50, 93–96.

Watt, I. & Penry, J. B. (1973) Cyst puncture in an unusual renal mass. *British Journal of Radiology*, 46, 1007–1009.

Weller, H. J. (1964) Macroradiography of the temporal bones. *Radiography*, 30, 49.

Wells, P. N. T. (1977) *Ultrasonics in Clinical Diagnosis*. 2nd edition. Edinburgh: Churchill Livingstone.

Weston, W. J. (1972) Soft tissue signs in recent subluxation and dislocation of the acromio-clavicular joint. *British Journal of Radiology*, **45**, 832.

White, T. C., Gardiner, J. H. & Leighton, B. C. (1967) *Orthodontics for Dental Students*, p. 150. London: Staples Press.

Woesner, M. E. & Saunders, I. (1972) Xeroradiography. A significant modality in the detection of non-metallic foreign bodies in soft tissue. *American Journal of Roentgenology, Radium Therapy and Nuclear Medicine*, **115**, 636.

Wolfe, J. N. (1969) Xeroradiography of the joints, bones and soft tissues. *Radiology*, **93**, No. 3, 583.

Wood, E. H. (1964) Thermography in the diagnosis of cerebro-vascular disease. *Radiology*, **83**, 540.

Wright, F. W. (1972) Renal puncture. In *Practical Procedures in Diagnostic Radiology*, ed. Saxton, H. M. & Strickland, B. 2nd edition. London: Lewis.

Ziedes des Plantes, B. G. (1970) Subtraction. In *Modern Trends in Diagnostic Radiology*. 4th series, ed. McLaren, J. W. London: Butterworth.

Index